Chronic Diseases

Chronic Diseases

An Encyclopedia of Causes, Effects, and Treatments

Volume 2: I–Z

JEAN KAPLAN TEICHROEW, EDITOR

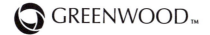 GREENWOOD™

An Imprint of ABC-CLIO, LLC

Santa Barbara, California • Denver, Colorado

Copyright © 2017 by ABC-CLIO, LLC

Library of Congress Cataloging-in-Publication Data

Names: Teichroew, Jean Kaplan, editor.
Title: Chronic diseases : an encyclopedia of causes, effects, and treatments / Jean Kaplan Teichroew, editor.
Other titles: Chronic diseases (Teichroew)
Description: Santa Barbara, California : Greenwood, [2017] | Includes bibliographical references and index.
Identifiers: LCCN 2016025459 (print) | LCCN 2016026316 (ebook) |
    ISBN 9781440801037 (hard copy (set) : alk. paper) | ISBN 9781440846205
    (v. 1 : alk. paper) | ISBN 9781440846212 (v. 2 : alk. paper) | ISBN 9781440801044
    (set EISBN) | ISBN 9781440801044 (ebook (set))
Subjects: | MESH: Chronic Disease | Encyclopedias
Classification: LCC RC41 (print) | LCC RC41 (ebook) | NLM WT 13 | DDC 616.003—dc23
LC record available at https://lccn.loc.gov/2016025459

ISBN: 978-1-4408-0103-7 (set)
      978-1-4408-4620-5 (vol. 1)
      978-1-4408-4621-2 (vol. 2)
EISBN: 978-1-4408-0104-4

21 20 19 18 17   1 2 3 4 5

This book is also available as an eBook.

Greenwood
An Imprint of ABC-CLIO, LLC

ABC-CLIO, LLC
130 Cremona Drive, P.O. Box 1911
Santa Barbara, California 93116-1911
www.abc-clio.com

This book is printed on acid-free paper (∞)
Manufactured in the United States of America

Contents

Alphabetical List of Entries

Guide to Related Topics

Following are the entries in this encyclopedia, arranged under broad topics for enhanced searching. Readers should also consult the index at the end of the encyclopedia for more specific subjects. Some entries are listed more than once.

ADDICTION

Alcoholism
Fetal Alcohol Syndrome

Substance Abuse
Tobacco Addiction

ARTHRITIS

Adult Onset Still's Disease
Gout
Juvenile Arthritis

Osteoarthritis
Reactive Arthritis

BLOOD, HEART, AND CARDIOVASCULAR DISORDERS

Aneurisms
Angina
Angiogram
Arrhythmias/Dysrhythmias
Arteriovenous Malformations
Atherosclerosis
Atrial Fibrillation
Bleeding Disorders
Blood Cancers
Blood Disorders
Blood Pressure
Bradycardia
Cardiomyopathy
Cardiovascular Disease
Cholesterol
Circulation Disorders
Congenital Heart Disease
Congestive Heart Failure
Cor Pulmonale
Deep Vein Thrombosis
Endocarditis
Familial Hypercholesterolemia
Gangrene

Heart Diseases
Heart Murmur
Heart Valve Disorders
Hemochromatosis
Hemophilia
Hyperlipidemia
Hypertension (High Blood Pressure)
Hypoglycemia
Hypotension (Low Blood Pressure)
Iron Overload Disease
Kawasaki Disease
Leukemia
Multiple Myeloma
Pericardial Disorders/Pericarditis
Peripheral Arterial Disease
Platelet Disorders
Raynaud's Phenomenon
Rheumatic Fever and Rheumatic Heart
    Disease
Tachycardia
Thrombophlebitis
Vascular Disorders
Venous Disorders

BREAST DISORDERS

Breast Cancer
Breast Diseases

Male Breast Cancer
Paget's Disease of the Breast

CANCER

Anal and Rectal Diseases
Basal Cell Carcinoma
Bile Duct Cancer
Bladder Cancer
Blood Cancers
Bone Cancer
Brain Cancer
Breast Cancer
Cancer Survivorship
Cancer
Cancers, Childhood
Cancers, Occupational
Cervical Cancer
Colon Cancer
Esophageal Cancer
Eye Cancer
Gastric Cancer
Head and Neck Cancer
Hodgkin Disease
Kidney Cancer

Laryngeal Cancer
Leukemia
Liver Cancer
Lung Cancer
Male Breast Cancer
Melanoma
Neoplasms
Non-Hodgkin Lymphoma
Oral Cancer
Ovarian Cancer
Pancreatic Cancer
Prostate Cancer
Skin Cancer
Squamous Cell Children
Testicular Cancer
Throat Cancer
Thyroid Cancer
Urethral Cancer
Uterine Cancer

CHILDREN AND YOUTH

Asthma, Children and Youth
Cancers, Childhood
Failure to Thrive
Fetal Alcohol Syndrome

Juvenile Arthritis
Overweight and Obesity in Children
Phenylketonuria
School Wellness Programs

DIABETES

Diabetes, Type 1
Diabetes, Type 2

Prediabetes
Sugar Diabetes

DIGESTIVE SYSTEM/EXCRETORY SYSTEM

Abdominal Diseases
Anal and Rectal Diseases
Bile Duct Cancer
Biliary Cirrhosis
Biliary Diseases
Bowel Incontinence
Crohn's Disease

Cyclic Vomiting Syndrome
Cystic Fibrosis
Digestive Diseases
Diverticular Disease
Esophageal Cancer
Gall Bladder Disease
Gastric Cancer

Gastroesophageal Reflux Disease (GERD)
Inflammatory Bowel Disease
Intestinal Obstruction
Irritable Bowel Syndrome
Lactose Intolerance

Malaria
Peptic Ulcers
Peritoneal Disorders
Swallowing Disorders
Ulcerative Colitis

EAR DISORDERS

Ear Diseases
Tinnitus

Vestibular Diseases

EYE DISORDERS

Color Blindness
Eye Cancer
Eye Diseases
Glaucoma

Hyperopia
Macular Degeneration
Myopia
Retinopathy

GENETICS

Cystic Fibrosis
Ehlers-Danlos Syndrome
Genetics and Genomics

Phenylketonuria
Sickle-Cell Disease
Tay-Sachs Disease

GLANDULAR AND ENDOCRINE SYSTEMS

Addison's Disease
Adrenal Diseases
Diabetes, Type 1
Diabetes, Type 2
Graves' Disease
Hashimoto's Disease
Hypothyroidism

Pancreatic Cancer
Pancreatitis
Pituitary Disorders
Prediabetes
Sugar Diabetes
Thyroid Cancer
Thyroid Disease

HEALTH

Body Mass Index (BMI)
Global Health
Health
Health Disparities
Healthy Lifestyles and Risky Behaviors
Healthy People 2020
Occupational Health
Physical Activity

Physical Therapy
Public Health
Risk Factors
School Wellness Programs
Self-Management
Sleep Disturbances and Sleep Disorders
Spirituality

IMMUNE SYSTEM DISORDERS

AIDS (Acquired Immune Deficiency
   Syndrome)

Autoimmune Disease
Celiac Disease

Diabetes, Type 1
Diabetes, Type 2
Failure to Thrive
Hashimoto's Disease
Immune System Disorders

Kaposi's Sarcoma
Lupus
Neoplasms
Sjögren's Syndrome

INFLAMMATORY DISORDERS

Adult Onset Still's Disease
Allergies
Amyloidosis
Ankylosing Spondylitis
Arthritis
Autoimmune Disease
Behcet's Syndrome
Buerger's Disease
Bursitis
Crohn's Disease
Felty Syndrome

Gout
Inflammation
Inflammatory Bowel Disease
Kawasaki Disease
Lupus
Myopathies
Pelvic Inflammatory Disease
Peritoneal Disorders
Polymyositis
Rheumatoid Arthritis
Thrombophlebitis

INFORMATION

Centers for Disease Control and
   Prevention (CDC)
Epidemiology
Etiology

Health Literacy
National Institutes of Health (NIH)
World Health Organization

ISSUES

Environment
Health Disparities
Minority, Chronic Disease
Pollution

Poverty
Public Health
School Wellness Programs

KIDNEY AND URINARY DISORDERS

Addison's Disease
Bladder Cancer
Bladder Diseases
Kidney Cancer
Kidney Disease
Kidney Failure
Kidney Stones

Nephritis
Urethral Cancer
Urethral Disorders
Urinary Incontinence
Urinary Tract Infections
Uterine Cancer
Uterine Diseases

LIFE STAGES

Adolescence and Chronic Disease
Aging, Healthy

Family Health

LIVER DISORDERS

Bile Duct Cancer
Biliary Cirrhosis
Biliary Diseases

Hepatitis
Liver Cancer
Liver Diseases

LYMPHATIC DISORDERS

Hodgkin Disease
Lymphatic Disorders

Lymphoma
Non-Hodgkin Lymphoma

MEN'S HEALTH

Male Breast Cancer
Men's Health

Prostate Cancer
Testicular Cancer

MENTAL HEALTH DISORDERS

Anxiety Disorders
Attention Deficit Hyperactivity Disorder
  (ADHD)
Cutting and Self-Harm
Depression
Eating Disorders
Mental Health Disorders

Obsessive Compulsive Disorder
Psychotic Disorders
PTSD (Post-Traumatic Stress Disorder)
Schizophrenia
Seasonal Affective Disorder
Stress

METABOLIC DISORDERS

Addison's Disease
Cystic Fibrosis
Diabetes, Type 1
Hypothyroidism

Metabolic Disorders
Metabolic Syndrome
Phenylketonuria
Tay-Sachs Disease

MUSCULOSKELETAL

Arthritis
Back Pain
Bursitis
Carpal Tunnel Syndrome
Ehlers-Danlos Syndrome
Joint Disorders
Juvenile Arthritis

Legg-Calve-Perthes Disease
Muscle Cramps
Musculoskeletal Disorders
Myopathies
Osteoarthritis
Reactive Arthritis
Rheumatoid Arthritis

NEUROLOGICAL DISORDERS

ALS (Amyotrophic Lateral Sclerosis)
Alzheimer's Disease
Autism
Autonomic Nervous System Disorders

Bell's Palsy
Bipolar Disorder
Brain Cancer
Brain Diseases

ORAL PHARYNGEAL DISORDERS

OVERWEIGHT AND OBESITY

PREVENTION AND CARE

REPRODUCTIVE SYSTEM DISORDERS

Pelvic Inflammatory Disease
Reproductive Disorders
Sexually Transmitted Diseases

Testicular Cancer
Vaginal Diseases

RESPIRATORY, LUNG, AND NASAL DISORDERS

Allergies
Asthma
Asthma, Children and Youth
Black Lung Disease
Bronchiectasis
Bronchitis
COPD (Chronic Obstructive Pulmonary
    Disease)
Cystic Fibrosis
Emphysema
Inhalers
Legionnaires' Disease

Lung Cancer
Lung Diseases
Nasal Disorders
Pleural Disorders
Pneumonia
Pneumothorax
Respiratory Diseases
Secondhand Smoke
Sinusitis
Tuberculosis
Whooping Cough

SEXUALLY TRANSMITTED DISEASES

AIDS (Acquired Immune Deficiency
    Syndrome)
Gonorrhea

HPV (Human Papillomavirus)
Sexually Transmitted Diseases

SKELETAL (BONE) DISORDERS

Ankylosing Spondylitis
Bone Cancer
Bone Diseases
Osteomyelitis

Osteonecrosis
Osteoporosis
Paget's Disease of the Bone
Rickets

SKIN

Basal Cell Carcinoma
Cellulitis
Dermatitis
Eczema
Hansen's Disease (Leprosy)
Herpes

Melanoma
Psoriasis
Rosacea
Skin Cancer
Squamous Cell Carcinoma

VIRAL, BACTERIAL, AND CONTAMINANT DISORDERS

Environment
Herpes
Lead Poisoning

Malaria
Occupational Health
Parasitic Diseases

WOMEN'S HEALTH

Atrophic Vaginitis
Breast Diseases
Cervical Cancer
Dysmenorrhea
Fetal Alcohol Syndrome

Osteoporosis
Ovarian Cancer
Vaginal Diseases
Women's Health

IMMUNE SYSTEM DISORDERS

The function of the immune system—a vast network of cells, tissues, and organs—is to help the body fight off bacteria, parasites, microbes, and other foreign invaders. Disorders affecting the immune system can cause the body to respond or overreact to substances that are not usually harmful, as with allergies and asthma; malfunction, as with immune deficiency diseases, in which the part of the immune system is missing; and mistakenly attack the body's cells and tissues, as in autoimmune diseases.

In an overactive immune system, certain genes can cause the immune system to overreact to allergens, such as dust, mold, foods, and other substances that are usually harmless. Common conditions include asthma, triggered by an allergen or an irritant; eczema, when an allergen causes an itchy rash; and allergic rhinitis, the sneezing and nasal passage swelling caused by allergens.

Immune deficiency diseases that weaken or suppress the immune system can be caused by pregnancy, chemotherapy or other drugs, smoking, alcohol, and poor nutrition, as well as influenza, mononucleosis, and other infections; opportunistic infections such as HIV/AIDS destroy white blood cells and weaken the immune system. Primary immune deficiency diseases, in which part of the immune system is missing or functions improperly, include a group of more than 250 chronic inherited genetic disorders that put children in constant danger of infections. Although there are more than 150 of these diseases, they are considered rare.

Autoimmune diseases, in which the immune system attacks one organ or a whole system, have strong genetic and environmental components. Of the more than 80 such diseases identified, common ones include Type 1 diabetes, where the immune system attacks insulin-producing cells in the pancreas; rheumatoid arthritis, which causes swelling and joint deformities; lupus, which attacks the lungs, kidneys, and skin; psoriasis, a skin condition that causes redness and irritation and thick, flaky, silver-white lesions; inflammatory bowel diseases that affect the colon and small intestine; celiac disease, a reaction to gluten that damages the small intestine's lining; and Sjögren's syndrome, which destroys the glands that produce tears and saliva and may affect kidneys and lungs. Women, especially African Americans, Hispanics, and Native Americans, face a slightly increased risk for some autoimmune diseases, which are often inherited.

Symptoms

Scientists have identified around 100 types of immune system disorders, with symptoms that can range from mild to severe. Common symptoms of an overactive immune system causing allergic rhinitis include sneezing; a runny, itchy or congested nose; and watery or swollen eyes. Food allergies can cause hives; swelling of the throat, lips, tongue; or anaphylaxis (severe reaction that can lead to unconsciousness or death). Eczema can cause itching, redness, flaking, or peeling.

Repeated and chronic infections, especially affecting the respiratory and digestive systems, are common symptoms suggesting an immune deficiency disorder, as does the development of severe bacterial infections that persist, recur, and lead to complications such as pneumonia.

The symptoms of autoimmune diseases depend on the part of the body affected, and initial symptoms may not appear specific until a disease grows more severe. Each autoimmune disease has unique symptoms, which may worsen with flareups and lessen in remission; any part of the body can be affected. The skin, joints, digestive system, muscles, red blood cells, connective tissue, and endocrine glands often experience inflammation and tissue damage that can lead to pain, deformed joints, weakness, jaundice, itching, difficulty breathing, fluid accumulation, delirium, and death. Some symptoms shared by many autoimmune diseases include fatigue, fever, muscle ache, and a general feeling of illness.

Causes

Causes of immune system disorders are many but can include inherited genetic predispositions to a weak immune system, acquiring a disease or condition that weakens the immune system infections, or environmental factors. Exposure to allergens mistaken as harmful by the body cause allergic reactions. Immune deficiency diseases differ, but they are the result of a defect in the function of the body's immune system, which may be caused by medications, chemicals, infection, burns, radiation therapy, poor nutrition, and many other contributing factors. No clear cause is known for autoimmune diseases, but genetics and environment contribute to their development; most likely, a combination of genes, infections, and elements in the environment trigger the genes.

Diagnosis

Medical and family histories, examination of symptoms, and a physical examination help diagnose an immune system disorder. Allergies are diagnosed with skin and blood tests. Diagnostic tools for immune deficiency disorders may include blood tests to determine the white blood cell count, skin tests for T-cell abnormalities, vaccines to test an immune response, and genetic testing. For autoimmune disorders, blood tests indicating the presence of inflammation may suggest an autoimmune disorder; further blood tests can detect specific antibodies, the proteins that recognize and fight specific substances.

Treatments

Medications that control immune system overreactions and immunotherapy, or allergy shots, are effective treatments for allergies and asthma. Immune deficiency disorders can be treated with antibiotics to fight bacterial infection, antiviral drugs to reduce the risk of viral infections, and vaccines to stimulate the production of antibodies that can attack specific bacteria or viruses. Occasionally for some conditions, a bone marrow transplant may be performed. Treatment for autoimmune disorders depends on the specific disease; it usually includes medications such as corticosteroids to relieve inflammation or others to reduce the immune system, although these increase the risk of certain infections and cancers. Blood transfusions may be given if the disorder affects the blood, and physical therapy may be prescribed for affected joints and muscles.

Prognosis and Outcomes

Treatment for allergic rhinitis lessens or eliminates symptoms, which usually lessen with age; although asthma is chronic and should be treated, it often goes into remission. Some immune deficiency disorders are mild, while others severe and may be life-threatening. If caused by medications or other modifiable factors, symptoms can disappear after those substances are removed. Most autoimmune disorders are chronic and require lifetime use of medication to manage or control symptoms. Prognosis depends on each specific disorder.

Ray Marks

See also: AIDS; Allergies; Asthma; Dermatitis; Diabetes, Type 1; Eczema; Failure to Thrive; Neoplasms; Psoriasis; Rheumatoid Arthritis; Sjögren's Syndrome; Skin Conditions

Further Reading

Healthline. (2015, July 22). Autoimmune disorders. Retrieved from www.healthline.com /health/autoimmune-disorders#Overview1.

Healthline. (2012, August 29). Immunodeficiency disorders. Retrieved from http://www .healthline.com/health/immunodeficiency-disorders#Overview1.

MedlinePlus. (2015, October 1). Immune system and disorders. Retrieved from http://www .nlm.nih.gov/medlineplus/immunesystemanddisorders.html.

MedlinePlus. (2015, September 18). Autoimmune diseases. Retrieved from https://www.nlm .nih.gov/medlineplus/autoimmunediseases.html.

Merck Manual. (2015). Overview of immunodeficiency disorders. Retrieved from http:// www.merckmanuals.com/home/immune-disorders/immunodeficiency-disorders /overview-of-immunodeficiency-disorders.

National Institute of Allergy and Infectious Diseases. (2014, January 14). Disorders of the immune system. Retrieved from http://www.niaid.nih.gov/topics/immuneSystem/Pages /immuneDisorders.aspx.

INFLAMMATION

Inflammation is the body's biological response through its immune system to protect against infections or remove irritants, damaged cells, and other harmful substances and to heal itself. It is the body's natural reaction, not an infection, although an infection can cause inflammation. Without inflammation, infections, wounds, and other tissue damage would never heal. But inflammation can take place without any foreign substances to fight, causing the body to damage itself, as in autoimmune diseases. Acute inflammation is a rapid onset that lasts for days or, occasionally, weeks. Chronic inflammation is an overresponse that can last for years, and it is linked to many diseases. A rare, but very dangerous, complication of inflammation, is sepsis, which occurs if large amounts of bacteria enter the bloodstream and multiply quickly. Many types of inflammation respond to treatment with medication.

Symptoms

Sometimes, an inflammation causes no symptoms as it heals the body. But usually, the inflammation process starts with irritation, then discharges pus, followed by the formation of wounds as small rounded masses of tissue. Symptoms of acute inflammation, which may start and become serious very quickly, may include redness; joint pain, swelling, stiffness, or loss of function; muscle stiffness; fever; chills; headache; and loss of appetite.

Chronic, or long-term, inflammation may last for months or even years. It is associated with hundreds of diseases and conditions that are considered autoimmune; among them are rheumatoid arthritis, Celiac disease, fibromyalgia, lupus, Type 1 diabetes, atherosclerosis, periodontitis, asthma and other allergies, ulcerative colitis, Crohn's disease, and active hepatitis. Inflammation may be caused by the failure to eliminate the original harmful substance, by an autoimmune response where the immune system attacks its own tissues mistakenly, or if a chronic irritant persists.

Causes and Risk Factors

In its attempt to protect and heal the body from harmful foreign substances, white blood cells release chemicals to the affected tissues. This increases blood flow, which can appear as redness or warmth in the area. Swelling takes place when the chemicals leak into the tissues, which can also cause pain, which may cause further joint irritation that eventually wears down bone cartilage.

The most common of the many different causes of inflammation are bacteria, viruses, and fungi, which may come about from a scrape or other external injury. Chemicals, severe burns, and radiation can also be causes. Conditions and diseases that cause inflammation include cystitis (in the bladder), bronchitis, otitis media (middle ear), and dermatitis (skin).

Research conducted at Emory University School of Medicine suggests that sleep deprivation or poor quality sleep raises inflammation, increasing the risk of heart disease and stroke (Medical News Today 2010). Inflammation risk is also greater for obese men, who have more white blood cells than men who are not obese or overweight (Medical News Today 2008).

Diagnosis

An inflammatory disease is diagnosed with a complete medical history and physical exam. A doctor will examine joints for evidence of stiffness, inflammation, or other symptoms, often using x-rays and a blood test for C-reactive protein (CRP), which increases with inflammation.

Treatments

Because inflammation is a natural healing process, it is not always necessary to reduce it. But it can be treated with variety of different medications, including naproxen, ibuprofen, and aspirin, which are nonsteroidal anti-inflammatory drugs (NSAIDs), and the corticosteroids prednisone and cortisol. Medications that are also used to treat other conditions may be prescribed in combination. Some herbs are known to have anti-inflammatory responses, including ginger, turmeric, and hyssop. The application of ice, in combination with rest, compression, and elevating the affected area (such as a swollen ankle) is a well-known treatment to reduce inflammation. Foods with omega-3 fatty acids (fish oil), green tea, and tart cherries have been shown to have anti-inflammatory effects, also.

Prognosis and Outcomes

Inflammation, unless it becomes acute or chronic, is a natural healing process. The chronic inflammatory diseases that may last for years or a lifetime can be treated with medications, which improve the outcomes depending their severity and frequency.

Ray Marks

See also: Arthritis; Asthma; Atherosclerosis; Autoimmune Disease; Celiac Disease; Crohn's Disease; Diabetes, Type 1; Endocarditis; Fybromyalgia; Gastroesophageal Reflux Disease; Hepatitis; Lupus; Rheumatoid Arthritis; Ulcerative Colitis

Further Reading

Groopman, J. (2015, November 30). Inflamed: The debate over the latest cure-all craze. *New Yorker, 91*(38), 36–41.

Medical News Today. (2001, November). Poor sleep tied to inflammation, a risk factor for heart disease, stroke. Retrieved from http://www.medicalnewstoday.com/articles/207877.php.

Medical News Today. (2008, October 20). Being fat and unfit linked to inflammation risk. Retrieved from http://www.medicalnewstoday.com/articles/126013.php.

Medical News Today. (2015, May 25). Inflammation: Causes, symptoms and treatments. Retrieved from http://www.medicalnewstoday.com/articles/248423.php.

PubMed Health. (2015, January 7). What is an inflammation? Retrieved from http://www.ncbi.nlm.nih.gov/pubmedhealth/PMH0072482/.

INFLAMMATORY BOWEL DISEASE

Background

Inflammatory bowel disease (IBD) is a chronic, long-lasting health condition often diagnosed in early adulthood. It involves chronic inflammation of the digestive tract, including the lining, and sometimes the walls of the small and large intestines, which become red and swollen. The condition can produce life-threatening complications, and is often accompanied by pain and some form of disablement. In certain cases, the inflammation occurs slowly over time, rather than suddenly, and can occur anywhere within the digestive tract or within different parts of the tract. The inflammation can spread from the digestive tract through its walls to neighboring tissues.

Up to 1 million Americans have IBD, and this group has a slightly increased mortality rate compared to healthy people. They are also more prone to developing cancer.

Conditions

Crohn's disease involves inflammation and ulcering of the lining and wall of any part of the digestive tract, especially the part known as the ileum.

Ulcerative colitis involves inflammation and ulcering in the lining of the colon and rectum.

The occurrence rates of these diseases is approximately the same in the United States, 70 to 150 cases per 100,000 people for ulcerative colitis and 133 cases per 100,000 people for Crohn's disease.

Causes

The causes of IBD include genetic factors, diet and stress, abnormal immune system reactions to an infection, and smoking.

Risk factors include age; ethnicity, especially being white or of Ashkenazi Jewish descent; family history; use of some types of pain relievers; and living in an industrial area or in a developed country.

Symptoms

Symptoms vary from mild to severe depending on the site of the condition and can include:

Abdominal cramping and pain, which can be severe and occur daily
Appetite loss
Arthritis or joint pain
Bleeding
Bloating
Constipation
Diarrhea

Eye inflammation
Fatigue
Fever
Inflammation of the liver or bile ducts
Nausea
Skin disorders or problems
Ulcers or small sores on the surface of the intestine
Vomiting
Weight loss that is unexplained

Diagnosis

Tests for digestive disorders may be noninvasive and involve use of ultrasound or x-rays, blood tests, stool exams, or they may be invasive exploratory investigations such as colonoscopy; endoscopy, which involves swallowing a capsule containing a camera; and sigmoidoscopy, or surgical approaches. Medical examinations may also be helpful.

Treatments

Treatment includes prescription and nonprescription medications to reduce inflammation and pain, surgery, dietary changes, and exercise. Nutrition education and nutritional supplements may also be indicated, as may giving up smoking and surgery, including removing the affected intestine and allowing intestinal wastes to empty into a pouch in the front of the abdomen or internally. Antibiotics, biologic therapies, immunomodulators, and corticosteroid drugs may be used.

Prognosis

The outcome will depend on the problem, its duration, and severity, as well as the age of the individual and his or her overall health status.

Complications may include ulcers; fistulas, or abnormal outgrowths between the skin and intestine or another organ; malnutrition; colon cancer; gallstones; arthritis; and inflammation of the bile ducts. The typical course of the disease consists of periods of flare-up interspersed with remission.

Prevention

A healthy diet, avoiding smoking, stress control and exercise are standard health practices that may offset the onset of an inflammatory bowel disorder.

Future

Researchers are examining new treatment approaches, including biologic therapies. Others are examining the use of fish or flaxseed oils in fighting inflammation of the bowel. Probiotics or good bacteria are also being examined to see if they can help reduce bowel inflammation.

Ray Marks

See also: Abdominal Disease; Crohn's Disease; Digestive Diseases; Ulcerative Colitis

Further Reading

Centers for Disease Control and Prevention. (2014, May 5). What is inflammatory bowel disease? Retrieved from http://www.cdc.gov/ibd/ http://www.cdc.gov/ibd/what-is-ibd .htm.

Mayo Clinic. (2015, February 18). Inflammatory bowel disease (IBD). Retrieved from http://www.mayoclinic.org/diseases-conditions/inflammatory-bowel-disease/basics /definition/con-20034908.

MedlinePlus. (2015, September 30). Irritable bowel syndrome. Retrieved from https://www .nlm.nih.gov/medlineplus/irritablebowelsyndrome.html.

WomensHealth.gov (2012, July 6). Inflammatory bowel disease fact sheet. Retrieved from http://womenshealth.gov/publications/our-publications/fact-sheet/inflammatory -bowel-disease.html.

INHALERS

According to Kalorama Information (2012), a health care marketing research publisher, estimates released as part of a report on the World Market for Respiratory Devices show that the sale of inhaled medications and other respiratory therapies reached more than $44 billion in 2011, driven by an aging population and an increased incidence (newly diagnosed cases) of respiratory diseases.

Inhaled medications are often prescribed for children and adults suffering from a number of respiratory illnesses, including asthma, bronchitis, and chronic obstructive pulmonary disease (COPD), a lung disease that narrows the airways and decreases the flow of oxygen throughout the body. This method of administering medication is highly preferred because inhaled medications go directly into the lungs and have been found to lead to fewer negative effects to the body overall (Hess 2005).

Effectiveness in treating respiratory disease depends on the extent of the illness and the regularity and correct use of the inhaler. Nadi and Zeraati (2005) discuss the importance of good technique in taking the medications. They state that failure to use inhalers appropriately has posed a problem for proper control of respiratory illnesses. Doctors throughout the world are recognizing how valuable inhalers have become globally.

Inhaled medications come in two forms, either dry-powder inhalers or mist inhalers packaged as metered-dose inhalers (also known as pumps). Advair and Flovent are two commonly used dry-powder inhalers used to prevent asthma or other respiratory symptoms. They are referred to as controller medications or anti-inflammatory medicines because they reduce the amount of swelling and mucus within the airways. Pulmicort, Serevent, and Q-var are other medications with the same function.

Unlike controller medications, the primary function of reliever medications is to release the muscles around the airway that are squeezing out the oxygen and making it difficult to breathe. They are used when symptoms are present or when conditions or known triggers for symptoms are expected. It is known as a bronchodilator or rescue medication because it quickly opens the airways during an episode. Use of these medications can be life-saving.

According to the Asthma and Allergy Foundation of America (2016), inhalers, also called puffers, help supply medication into the lungs, providing quick and effective relief, and for about 24 million Americans with asthma, this is an important medication.

Inhaler medications are not recommended for children younger than two years of age because respiratory diseases are difficult to diagnose in children of this age, due to their many respiratory infections and still developing immune system (Lenney 2008). The author reveals significant risk of death or damage to the airways. Lenney otherwise notes that prescription of inhaled medications to all other age groups is effective and safe.

While inhaler medications have been known to produce side effects such as headaches, throat irritation, dizziness, loss of appetite, altered taste, and vomiting, these side effects have been found to be mild and not have serious or long-term health implications. Children have been noted to become hyperactive or experience some weight gain. Thrush (a yeast infection in the mouth) is another side effect of using inhaler medications as a result of residue of the medicine staying in the mouth. A quick solution for this side effect is to rinse the mouth thoroughly after taking the medicine.

The benefits of using these medications have been found to far outweigh the negative side effects. While some studies suggest that inhaled medications can slow down rates of growth during preadolescence and adolescence, this is only temporary, and eventually growth normalizes so that there is no difference between those who use the medications and those who do not (Pedersen 2001).

While the use of inhaled medications has been highly studied and recommended as an effective treatment for prevention of acute attacks, administration of these medications—particularly controller medications for those with poorly controlled disease—is still not standard practice. It is not generally common practice for doctors in emergency rooms to prescribe this type of inhaler for patients coming in for acute care.

New York City Department of Health and Mental Hygiene recommendations through their East Harlem Asthma Center of Excellence have increased prescription of inhaled medications in the emergency rooms of two local hospitals, with the expectation that it will become standard practice throughout the state and part of best practices throughout the country, one of the main goals of the Institute of Education for the Care of Chronic Diseases as it works to establish new guidelines and perspectives in the treatment of chronic diseases.

Papi and colleagues (2011) recommend a "call to action" to inform providers of the importance of prescribing and demonstrating the proper use of inhaled medications to treat respiratory illnesses. There are several methods for taking these medications; one is putting your mouth directly onto the device. Nebulizer machines have been used for both children and adults to deliver mist medications as well. Another popular and preferred method for taking the medication is using the inhaler with a spacer.

Until recently, children within the school system were unable to take any type of medication on their own. This included inhaled medications for asthma symptoms. According to a ruling in 2004, asthmatic children were granted permission to carry and self-administer asthma medications as long as it had been established that they knew how to properly take their medicine. This also required that school personnel, especially school nurses, were informed of an asthma or respiratory disease diagnosis and that the proper documents with doctor recommendations were made available. In addition to the nation's capital, this law has been adopted by 40 states.

Over-the-counter inhaler medications were common use. They were considered safe for occasional use to help people with mild forms of a respiratory disease (Dickinson et al. 2000). Excessive use, however, could lead to severe reactions including death. In December 2011, Primatene Mist, the only over-the-counter reliever medication, was removed from the market after the negative environmental effects were discovered.

According to the Allergy and Asthma Network (2011), this and other prescribed inhaled medications containing chlorofluorocarbon propellants were all banned because they were found to cause damage to the ozone layer of the earth's atmosphere, a layer critical to filtering the harmful UV rays of the sun. New forms of inhaler medications have since been manufactured. These do not contain the harmful chemical and have been found to be equally effective in the treatment of respiratory illnesses.

Betty Perez-Rivera

See also: Allergies; Asthma; COPD (Chronic Obstructive Pulmonary Disease); Immune System Disorders; Respiratory Diseases

Further Reading

Allergy and Asthma Network. (2011). Primatene mist: Going, going, gone. Retrieved from http://www.aanma.org/2011/12/primatene-mist-going-going-gone/.

Asthma and Allergy Foundation of America. (2016). Retrieved from http://www.aafa.org /display. cfm?id=8&sub=17&cont=171.

Asthmatic School Children's Treatment and Health Management Act of 2004. Retrieved from http://www.gpo.gov/fdsys/pkg/PLAW-108publ377/pdf/PLAW-108publ377.pdf.

Dickinson, B. D., Altman, S. D., & Deitchman, H. C. (2000). Safety of over-the-counter inhalers for asthma: Report of the Council on Scientific Affairs. *Chest, 118,* 522–526.

Hess, D. R. (2005, October). Metered-dose inhalers and dry powder inhalers in aerosol therapy. *Respiratory Care, 50*(10), 1376–1383.

Jones, S. E., & Wheeler, L. (2004). Asthma inhalers in schools: Rights of students with asthma to a free appropriate education. *American Journal of Public Health, 94,* 1102–1108.

Kalorama Information. (2012). Press release on world market for respiratory devices. Retrieved from http://finance.yahoo.com/news/sales-inhalers-driving-respiratory-device -163300145.html;_ylt=A2KJ3CcOxMpPyncAjxXQtDMD.

Lenney, W. (2008). Pro-con debate: Inhaled corticosteroids should not be prescribed in primary care to children under two years of age—the case against. *Primary Care Respiratory Journal, 17*(3), 181–184.

Nadi, E., & Zeraati, F. (2005). Evaluation of the metered-dose inhaler technique among healthcare providers. *Acta Medica Iranica, 43*(4), 268–272.

Papi, A., Hughney, J., Virchow, J. C., Roche, N., Palkonen, S., & Price, D. (2011). Editorial: Inhaler devices for asthma: A call for action in a neglected field. *European Respiratory Journal, 37,* 982–985.

Pedersen, S. (2005, August 15). Do inhaled corticosteroids inhibit growth in children? *American Journal of Respiratory Critical Care Medicine, 164*(4), 521–535.

INTESTINAL OBSTRUCTION

The term *intestinal obstruction* refers to the complete or partial blockage of the bowel. This causes the intestinal contents to be unable to move through the intestine in the normal way and can occur readily, especially in individuals with Crohn's disease, a chronic disease.

Symptoms

An intestinal obstruction can result in complete absence of gas or stool passage and, on occasion, diarrhea. Other symptoms are pain, cramping, abdominal bloating, and fullness. In addition, other related symptoms include bad breath and vomiting.

Causes

Research shows an obstruction of the bowel may arise as a result of a mechanical blockage, in the absence of any structural damage. These mechanical blockages can be caused by abnormal tissue growth, scar tissue after surgeries such as appendectomies, fibrous bands of tissue in the abdomen called adhesions, colorectal surgery, and upper gastrointestinal procedures, as well as by the ingestion of foreign bodies that obstruct the intestine or hernias and abnormal twisting or narrowing of the intestines. A blockage can occur if one part of the intestine collapses like a telescope into another—a process known as *intussusception*. Other causes are diverticulitis or inflammatory bowel disease.

Another major cause of intestinal obstruction in infants and children is known as *paralytic ileus*. This condition, also called pseudo-obstruction, is caused by multiple factors, including chemical, electrolyte, or mineral disturbances; injury to the abdominal blood supply; intra-abdominal infection; complications of abdominal surgery; use of certain medications, particularly narcotics; and the presence of kidney or lung disease. In older children, the condition may be caused by bacterial, or viral, infections or food poisoning.

Risk factors for intestinal obstruction include previous abdominal or pelvic surgery, abdominal cancer, and Crohn's disease.

Treatment

The person who is suffering from an obstruction of the intestine may have to be hospitalized to decompress the intestine through a tiny tube called a nasogastric tube passed through the nose to the stomach because this is a dangerous condition. This procedure may relieve the blockage, and if not, surgery may be needed if some of the intestinal tissue has died due to the blockage.

For a partial obstruction, a special low-fiber diet may be recommended.

Diagnosis

The diagnosis of an intestinal obstruction involves a physical as well as a diagnostic or imaging exam. The physician can assess bowel sounds and order abdominal radiographs or abdominal CT scans.

Prevention

Some causes are not preventable. However, in the case of conditions such a tumor, diverticulitis, or hernias that can block the intestinal, treatment directed at these conditions may be helpful.

Prognosis and Outcome

With proper diagnosis and treatment, the outcome is good. If untreated, the condition may lead to the death of some related intestinal tissues. This could also result in an infection or gangrene. A hole or perforation in the wall of the intestine is another possible complication of intestinal obstruction. This situation would require immediate surgery to prevent severe infection in the abdominal cavity or peritonitis, shock, and the risk of death. Paralytic ileus is often a temporary condition that recovers on its own. If not, medications to produce muscle contractions can help to move fluid and solids through the intestine.

Ray Marks

See also: Abdominal Diseases; Crohn's Disease; Digestive Diseases; Diverticular Disease

Further Reading

Mayo Clinic. (2012, December 18). Intestinal obstruction. Retrieved from http://www .mayoclinic.org/diseases-conditions/intestinal-obstruction/basics/definition/con -20027567.

MedlinePlus. (2015, September 3). Intestinal obstruction. Retrieved from https://www.nlm .nih.gov/medlineplus/intestinalobstruction.html.

National Institute of Diabetes and Digestive and Kidney Diseases. (2013, July 10). Anatomic problems of the lower GI tract. Retrieved from http://www.niddk.nih.gov /health-information/health-topics/digestive-diseases/anatomic-colon/Pages/facts .aspx.

University of Maryland Medical Center. (2014, August 11). Intestinal obstruction. Retrieved from http://umm.edu/health/medical/ency/articles/intestinal-obstruction.

IRON OVERLOAD DISEASE

Iron overload disease is a common metabolic health condition in which there is an excessive amount of iron absorbed from foods and drinks into the body. The presence of excess iron, which is not removed and is stored in the tissues of major organs of the body, may damage the liver and other organs and give the skin a bronze color. If the condition is not resolved, the pancreas may become involved, and the person may develop diabetes. Other health conditions that can arise if the condition is genetic are hemochromatosis, heart disease, cirrhosis, and cancer.

The condition is more common in men than women and involves a 25-amino acid peptide hormone that regulates iron metabolism, called *hepcidin*. It affects millions of people worldwide.

Types

Juvenile iron overload disease starts early on in life, between ages of 25 and 30 years, and is the most severe form of the disease. Neonatal iron overload disease occurs if iron accumulates in the infant's liver too rapidly, and it can cause death before or after birth.

Symptoms

The key symptoms are the presence of abdominal pain, fatigue, high blood sugar levels, low thyroid function, joint pain, skin taking on a bronze color, shortness of breath, tiredness, weakness, and weight loss, although no symptoms may prevail.

Causes

The condition may be genetic, due to a deficiency in hepcidin if an individual inherits abnormal genes from both parents, in which case it is called *primary iron overload disease* or *classic iron overload disease*. This is a common disease among U.S. Caucasians, affecting 240 to 300 individuals. If the disease is caused by some other health condition, such as chronic liver disease, where excess iron may be absorbed, the condition is known as *secondary iron overload disease*. It can also result from taking large doses of iron orally, by injection, or via blood transfusions and by long-term kidney dialysis.

Treatment

The main treatment may involve removing iron-rich blood from the patient regularly, called *phlebotomy*, along with medications that bind iron so it can be excreted from the body.

Eating iron-rich foods such as red meat, as well as vitamin C–rich foods should be avoided, as should raw seafood and alcohol.

Diagnosis

The main tests used for diagnosing this condition are blood tests to examine ferritin levels that are high in patients with iron overload disease; serum iron testing, a measure of iron content of the serum; and a careful medical history. Other tests include genetic tests and biopsies of the liver.

Prognosis and Outcome

The condition can occur with no symptoms or with severe symptoms. Effective treatment can improve most related health conditions, except cirrhosis, and the risk of developing liver cancer. As the condition progresses, patients can develop arthritis, liver cirrhosis, diabetes, an enlarged liver, heart disease, and pancreatitis.

Future

In efforts to treat iron overload, researchers at the University of California, Los Angeles (UCLA) have developed a new form of therapy based on small molecules that mimic the effects of hepcidin in mice. Hepcidin works by interacting with a receptor protein called ferroportin to change iron flow in the body. The UCLA scientists tried to understand how these proteins interlock and which aspects of this process are most important. After they found the first third of the molecule of hepcidin provided the best fit to link to ferroportin, they reengineered this portion to produce new molecules called "minihepcidins." These minihepcidins were effective in healthy mice, where they prevented iron overload in mouse models of hereditary iron overload. The minihepcicins were more effective than the regular, naturally occurring hormone. In the future, optimal forms of minihepcidens will be investigated and introduced into human preclinical and clinical trials.

Ray Marks

See also: Genetic Diseases; Hemochromatosis

Further Reading

Fleming, R. E., & Ponka, P. (2012). Iron overload in human disease. *New England Journal of Medicine, 366,* 348–359. Retrieved from http://www.nejm.org/doi/full/10.1056/NEJMra1004967.

Iron Disorders Institute. (2012). Iron overload. Retrieved from http://www.irondisorders.org/iron-overload.

Lee, D. (2007). Hereditary hemochromatosis (iron overload). MedicineNet.com. Retrieved from http://www.medicinenet.com/iron_overload/article.htm.

Lee, P. L., & Beutler, E. (2009). Regulation of hepcidin and iron-overload disease. *The Annual Review of Pathology Mechanisms of Disease.* Retrieved from http://www.annualreviews.org/doi/pdf/10.1146/annurev.pathol.4.110807.092205.

Nordqvist, C. (2009, October 7). What is iron overload disorder? What is hemochromoto-sis? What causes iron overload disorder? *Medical News Today*. Retrieved from http://www.medicalnewstoday.com/articles/166455.php.

Science Daily. (2012). Scientists design experimental treatment for iron-overload diseases. Retrieved from http://www.sciencedaily.com/releases/2011/11/111101125544.htm.

IRRITABLE BOWEL SYNDROME

Irritable bowel syndrome (IBS) is a functional gastrointestinal disorder affecting the function of the large intestine or colon. It is a common health condition, affecting about 10 to 20 percent of the population, but one that is generally manageable. Risk factors for irritable bowel syndrome include being young or under age 35, being female, and having a family history of the condition. The condition is characterized by fluctuating episodes of abdominal pain and bowel habits in the absence of specific and definitive organic pathology.

History

According to Lehrer and Lichtenstein (2012), the original term *mucous colitis* was framed by Osler in 1892 to describe a disorder of mucorrhea and abdominal colic that occurred at high rates in patients with psychopathology. After that, the syndrome was referred to as spastic colon, irritable colon, colitis, or nervous colon.

Types

Irritable bowel syndrome is often divided into four subtypes:

IBS with constipation
IBS with diarrhea
Mixed IBS
Unclassifiable subtypes IBS

Symptoms

Key symptoms associated with irritable bowel syndrome are abdominal pain or cramps, feeling bloated, excessive flatulence or gas, constipation or diarrhea, and mucus in the stool. Other possible symptoms are fever, weight loss, anemia, and rectal bleeding.

The symptoms may vary from mild to severe. They may also fluctuate, as with any chronic condition, and come and go.

Causes

The key cause of irritable bowel syndrome is not known, but it is being actively researched. However, abnormalities in the nervous system—including abnormal signaling between the brain and nerves of the small and large intestine or colon, as well as psychopathology, or psychological illnesses, that create a proinflammatory state and some forms of bowel infection—may play a role. Certain foods, too, may act as triggers for some people, such as milk, chocolate, and alcohol. Stress may cause the symptoms to worsen, and in women, hormonal changes related to the menstrual cycle may play a role. The bowel may exhibit muscle or movement problems or hypersensitivity to stretching. Another theory is that individuals with irritable bowel syndrome have altered levels of neurotransmitters, chemicals that transmit nerve signals, and gastrointestinal hormones.

Treatment

Treatment involves stress management, counseling, and dietary and lifestyle changes. Medications and avoiding carbonated beverages, salads, and raw fruits and vegetables—especially cabbage, cauliflower, beans, fatty foods, and broccoli—may help. Drinking plenty of water and exercising may help. Patient education is thus very important in this health condition.

Diagnosis

A diagnosis of irritable bowel syndrome can include a medical examination and a physical exam. A diagnosis may be made if abdominal pain and discomfort have lasted for at least 12 weeks and fulfill available guidelines. Additional tests include stool studies, computerized tomography scans, blood tests, lactose intolerance tests, colonoscopy, or flexible sigmoidoscopy.

Prevention

Reducing stress may be helpful in preventing irritable bowel syndrome.

Prognosis and Outcome

Irritable bowel syndrome is not life-threatening, but it can reduce the quality of life because it a chronic or long-standing relapsing disorder.

Ray Marks

See also: Abdominal Diseases; Diet and Nutrition; Stress; Women's Health

Further Reading

About Irritable Bowel Syndrome. (2015). Irritable bowel syndrome. Retrieved from http://www.about-irritablebowelsyndrome.com/.

HealthLine. (2014, September 29). What do you want to know about IBS? Retrieved from http://www.healthline.com/health/irritable-bowel-syndrome.

International Foundation for Functional Gastrointestinal Disorders, Inc. (2014, September 15). Intro to IBS. Retrieved from http://www.aboutibs.org/site/what-is-ibs/intro-to-ibs/.

Lehrer, J. K., & Lichtenstein, G. R. (2011). Irritable bowel syndrome. *Medscape*. Retrieved from http://emedicine.medscape.com/article/180389-overview.

Mayo Clinic. (2014, July 31). Irritable bowel syndrome. Retrieved from http://www.mayoclinic.org/diseases-conditions/irritable-bowel-syndrome/basics/definition/con-20024578.

National Institute of Diabetes and Digestive and Kidney Diseases. (2015). Irritable bowel syndrome. Retrieved from http://www.niddk.nih.gov/health-information/health-topics/digestive-diseases/irritable-bowel-syndrome/pages/overview.aspx.

J

JOINT DISORDERS

Throughout the body, two or more bones come together as *joints*, such as at the knee, hip, elbow, and shoulder. Joint disorders, which cause pain or restricted range of motion, can be the result of inflammation due to infection, degeneration, diseases, and injuries. Chief among them is arthritis, which generally describes the many disorders affecting the joints that can lead to pain, stiffness, and swelling and can cause severe damage over time. Another is bursitis, which takes place when the small fluid-filled sacs that cushion the joints become inflamed. Joints can also become injured from sprains and dislocations.

Arthritis generally describes more than 100 disorders that affect the joints, and it affects more than 52.5 million adults and 1 in 250 children in the United States. The most common type of arthritis is osteoarthritis, which most often affects the fingers, knees, and hips. Rheumatoid arthritis is the most common type of autoimmune arthritis, which takes place when the body mistakenly attacks healthy tissues in the joints. Other arthritis types include juvenile arthritis, which affects children; infectious arthritis, an infection that spreads from somewhere in the body to a joint; psoriatic arthritis, which affects people the chronic skin condition psoriasis; and gout, the buildup of uric acid in the body.

Common in the shoulders, knees, elbows, fingers, and jaw, dislocations are injuries to a joint that force the ends of the bones from their natural positions. Sprains can damage joints when their connective tissues, tendons, and ligaments are overstretched or torn.

Symptoms

Pain is the foremost symptom, regardless of how a joint has been affected. In general, the various forms of arthritis are characterized by pain and stiffness, often in the back, hands, knees, or shoulders, as well as soreness and trouble moving the joints. Signs of this type of inflammation include joint swelling and tenderness, skin hot to the touch, redness around the joint, muscle spasm, limited range of motion, fatigue, and weakness. Symptoms of rheumatoid arthritis, which can affect other organs in the body, may include fever, unintended weight loss, trouble breathing, and rashes or itches. Osteoarthritis that occurs in the spine may cause numbness, pain, and weakness in the arms or legs.

Symptoms of bursitis may include ache or stiffness around the affected joint, as well as swelling and redness and pain to the touch. When a joint becomes dislocated, pain, swelling, and discoloration are primary symptoms. The joint may also appear to be out of place or deformed and may not move properly, causing tingling or numbness. A joint affected by a sprain is also very painful, swollen, and restricted in its range of motion.

Causes and Risk Factors

The causes remain unknown for many types of arthritis, but genetics, lifestyle, and certain types of bacteria, as well as a combination of genetics and an environmental trigger such as a virus or toxin may be contributing factors.

The most common type of arthritis, osteoarthritis, occurs as people age and the cartilage at the ends of the joints gets worn down, but it can also result from an injury or an infection. Rheumatoid arthritis is the immune system mistakenly attacking the membrane or lining around the joint parts, destroying the cartilage and bone over time. A family history of arthritis, including genes specifically associated with certain types of arthritis; age; being overweight; and previous injury to a joint are risk factors for arthritis. Women are more likely to experience arthritis, including rheumatoid arthritis, while men more often have gout.

Most bursitis is caused by the overuse of a joint or an injury, often at the shoulder, knee, hip, or elbow, which irritate the fluid-filled cushions around a joint. Aging and work or activities that require repetitive motion or pressure, as well as rheumatoid arthritis, gout, and diabetes are risk factors.

A fall, an injury from a contact sport, a sudden impact on a joint, or other unusual body movements are the causes of most joint dislocations. Hereditary loose ligaments, falling, playing high-impact or contact sports, as well as involvement in a motor vehicle accident are risk factors for joint dislocations. Sprains are the result of overstretching or tearing the connective tissues, tendons, and ligaments that are associated with a joint. Risk factors for sprains include poor muscle conditioning, fatigue, walking or running on dangerously slippery or uneven surfaces, and ill-fitting shoes and improper warm-ups before physical activity.

Diagnosis

Diagnosing arthritis involves taking a medical history, including all current and previous symptoms, and a physical examination of symptoms; x-rays and blood work may also be examined. X-rays can show cartilage loss, bone damage, and bone spurs but may not reveal joint damage from arthritis; they may be used to track progression of the disease. Imaging tests of the bones, ligaments, tendons, and cartilage may include CT scans, MRIs, and ultrasound. Arthroscopy, or the insertion of an arthroscope (small flexible tube), through an incision near the joint may be used to look for joint damage.

No one blood test exists for osteoarthritis, a diagnosis is based on symptoms, a physical examination, and occasionally x-rays to track the progression of rheumatoid arthritis in the joints over time. A sample of joint fluid may be examined to differentiate osteoarthritis from an infection, gout, or other joint disorders. Visible symptoms, x-rays, and a blood test can confirm the diagnosis of rheumatoid arthritis; those who have rheumatoid arthritis usually have an elevated erythrocyte sedimentation rate, indicating inflammation in the body.

A diagnosis of bursitis is based on a medical history and physical exam but may include imaging tests to exclude other disorders or if the physical exam is inconclusive. Blood tests or fluid analysis also help determine the cause of this joint pain. In addition, a physical examination of a dislocation injury, an x-ray, and MRI can confirm and assess damage to the joint and surrounding soft tissues. Sprains are diagnosed based on the symptoms present in a physical examination, including swelling, location of tenderness, and intensity of pain. X-rays can help rule out a fracture, and an MRI may help determine the extent of the injury.

Treatments

Treatment of joint problems depends on the cause. Arthritis treatment focuses on controlling pain, reducing joint damage, improving function, and controlling inflammation where appropriate. No cure exists for rheumatoid arthritis, but as for other forms of arthritis, medications may include analgesics to reduce pain; nonsteroidal anti-inflammatory drugs (NSAIDs) to reduce pain as well as inflammation; creams and ointments containing menthol or capsaicin that interfere with the transmission of pain signals from the joint; disease-modifying antirheumatic drugs for rheumatoid arthritis, which work to keep the immune system from attacking joint tissues; biologics, which are genetically engineered drugs that target proteins in the immune response; and corticosteroids, which reduce inflammation and suppress the immune system. Physical therapy, splints or joint assistive aids, and weight loss may be recommended as needed. Types of arthritis surgery include joint replacement, which replaces damaged joints, such as knees and hips, with artificial joints; joint fusion, which may lock together the ends of two joints in the wrist, ankle, or fingers so they can heal as one unit; and tendon repair for rheumatoid arthritis.

Bursitis is treated with rest, ice, and pain relievers. But antibiotics, physical therapy, corticosteroid injections to relieve inflammation, a cane or other assistive device, and (rarely) surgery may be prescribed if more conservative measures are not effective.

A dislocated joint is a medical emergency. Treatment depends on the affected joint and may include repositioning the bones, medication, immobilization in a splint or sling, and rehabilitation. Sprains are usually treated with over-the-counter pain relievers and the application of ice to minimize swelling. Occasionally, a brace or splint is necessary to immobilize the affected joint. Surgery is rare but may be necessary if a ligament or muscle is torn.

Prevention

It is not possible to prevent arthritis, but steps can be taken to reduce some risk factors or delay the onset of some forms, including maintaining a healthy body weight and protecting joints from injuries or overuse, especially for osteoarthritis.

Other activities include regular exercise, warm showers in the morning, using medication as prescribed, and visiting doctors regularly.

Preventing bursitis or reducing the risk factors may be accomplished by protecting the joints with appropriate padding (such as knee pads), as well as by lifting properly and taking breaks when performing repetitive tasks. As with arthritis, maintaining a healthy weight and exercise are effective preventive measures.

Wearing protective sports gear and taking precautions to avoid falls help prevent joint dislocations; a dislocated joint is more susceptible to recurrence. Similarly, regular strength-training exercises to condition muscles and warming up can reduce the risk of sprains, as can appropriate footwear offering support.

Prognosis and Outcomes

The prognosis for arthritis depends on the type, but those who receive an early accurate diagnosis, stick to their treatment plans, and follow preventive measures usually have the best outcomes. However, rheumatoid arthritis causes most people develop permanent joint abnormalities within 10 years and decreases life expectancy by three to seven years. Even with treatment, which is effective in three out of four people, at least 10 percent will become severely disabled. This disorder increases the risk of heart disease, infection, and gastrointestinal bleeding, which are the most common complications causing death.

The prognosis of bursitis is usually very good, usually after adjusting activities to prevent recurrence. With proper treatment and follow-up, most joint injuries recover within a few weeks or months.

Jean Kaplan Teichroew

See also: Arthritis; Bone Diseases; Bone Infections; Bursitis; Rheumatoid Arthritis

Further Reading

Arthritis Foundation. (2015). Understanding arthritis. Retrieved from http://www.arthritis.org/about-arthritis/understanding-arthritis/.

Mayo Clinic. (2014, October 9). Osteoarthritis. Retrieved from http://www.mayoclinic.org/diseases-conditions/osteoarthritis/basics/definition/con-20014749.

Mayo Clinic. (2014, January 25). Dislocations. Retrieved from http://www.mayoclinic.org/diseases-conditions/dislocation/basics/definition/con-20022264.

Mayo Clinic. (2015, January 24). Sprains and strains. Retrieved from http://www.mayoclinic.org/diseases-conditions/sprains-and-strains/basics/definition/con-20020958.

Merck Manual. (2015). Joint disorders. Retrieved from http://www.merckmanuals.com/home/bone-joint-and-muscle-disorders/joint-disorders/.

National Institute of Arthritis and Musculoskeletal and Skin Disease. (2014, July). Arthritis. Retrieved from http://www.niams.nih.gov/Health_Info/Arthritis/default.asp#b.

JUVENILE ARTHRITIS

Juvenile arthritis is also known as childhood arthritis. This condition can take the form of any kind of arthritis, or conditions related to arthritis, that occurs in persons under 16 years old. It is one of the most common childhood diseases in the United States. The term *childhood arthritis* is an umbrella term, which covers a number of types of arthritis with differing definitions.

It is estimated that approximately 294,000 children in the United States, or 1 in 250 children, have been diagnosed with arthritis or other conditions caused by inflammation, swelling, and pain in the muscles or joints.

Symptoms

Common symptoms include pain, swelling, tenderness, and stiffness in joints. Joints may also have a limited range of motion. Joint contracture may occur, which means that muscles, ligaments, or tendons have become shortened, preventing a joint from having full range of motion. Damage to cartilage and bone in the joint can lead to an observable deformity to a joint. A child experiencing arthritis may only grow to a short stature due to altered growth in the bone and joints. Depending on the type of arthritic condition, the skin, eyes, and internal organs may be affected by inflammation.

Types

It is commonly agreed that types of childhood arthritis include juvenile rheumatoid arthritis or juvenile idiopathic arthritis. In addition, there are other arthritic or rheumatic diseases affecting children. However, there remains some disagreement in the medical profession as to what specific conditions fall under the term.

JRA (juvenile rheumatoid arthritis), is the most common form of childhood arthritis. It is diagnosed in a child younger than 16 years after at least six weeks of persistent arthritis that is not attributed to any other type of childhood arthritis.

Children with juvenile rheumatoid arthritis may experience symptoms for just a few months; other may experience symptoms for the rest of their lives.

Complications can include growth problems and eye inflammation.

A child may experience pain in joins or limbs, especially shortly after sleep. Swelling is common in the joins. Stiffness may result in a child experiencing clumsy movement, particularly after sleep. These symptoms can occur in one or multiple joints; in some cases, the entire body is affected with swollen lymph nodes, rash, and fever. Should any of these symptoms occur for more than a week, the child should be seen by a doctor.

These other conditions include juvenile dermatomyositis, juvenile lupus, juvenile scleroderma, Kawasaki disease, and mixed connective tissue disease.

> *Juvenile lupus* is a disease affecting the immune system, the joints, skin, kidneys, and blood as well as other parts of the body. Symptoms may include a rash shaped like a butterfly that occurs on both nose and cheeks, a scale-like rash on the face or neck, sensitivity to sunlight, and pain in the joints or on the chest.
>
> *Juvenile scleroderma* is a group of conditions that causes the skin to tighten and become hard. The word *scleroderma* literally means "hard skin." There are two forms, one in which the whole body is affected and a second in which only a portion of the body

is affected. When the whole body is affected, the condition also affects internal organs and most affects the fingers, hands, face, and forearms.

Kawasaki disease is characterized by inflammatory symptoms followed by heart complication experiences by children in later years. Infants and young children are mostly affected. It is common for the child with condition to experience a succession of symptoms: the condition starts with a high fever, often followed by a rash; then there is swelling in hands and feet, followed by a few weeks by peeling of skin around the fingers and toes. It is common for the child to have arthritis in addition; however, the most serious symptom is inflammation of blood vessels requiring close monitoring for heart complications.

Mixed connective tissue disease may include characteristics of arthritis, lupus, dermatomyositis, and scleroderma. The condition is associated with particularly high levels of a specific type of antibody.

Juvenile dermatomyositis (JDMS) is an inflammatory condition that causes muscles to weaken and causes skin rashes on the eyelids and knuckles. It is common for children with this condition to also have mild rheumatoid arthritis; the disease affects approximately one in five children. Most commonly, muscle weakness occurs in the torso, shoulders, and upper legs. This weakness may limit capacity for physical activity like running and climbing stairs.

Diagnosis

JDMS can develop either over a long period of time or over a very short period. Diagnosis is accomplished by analysis of symptoms such as the appearance or description of the symptoms, when the symptoms began, what areas of the body are affected, and whether the symptoms improve or get worse, as well as other considerations.

In addition to considering symptoms, laboratory tests may assist the doctor in establishing a JDMS diagnosis. These tests measure the degree of inflammation in the body. Tests may be repeated over a period of time to determine if changes in the measure occur over time.

Certain muscle enzymes may be present in the blood that are not normally present. The measure of these enzymes provides indication of muscle damage.

A doctor may also measure antibodies and electrical activity in the muscles. A biopsy of the muscle may also be taken to examine the muscle and is surrounding tissue directly.

Lastly an MRI, a highly sophisticated x-ray, scan may be completed to identify inflammation or identify muscles suitable for biopsy.

Using all the preceding strategies in the physician's toolkit, the doctor may confirm a diagnosis of JDMS, or rule JDMS out as the cause to a patient's illness.

Cause

Childhood arthritis occurs when the body's cells and tissues are attacked by its own immune system. The root cause of this attack is unknown; however, evidence has shown that genetics and environmental conditions can play a role. Some gene mutations may make some more susceptible to environmental factors such as viruses that trigger the immune attack than others.

Risk Factors

Risk factors are not well known. However, it has been found that girls are more commonly affected by the condition.

Treatments

Because there is no cure for JDMS, one can only treat the illness, aiming to prevent the appearance of symptoms. Treatments include medication, exercise, adjustment of diet, as well as patient education.

The best care for a child with childhood arthritis is a care regime specifically tailored to each child and his or her condition. Treatment goals including control of symptoms, preventing damage to joints, and maintaining function.

Treatments typically involved anti-inflammatory drugs such as ibuprofen. As a second line of treatment—disease-modifying drugs—may be prescribed if there is little or no response to anti-inflammatories. These types of drugs can include side effects that will require close monitoring by the health care team.

If the child's condition is isolated to a single joint, a steroidal injection can be administered to the site before other drugs are provided. Typically, oral steroids are avoided due to their unacceptable side effects but, when necessary, are given in the lowest dose and shortest period possible.

Prevention

The cause of most forms of childhood arthritis are not known; however, it is not contagious, and foods, toxins, allergies or vitamin deficiency do not play any role in causing the condition. Therefore, means of prevention are unknown.

Prognosis

Children with arthritis attend school, play, and participate in normal activities like any other child. Positive environments and participating in normal activities are part of a successful treatment regime.

Bradley Lang

See also: Arthritis; Osteoarthritis; Rheumatoid Arthritis

Further Reading

American College of Rheumatology. (2012). Arthritis in children. Retrieved from http://www
.rheumatology.org/practice/clinical/patients/diseases_and_conditions/juvenilearthritis
.asp.

Arthritis Foundation. (2012). Juvenile arthritis fact sheet. Retrieved from http://www.arthritis .org/ja-fact-sheet.php.

Arthritis Foundation. (2012). Juvenile arthritis. Retrieved from http://www.arthritis.org /disease-center.php?disease_id=37&df=treatments.

Centers for Disease Control and Prevention (CDC). (2011). Childhood arthritis. Retrieved from http://www.cdc.gov/arthritis/basics/childhood.htm.

National Center for Biotechnology Information (NCBI). (2002). Treatment options for juvenile-onset systemic lupus erythematosus. Retrieved from http://www.ncbi.nlm.nih .gov/pubmed/11960513.

K

KAPOSI'S SARCOMA

Kaposi's sarcoma (KS) is a type of soft-tissue cancerous tumor that typically affects the mouth and skin, but it can also occur in the internal organs. It generally appears as a pink or red lesion; however, in those with darker skin, the tumor can appear dark brown or black. KS is rare in the mainstream population and most commonly affects people with compromised immune systems, such as the elderly or those whose bodies have already been weakened by HIV/AIDS. In the United States, some six cases of KS per 1 million people are reported per year, while in some parts of Africa, around 90 percent of the population show signs of the condition. Annually, around 34,000 new cases of KS are reported around the world.

KS is caused by an infection with the virus Kaposi's sarcoma herpes virus (KSHV), which is also known as human herpesvirus 8. This virus is common—about 1 in every 20 people carry it—but in the majority of cases, it remains dormant and does not create any detectable health issues. In a person with a comprised immune system, KSHV can multiply to high levels in blood and lymph cells, increasing the risk that the cells will turn cancerous. When KS forms, it usually first appears as red or purple bumps or lesions on the skin. These lesions often crop up in multiple locations and generally are not painful; though if they appear in the mouth, they may make it difficult to chew or swallow. KS may also affect such internal organs as the lymph nodes, stomach, intestines, or lungs. Symptoms of the condition will differ depending on which organs are affected. For example, KS lesions in the lungs can create coughing or bloody spittle, while KS lesions in the lymph nodes commonly create swollen glands, and KS issues in the digestive system may create such symptoms as nausea or diarrhea.

There are four main types of KS: epidemic or AIDS-related KS, classic KS, endemic (African) KS, and latrogenic KS. Epidemic or AIDS-related KS occurs in people who are infected with HIV. It is often considered a defining characteristic of AIDS because an HIV-infected person who develops KS is now thought to have full-blown AIDS and is no longer just HIV-positive. Endemic (African) KS occurs in those living in equatorial Africa and is one of the most common types of cancer in that region—approximately 1 in 10 cases of cancer in Africa is endemic KS. Classic KS mainly affects adults 40 and older who are of Mediterranean, Eastern European, or Middle Eastern descent. It is generally nonfatal, affecting the skin only, and is more common in men than women. Sometimes known as transplant KS, latrogenic KS occurs as a rare complication of an organ transplant surgery. People who receive a transplant organ typically have to take immunosuppressant medications to help their body accept the new organ, which increases the risk of developing KS in those who already have KSHV. About 1 in every 200 U.S. transplant patients develops KS. Although classic KS is a slow-developing disease, the other three types can be very aggressive, creating lesions that spread rapidly over the body in a matter of months.

KS develops in four stages: Stage 1 occurs when the lesions are limited to one or a few localized areas of the skin. Stage 2 is confirmed by the growth of deeper nodules that damage inner layers of the skin. Stage 3 happens when the lymph system is affected by KS but other internal organs are not yet compromised. Stage 4 means the cancer has spread internally. KS is commonly diagnosed through a biopsy, a procedure used to remove and analyze a small sample of cells. If a practitioner suspects that the condition is internal, an endoscopy procedure that places a flexible tube with a camera down into the lungs and digestive system may be performed to examine these organs up close. X-rays or magnetic resonance imaging (MRI) scans may also be recommended to provide more detailed images of the internal organs. Treatment of the disease depends on several factors, including how advanced the condition is and what type of KS has been contracted. Surgery, chemotherapy, radiotherapy (using high-energy rays to destroy cancerous cells), and antiretroviral medication are among the common forms of treatment for the disease. Some 30 percent of those with KS die within five years of diagnosis.

Hungarian dermatologist Moritz Kaposi first discovered KS in 1872, but it was not until the 1990s that the cause, KSHV, was pinpointed. With that, scientists began researching the ways the virus could be transmitted and developing tools to counteract it. While there is currently no vaccine against KSHV, new research on a potential vaccination strategy was released in 2012. However, according to the Centers for Disease Control and Prevention, the CDC (2016), "Pre-exposure prophylaxis, or PrEP, is a way for people who do not have HIV but who are at substantial risk of getting it to prevent HIV infection by taking a pill every day." The pill "contains two medicines (tenofovir and emtricitabine) that are used in combination with other medicines to treat HIV." People who are exposed to HIV through sex or injected drugs, can use these antiviral drugs to keep the virus from taking hold as a permanent infection.

Tamar Burris

See also: AIDS; Cancer; Head and Neck Cancer; Immune System Disorders

Further Reading

American Cancer Society. (2015). What is Kaposi sarcoma? Retrieved from http://www.cancer.org/cancer/kaposisarcoma/detailedguide/kaposi-sarcoma-what-is-kaposi-sarcoma.

Centers for Disease Control and Prevention (CDC). (2016, February 10). Pre-exposure prophylaxis (PrEP). http://www.cdc.gov/hiv/risk/prep/index.html.

Johns Hopkins Medicine. (2015). Kaposi's sarcoma. Retrieved from http://www.hopkinsmedicine.org/kimmel_cancer_center/types_cancer/kaposis_sarcoma.html.

Mount Sinai Hospital. (2015). Kaposi's sarcoma. Retrieved from http://www.mountsinai.org/patient-care/health-library/diseases-and-conditions/kaposis-sarcoma.

Pories, S. E., et al. (2009). *Cancer.* Westport, CT: Greenwood.

Stolley, K. S., & Glass, J. E. (2009). *HIV/AIDS.* Westport, CT: Greenwood.

KAWASAKI DISEASE

Kawasaki disease is a rare disease characterized by the sudden onset of fever of unknown cause in children younger than five years of age, usually boys, although it can occur at any age and in girls. The disease is not contagious and occurs worldwide, with the highest rates reported to occur in Japan. Kawasaki disease is the leading cause of acquired heart disease in children and may be a risk factor for adult ischemic heart disease; it involves generalized vasculitis or inflammation of the small and medium-sized arteries throughout the body that damages these blood vessels, especially those around the heart or coronary arteries, and suggests the immune system may play a role in this disease. In the United States, approximately 100,000 cases are diagnosed annually. It is also termed *infantile polyarteritis, infantile periarteritis nodosa, Kawasaki syndrome,* and *mucocutaneous lymph node syndrome.*

History

Kawasaki disease was initially described in 1967 by pediatrician Tomisaku Kawasaki, who reported 50 cases with distinct symptoms at the Tokyo Red Cross Medical Center in Japan. In 1976, the first cases outside of Japan occurred in Hawaii in a group of 12 children from Honolulu.

Symptoms

Kawasaki disease is characterized by the presence of a fever; swelling of the hands and feet; irritation and redness of the white areas of the eyes; swelling of the neck lymph glands; a cough and a runny nose; the presence of a bright red rash; peeling skin on the main part of the trunk and in the area of the genitals, especially on the palms and soles; irritability; abdominal pain; diarrhea and vomiting; joint pain, often on both sides of the body; ulcerative gum disease; and throat-, mouth-, and lip-related inflammation and irritation.

Causes

The causes of Kawasaki disease are unknown but are probably infectious in nature, involving microorganisms or toxins, and the disease tends to occur seasonally, in early spring and late winter. There may also be a genetic basis for the condition. Risk factors include age, gender, and ethnicity.

Diagnosis

There is no specific test for Kawasaki disease; however, the diagnosis is made on the basis of the presence of four out of five key clinical characteristics. Laboratory tests may be conducted where the clinical evidence is not clear and to rule out other conditions. Electrocardiograms and echocardiograms or ultrasound tests of the status of the heart may be conducted, as may blood tests to assess inflammation in efforts to monitor disease activity.

Treatment and Prevention

Early administration of immunoglobulin, together with fluids, delivered intravenously, and high doses of aspirin, is said to reduce the risk of cardiac involvement later on by approximately 5 percent. In cases that do not respond to therapy, corticosteroids and biological agents may be applied, as may plasmapheresis, where the patient's plasma is removed from the blood and replaced with protein-containing fluids; in the case of persistent joint pain, anti-inflammatory drugs may be applied. Early treatment within seven days of fever onset is indicated to reduce the risk of complications. There are, however, no preventive measures presently advocated for reducing the incidence of this disease, but parents should get prompt help if their child has symptoms of a fever or rash that lasts for several days. As the child recovers, periodic health checks may be useful to monitor the heart condition and the onset of any problems.

Prognosis and Outcomes

Although the disease was first thought to be self-limiting within four to eight weeks and benign, with full recovery if treatment is applied early enough, later evidence showed approximately 2 percent of cases died from the condition, and these children were mostly under the age of two. Serious complications of Kawasaki disease include coronary artery damage leading to heart muscle damage, heart failure and various forms of heart disease, and the widening of blood vessels or aneurysms, and these conditions are more likely to occur if the diagnosis is delayed initially.

Future

Elevated levels of filamen C, a protein, and meprin A, an enzyme related to inflammation, in blood or urine samples may allow clinicians to diagnose the disease more accurately. Medications that block the effect of tumor necrosis factor as a messenger in the inflammatory response cycle are being studied to examine their use in the treatment process. A substance called Trental is also being studied as a possible treatment agent for Kawasaki disease. Researchers are focusing on methods for detecting children at risk for later complications, especially aneurysms of the coronary arteries, and to investigate variants of Kawasaki disease that do not have a classical appearance.

Ray Marks

See also: Abdominal Diseases; Aneurisms; Coronary Artery Disease; Heart Diseases

Further Reading

American Academy of Pediatrics. (2015, August 20). Kawasaki disease. Retrieved from https://www.healthychildren.org/English/health-issues/conditions/heart/Pages/Kawasaki-Disease.aspx.

American Heart Association. (2015, October 22). Kawasaki disease. Retrieved from http://
www.heart.org/HEARTORG/Conditions/More/CardiovascularConditionsofChildhood
/Kawasaki-Disease_UCM_308777_Article.jsp#.VkXya2tKjwo.

Mayo Clinic. (2014, February 15). Kawasaki disease. Retrieved from http://www.mayoclinic
.org/diseases-conditions/kawasaki-disease/basics/definition/con-20024663.

MedicineNet.com. (2014, October 20). Kawasaki's disease. Retrieved from http://www
.medicinenet.com/kawasaki_disease/article.htm.

MedlinePlus. (2015, November 5). Kawasaki disease. Retrieved from https://www.nlm.nih
.gov/medlineplus/kawasakidisease.html.

National Heart, Lung, and Blood Institute. (2011, November 20). What is Kawasaki disease? Retrieved from http://www.nhlbi.nih.gov/health/health-topics/topics/kd/.

KIDNEY CANCER

Originating in a kidney, malignant cells that grow out of control and form a tumor are referred to as kidney, or renal, cancer. When kidney cancer spreads, it may go to the other kidney, the lungs, bones, liver, or lymph glands. Kidney cancer is most common in people over age 45 and among African Americans, and it occurs twice as often in males. About 50,000 to 60,000 cases are diagnosed in the United States each year.

The kidneys are two fist-size organs attached to the upper back wall of the abdomen, one to the left and one to the right of the spine. Protected by the rib cage, the purpose of the kidneys is to filter the blood coming in from the renal arteries and remove excess water, salt, and waste products, which become urine. The urine leaves the kidneys through the ureters, or tubes leading connecting the kidney to the bladder. The kidneys also aid in controlling blood pressure and produce a hormone that instructs the body to produce red blood cells.

Renal cell carcinoma is the most common, making up 85 percent of all kidney cancers. It affects the kidney's filtration system, including the cells lining the ureters. Transitional cell carcinoma affects the area of the kidney where urine collects before moving to the bladder, comprising about 10 to 15 percent of kidney cancers in adults. Sarcoma of the kidney is rare, and it usually does not spread. Wilms tumor is a form of kidney cancer in children.

The causes of kidney cancer are not known, but aging, smoking, certain genetic disorders, high blood pressure, family history, having lymphoma or kidney disease, exposure to chemicals, and long-term misuse of pain medications are risk factors that increase the likelihood of the disease. Treatment options include surgery, radiation, chemotherapy, or biologic or targeted therapies.

Symptoms

The most common symptoms of kidney cancer include the presence of blood in the urine, pain located on the side of the body or lower back that does not go away, a lump on the side of the body or in the abdominal area, unexplained weight loss, anemia, fatigue, and intermittent fever. If the cancer has spread to other parts of the body, bone pain, shortness of breath, and coughing up blood may be present.

Causes and Risk Factors

The precise causes of kidney cancer are not known, but the factors that contribute to a higher risk include smoking, obesity, high blood pressure, long-term kidney dialysis for kidney failure, some genetic diseases (von Hippel-Lindau syndrome, Birt-Hogg-Dube syndrome, tuberous sclerosis, and familial papillary renal cell carcinoma), exposure to asbestos or cadmium in the workplace, and being male. Using certain pain medications for prolonged periods, diets high in calories or fried meats, and having lymphoma increase the risk of kidney cancer; African Americans are at a slightly higher risk.

Diagnosis

Along with a complete medical history and physical exam, a doctor may order urine and blood tests, as well as imaging tests such as a CT scan, an MRI that gives a detailed picture of the kidneys, an ultrasound to detect the presence of a tumor, a positron emission tomography (PET) scan to spot small collections of cancer cells and detect spreading to lymph nodes near the kidney, and intravenous pyelogram (x-ray of the urinary system). Other tests may include biopsies and a renal arteriogram to examine the blood supply to the kidney and detect small tumors.

The extent of the cancer is described as stages: Stage I is early, where the tumor is only in the kidney and measures about seven centimeters; stage II is also early, but the tumor is larger than seven centimeters; stage III cancer cells have spread to one nearby lymph node or blood vessels; stage IV is when the tumor extends beyond the kidney, or where cells are found in more than one nearby lymph nodes or other organs.

Treatments

The stage of the disease helps inform the most effective treatment option. Surgery is the primary treatment—either the removal of the entire cancerous kidney or the tumor. Other treatments include chemotherapy, radiation therapy (x-rays to kill cancer cells), biologic therapy (to boost the body's own fighting abilities), targeted therapy (substances that attack cancer cells without harming other cells), cryoablation (freezing cancer cells), radiofrequency ablation (heating cancer cells), and arterial embolization, which blocks blood flow to the tumor and helps shrink it before surgery.

Prevention

Because the causes of kidney cancer are unclear, preventive measures are unknown. But lowering the likelihood based on known risk factors include quitting smoking, maintaining a healthy weight, managing blood pressure, and avoiding chemical exposure.

Prognosis and Outcome

Depending on the stage of the disease and a patient's age and overall health, kidney cancer detected in an early stage can be treated successfully with a good outcome.

Future

Researchers are studying different forms of treatment and combinations of treatment, such as chemotherapy and stem cell transplants. Others are studying cancer vaccines that could help the immune system attack kidney cancer cells.

Ray Marks

See also: Abdominal Diseases; Cancer; Kidney Diseases

Further Reading

American Cancer Society. (2015, March 3). Kidney cancer. Retrieved from http://www.cancer .org/cancer/kidneycancer/index.
Kidney Cancer Association. (2014, November 18). About kidney cancer. Retrieved from http://www.kidneycancer.org/.
Mayo Clinic. (2015, February 13). Kidney cancer. Retrieved from http://www.mayoclinic .com/health/kidney-cancer/DS00360.

KIDNEY DISEASE

Located in on each side of the spine, the kidneys clean the body's blood every 30 minutes by removing waste and excess fluid (which become urine), regulating blood pressure, maintaining its balance of salts and minerals, stimulating red blood cell production, and activating vitamin D. If they are damaged by genetic disorders, injuries, or medications, wastes and fluid accumulate, resulting in ankle swelling, nausea, weakness, and respiratory and sleep problems. Untreated diseased kidneys can stop functioning, leading to the serious and often fatal loss of kidney function.

If this happens suddenly, it is called acute kidney injury or failure, most often caused by trauma, diseases, medical conditions that slow blood flow to the organs or block the passage of urine from the body, and some over-the-counter pain medications. Although it can be fatal, the condition can be treated and may be reversible. Chronic kidney disease describes the slow loss of kidney function over time or decreased kidney function or damage lasting longer than three months. Affecting 26 million adults in the United States, it is the ninth leading causes of death; anyone of any age or race can develop kidney disease. It is especially dangerous because symptoms can occur so gradually that they go unnoticed until the disease is quite advanced. Diabetes and high blood pressure are the most common causes, so treatment focuses on managing the underlying illnesses and reducing damage.

Symptoms

Early kidney disease may present symptoms similar to other illnesses, including fatigue or weakness, headache, itching or dry skin, nausea, loss of appetite, and unexpected or unintended weight loss. As the disease progresses, symptoms can typically include changes in urination such as difficulty or pain, increased urge, or decreased amount; urine that is foamy, pink, dark, or bloody; swollen or puffy eyes, face, hands, feet, ankles, and stomach; pale skin; sleep problems; decreased mental sharpness; leg muscle cramps; hiccups; breath odor or metallic taste; chest pain, indicating fluid buildup around the heart; shortness of breath, indicating fluid in the lungs; and persistent or uncontrollable hypertension, or high blood pressure.

Causes and Risk Factors

In addition to direct trauma, acute damage to the kidneys can be caused by medical conditions that slow blood flow to the kidneys, such as heart disease or attack; infection; liver failure; severe allergic reactions, burns, or dehydration; and long-term use of over-the-counter nonsteroidal anti-inflammatory drugs. Other causes include conditions that block the passage of urine from the body, such as bladder, cervical, colon, or prostate cancer; urinary tract blood clots; kidney stones; and nerve damage to the bladder. Acute kidney failure is usually related to another illness or event; factors that increase the risk of acute kidney failure include hospitalization, advanced age, diabetes, high blood pressure, peripheral artery disease, heart failure, and liver and other kidney diseases.

Types 1 and 2 diabetes and hypertension, or high blood pressure, are the most common causes of chronic kidney disease. Other known causes include lupus, HIV/AIDS, hepatitis B and C; urinary tract infections and inflammation within the kidneys; polycystic kidney disease, an inherited condition where the kidneys develop fluid-filled cysts; birth defects resulting from a urinary tract obstruction or malformation; drugs and toxins, including long-term exposure to some over-the-counter nonsteroidal anti-inflammatory drugs and the illegal use of some intravenous drugs. Other risk factors for chronic kidney disease include cardiovascular disease, high cholesterol, smoking tobacco, age 60 or older, obesity, populations with high rates of diabetes or high blood pressure (African Americans, Hispanic Americans, Asian Americans, Pacific Islanders, and American Indians), and family history of kidney disease.

Diagnosis

Diagnosis of acute kidney failure and chronic kidney disease are based on the urine test called albumin-to-creatinine ratio (ACR), which estimates the amount of albumin and is a common indication of kidney damage, and the glomerular filtration rate (GFR), a blood test that measures how well the kidneys are removing wastes from the blood. Other diagnostic tools include blood pressure checks; urine tests that measure daily output and detect abnormalities; kidney biopsy for further lab tests; and imaging tests, such as abdominal or kidney CT or MRI scans or ultrasounds.

Treatments

Usually requiring hospitalization, acute kidney failure focuses on treatment of the underlying injury or illness. Treatment of chronic kidney disease also depends on the underlying condition; the goals include controlling symptoms, reducing complications, and slowing the progression of kidney damage. Medications may be prescribed to lower blood pressure or cholesterol, relieve fluid accumulation and swelling, treat anemia, and prevent bone weakness and lower the risk of fracture.

Diet can slow kidney disease; recommended steps include eating heart-healthy foods with less salt and sodium, small portions of protein, and those with less phosphorus and the right amount of potassium, and drinking small amounts of alcohol.

Prevention

Diabetes and high blood pressure account for most chronic kidney disease, so careful and diligent management of those illnesses with diet, exercise, and medication may help prevent kidney disease. Acute kidney failure may be difficult to prevent other than by reducing risk factors, including limiting overexposure to pain medications known to increase kidney failure, managing symptoms of diabetes and high blood pressure, and making lifestyle and diet changes as necessary. Measures to prevent the development of chronic kidney disease also include the prevention of high blood pressure and diabetes: keeping blood pressure and blood cholesterol level within prescribed target ranges, reducing daily sodium ingestion, avoiding cigarette smoking, following medication prescriptions, getting regular physical activity, and maintaining a healthy body weight.

Prognosis and Outcomes

People can live productive lives after early detection, diagnosis, and treatment of any underlying causes of kidney disease. Untreated kidney disease does not disappear on its own, and it usually worsens over time and leads to loss of kidney function, or kidney failure, and the need for dialysis or transplant.

Ray Marks

See also: Diabetes, Type 1; Diabetes, Type 2; Hypertension; Kidney Cancer; Kidney Failure; Nephritis

Further Reading

Hunt, W. A. (2011). *Kidney disease: A guide for living.* Baltimore, MD: The Johns Hopkins University Press.

Mayo Clinic. (2015, June 5). Acute kidney failure. Retrieved from http://www.mayoclinic .org/diseases-conditions/kidney-failure/basics/definition/CON-20024029.

Mayo Clinic. (2015, January 30). Chronic kidney disease. Retrieved from http://www .mayoclinic.org/diseases-conditions/kidney-disease/basics/definition/con-20026778.

National Institute of Diabetes and Digestive and Kidney Diseases. (2014, September 17). Learn about kidney disease. Retrieved from http://www.niddk.nih.gov/health -information/health-communication-programs/nkdep/learn/Pages/learn.aspx.

National Kidney Foundation. (2015). Kidney disease. Retrieved from http://www.kidney .org/kidneyDisease/.

KIDNEY FAILURE

Description

Chronic kidney disease is a condition in which, most commonly, the kidneys gradually lose their function of removing body wastes and water from the body. Chronic kidney disease can also come on suddenly rather than slowly over time. In either case, this condition produces a dangerous buildup of excess fluid, toxic substances, and waste products that can influence blood pressure, red blood cell production, and bone health negatively, and the disease is an important public health problem.

When the kidneys actually fail to carry out their intended their function of filtering wastes and excess fluids from the blood, and excreting this in the form of urine, this condition is known as kidney failure or renal failure. This final stage is termed end-stage renal disease (ESRD) or chronic renal failure, and the person with this condition may require either dialysis or a kidney transplant.

More than 2 out of every 1,000 persons, or 20 million people, in the United States are said to have chronic kidney disease.

In the early stages of kidney disease, there may be no symptoms. However, as kidney function begins to be impaired, a variety of symptoms, signs, and complications may be observed. The first symptoms that usually occur as a result of kidney failure include decreased urination, fatigue, nausea, confusion, drowsiness, fluid retention, and chest pain. It can take anywhere from a couple of hours to a few days after the kidneys begin to fail for symptoms to start appearing. If the condition progresses, more severe symptoms such as vomiting, excessive thirst, muscle cramps and swelling, bone pain, and seizures may occur. If left untreated, kidney failure can lead to permanent kidney damage or death.

Causes and Risk Factors

Two very common causes of chronic kidney disease are diabetes and high blood pressure.

Other common causes or risk factors are:

Age 65 and above
African American, American Indian, or Asian American race
Autoimmune disorders
Birth defects involving the kidneys
Bladder cancer
Blockage of the renal artery carrying blood to the kidneys
Certain drugs and long-term use of medications
Certain toxic chemicals
Enlarged prostate gland
Family history of kidney disease
Heart disease
High cholesterol
Infections

Injury or trauma
Kidney cancer, kidney diseases, kidney stones, or kidney inflammation or infection
Obesity
Smoking
Urinary blockages
Vasculitis

Diagnosis

In order to diagnose kidney failure, a medical professional will conduct a physical examination for signs of kidney failure, as well as ask about any symptoms being experienced that typically occur as a result of the disease. If the doctor believes that kidney failure is a possibility, several tests can be conducted to get a more accurate diagnosis. One test is a urine output measurement, which tracks how much urine the patient has released during the day. Such a test can be used to determine the cause of the kidney failure. The urine sample can also be analyzed using a process called urinalysis in order to determine if kidney function is normal or failing. Blood samples may also be taken in order to measure creatinine and urea levels, both of which generally rise rapidly if the kidneys begin to fail. Image tests such as a CT scan or ultrasound can also be used in order check the kidneys for any damage that could cause kidney failure. If these tests cannot produce a clear diagnosis, a kidney biopsy may need to be performed in order to gain a clearer picture of the health of the kidney.

Other tests include abdominal or kidney CT scans or MRI scans, abdominal or kidney ultrasound, urinalysis, kidney biopsy, and kidney function tests.

Laboratory tests conducted at regular intervals to assess albumin, calcium, cholesterol, blood cell levels, and electrolytes may be helpful, as may bone density tests and vitamin D tests.

Treatment

One way of reducing the symptoms and progression of kidney disease may be efforts to control blood pressure.

Treatment options for kidney failure vary depending on what caused the condition, though a hospital stay is typically required. If the kidney failure is caused by a lack of fluids and nutrients in the blood, an IV will be inserted into a vein to resupply the kidneys with fluids and nutrients. If the body has so much fluid that the appendages are beginning to swell, a medication such as a diuretic may be prescribed in order to relieve the body of excess fluids. If potassium is not being properly filtered by the kidneys, supplements such as calcium, sodium polystyrene sulfonate, or glucose may be prescribed in order to prevent the blood's potassium content from becoming too high. If there is too much potassium, it can lead to muscle weakness and irregular heartbeat. If the kidneys can no longer filter waste out of the blood, then dialysis—a process in which a machine pumps blood through an artificial kidney, or dialyzer, in order to filter out waste—is usually required. Once the blood has been cleaned of waste products, it is transferred back into the body. While dialysis is sometimes only used until the kidneys heal and can once again filter blood, the process can become a permanent part of the lives of patients with severely damaged kidneys.

Prevention

While renal, or kidney failure is often difficult to prevent because it is usually caused by other diseases and conditions, some steps can be taken to reduce the risk of acquiring the condition. Eating a healthy diet, exercising regularly, and not smoking can help to prevent the onset of conditions such as high blood pressure, diabetes, and heart disease, which can cause kidney failure.

Prognosis and Outcomes

Controlling blood pressure and diabetes may prove helpful in preventing chronic kidney failure. Treatment of the underlying condition may help restore kidney function. Usually, however, the kidney function decreases over time, and the only options are permanent dialysis or kidney transplantation. For people with kidney failure who require dialysis or transplant of a healthy kidney, support groups may be helpful.

Ray Marks and Renee Dubie

See also: Abdominal Diseases; Kidney Cancer; Kidney Diseases; Kidney Stones; Nephritis

Further Reading

American Diabetes Association. (2013). Kidney disease (nephropathy). Retrieved from http://www.diabetes.org/living-with-diabetes/complications/kidney-disease-nephropathy.html.

Centers for Disease Control and Prevention. (2015). Info cards/memes on diabetes and chronic kidney disease. Retrieved from http://www.cdc.gov/diabetes/library/socialmedia/infocards.html.

Daugirdas, J. T. (2011). *Handbook of Chronic Kidney Disease Management*. New York: Lippincott Williams & Wilkins.

Family Doctor. (2012). Chronic kidney disease. Retrieved from http://familydoctor.org/familydoctor/en/diseases-conditions/chronic-kidney-disease.html.

Hunt, W. A., & Perrone, R. D. (2011). *Kidney Disease: A Guide for Living*. Baltimore, MD: Johns Hopkins University Press.

Kausz, A. T., & Levey, A. S. (2002). The care of patients with chronic kidney disease. What must we do and who should do it? *Journal of General Internal Medicine, 17,* 659–663.

Lin, H. Y. (September, 2011). Chronic kidney diseases. MedlinePlus. U.S. National Library of Medicine. National Institutes of Health. Retrieved from http://www.nlm.nih.gov/medlineplus/ency/article/000471.htm.

Mayo Clinic. (2015). Acute kidney failure. Retrieved from http://www.mayoclinic.org/diseases-conditions/kidney-failure/basics/definition/con-20024029.

Mayo Clinic. (2012). Chronic kidney disease. Retrieved from http://www.mayoclinic.com /health/kidney-failure/DS00682.

National Kidney Foundation. (2016). Chronic kidney disease. Retrieved from http://www .kidney.org/kidneydisease/ckd/index.cfm.

KIDNEY STONES

Overview

Kidney stones commonly comprise a hard, crystalline mineral compound known as calcium oxalate and occur as a result of an excess buildup of dissolved minerals within the kidney. Other chemicals that can form stones in the urinary tract are uric acid, magnesium ammonium phosphate, struvite, and cystine. Located in the kidney, bladder, or ureter, these deposits can grow as large as a golf ball or may be very small and pass unnoticed through the urinary tract (the tract that extends from your kidneys to the bladder). They can cause immense pain as a result, occur more commonly in men than women between the ages of 30 and 50, and are more common in Caucasians than African Americans. Approximately 7 to 12 out of every 10,000 persons in the population will present with a kidney stone attack each year. Kidney stones can also occur in children, and in premature babies, the rates of childhood kidney stones is rising. Kidney stones are also termed *nephrolithiasis, renal calculi,* or *renal lithiasis.*

Symptoms

Blood in the urine
Burning sensation during urination
Fever and chills
Infected urine
Nausea and vomiting
Reduced amount of excreted urine
Severe groin pain
Urinating more than usual

Causes

Among the leading cause of kidney stones is a deficient intake of water or kidney obstruction. As a result of a limited amount of water, the internal environment of the kidneys can become acidic, and this can promote the development of stones.

Other causes include health conditions such as Crohn's disease, urinary tract infections, hypercalciuria, hyperparathyroidism, gout, and a problem known as Dent's disease. Other related causes include a family history of kidney stones and increased risk due to the drug Topamax, which is used to treat seizures and migraines. Additional risk factors are diets high in protein and sodium but low in calcium, a sedentary lifestyle, obesity, high blood pressure, diabetes, gastric bypass surgery, and chronic diarrhea.

Treatment

Treatment is focused on symptom management and passing the stone. Hospital treatment may be needed to hydrate the individual and to administer pain and anti-inflammatory medications intravenously and to manage any nausea and vomiting that may occur.

In selected cases, a form of therapy known as lithotripsy or shock wave therapy may be used to fragment the stone and allow the smaller pieces to pass. Those patients with large stones may undergo surgical procedures involving the removal of stones through an incision in the back, or the removal of the stone via a thin tube passed into the urethra, termed ureteroscopic stone removal.

If kidney stones are caused by an overactive parathyroid gland, removing the growth from the gland may stop the formation of kidney stones.

Diagnosis

Several tests can be used to verify the presence of kidney stones, including a physical examination, an analysis of urine, and blood tests. A helical CT scan of the abdomen is the best way to verify the presence and location of a kidney stone, as well as its size and the state of adjacent organs. If a kidney stone is diagnosed, regular x-rays can be used to examine its state as a result of treatment.

Prevention

Some research indicates drinking diet sodas and a daily glass of orange juice, while reducing caffeine usage, may be beneficial in the treatment of kidney stones. Staying hydrated is especially important. Individuals at risk for kidney stones may be given prescription medication by their doctors.

Prognosis and Outcome

If kidney stones are not treated adequately, they can lead to kidney failure, which is life-threatening. A kidney stone can also rupture the collection system of the kidney. However, chances of recovering are good, and stones usually cause no permanent damage, although about 70 to 80 percent of cases will experience a recurrent attack.

Research

Scientists have found calcium and vitamin D supplements may increase the risk of developing kidney stones, and they believe kidney stones may become more common as temperatures rise in North America, which may cause more people to become dehydrated.

Ray Marks

See also: Kidney Cancer; Kidney Diseases; Kidney Failure

Further Reading

Kidney Stone Website. (2015, November 1). Why be concerned about kidney stones? Retrieved from http://kidneystonewebsite.com/.

Mayo Clinic. (2015, February 26). Kidney stones. Retrieved from http://www.mayoclinic.org/diseases-conditions/kidney-stones/basics/definition/con-20024829.

Medical News Today. (2015, July 17). Kidney stones: Causes, symptoms and treatments. Retrieved from http://www.medicalnewstoday.com/printerfriendlynews.php?newsid=154193.

National Institute of Diabetes and Digestive and Kidney Diseases. (2013, February). What I need to know about kidney stones. Retrieved from http://www.niddk.nih.gov/health-information/health-topics/urologic-disease/kidney-stones-in-adults/Pages/ez.aspx.

Rodman, J. S., Sosa, R. E., Seidman, C., & Jones, R. (2007). *No More Kidney Stones*. Hoboken, NJ: Wiley.

LACTOSE INTOLERANCE

The term *lactose intolerance* refers to the inability of the body to digest lactose, a form of natural sugar found in milk and dairy products. Some people cannot tolerate any form of lactose and others can tolerate small amounts. The problem is common, especially among people from Asia, Africa, and South America, as well as Native Americans. The condition commonly runs in families and develops during the teen or adult years, with a higher incidence among older adults. More than 30 million Americans suffer from this condition by age 20.

Symptoms

A person who experiences lactose intolerance may feel bloated or experience belly pain and cramps, diarrhea, nausea or vomiting, and gas after eating products containing lactose, and these symptoms can range from mild to severe, depending on how much lactase they produce and the extent of their consumption of milk and other dairy products. Dehydration may occur if symptoms are severe. These symptoms may last from 30 minutes to two hours after eating or drinking milk products.

Causes

Lactose intolerance develops when the small intestine of the digestive tract fails to make enough of the enzyme called lactase. This can occur temporarily as a result of flu, other illnesses, and injury. It can also occur secondarily as part of the health condition known as cystic fibrosis as well intestinal diseases such as celiac disease. Surgery to the small intestine may produce a temporary or permanent reduction in the lactase requirement of the body. Premature babies with lactose intolerance may be able to produce lactase as they mature, and lactose intolerance may occur as a normal result of aging. Certain treatments for cancer, such as radiation of the abdominal region, or intestinal problems from chemotherapy can increase the risk for lactose intolerance.

Treatment

People with lactose intolerance need to adjust their diets and also need to make sure they take in enough calcium that would otherwise be found in milk and dairy products. Substitute products such as soy milk and soy cheese may be helpful. Some dairy products contain lactase, and this may help to digest the product. Calcium can be obtained from other foods, such as broccoli, canned tuna and sardines, calcium-fortified cereals and juices, and calcium-fortified soy products. Lactase enzyme tablets or drops containing lactase enzyme may aid some sufferers to better digest the dairy product. Lactase-free milk products may also be helpful, as is working with a dietician.

Diagnosis

The doctor may be able to diagnose lactose intolerance by taking a careful history and performing a physical examination. A hydrogen breath test or blood sugar test may be performed to confirm the diagnosis. In children, a stool acidity test may be conducted. Doctors can also use endoscopy tests where they examine the interior of the intestines through a long tube with a light and tiny camera attached to its end. They can also take tissue samples from the inside of the intestine and measure the amount of lactase enzyme in these samples.

Prevention

There is no way to prevent lactose intolerance. Symptoms can be prevented by reducing the intake of dairy products and using products indicated for this condition. People with lactose intolerance should be aware of milk and milk products added to processed foods. It is also present in some prescriptions, including birth control pills, and medicines designed to treat stomach acid or gas, so reading and interpreting labels is important in preventing signs and symptoms.

Prognosis and Outcome

Lactose intolerance is not life-threatening but may prove uncomfortable unless lactose products are avoided. Treatment of any underlying disorder may help improve the signs and symptoms.

Future

Researchers have identified a possible genetic cause of lactase deficiency. It appears some people inherit a gene causing this condition from their parents. This finding may help researchers to develop genetic tests to better identify people at risk for lactose intolerance.

Ray Marks

See also: Allergies; Celiac Disease; Cystic Fibrosis; Digestive Diseases

Further Reading

Del Rosario, J. F. (2015). Lactose intolerance. *KidsHealth*. Retrieved from http://kidshealth .org/PageManager.jsp?dn=KidsHealth&lic=1&ps=207&cat_id=20132&article_set =21033.

MedlinePlus. (2014). Lactose intolerance. U.S. National Library of Medicine. National Institutes of Health. Retrieved from https://www.nlm.nih.gov/medlineplus/lactoseintolerance.html.

National Digestive Diseases Information Clearinghouse (NDDIC). (2012). Lactose intolerance. Retrieved from http://digestive.niddk.nih.gov/ddiseases/pubs/lactoseintolerance/.

New York Times. (2015). Lactose intolerance overview. Retrieved from http://health.nytimes.com/health/guides/disease/lactose-intolerance/overview.html?print=1.

Nordqvist, C. (2010). What is lactose intolerance (lactase deficiency)? What causes lactose intolerance? *Medical News Today.* Retrieved from http://www.medicalnewstoday.com/articles/180120.php.

LARYNGEAL CANCER

Laryngeal cancer is a rare disease of the larynx or voice box in which cancer cells grow in the larynx. The estimated number of new cases and deaths from laryngeal cancer in the United States in 2013 is 12,260 new cases and 3,630 deaths. For survivors, this form of cancer can be severe because it affects breathing, speaking, and swallowing functions negatively. More than 90 percent of laryngeal cancers are of the squamous cell type. It is also termed *cancer of the glottis, larynx cancer, throat cancer, voice box cancer,* and *vocal cord cancer.*

Symptoms include difficulty swallowing, having a persistent cough, sore throat, or hoarseness; having an abnormal lump in the throat to neck regions; pain when swallowing; and frequent choking on food. Other symptoms include noisy or difficult breathing, unplanned or significant weight loss, persistent ear pain, or unusual sensations around the ear and in the ear.

Causes and Risk Factors

Why laryngeal cancer occurs is unknown. However, risk factors include smoking, excessive alcohol use, poor diet, weakened immune system, being black, being 55 years or older, and being male. Other factors involve exposure to certain chemicals, wood dust, and asbestos; having a weakened immune system; having a precancerous condition called laryngeal dysplasia; and having gastrointestinal reflux disorder.

Diagnosis

Diagnosis includes the use of a medical history and physical exam of the throat and neck, as well as a variety of tests.

These tests include the use of biopsies or removal of a small sample of tissue from the larynx through an endoscope and testing them for the presence of cancer cells. Additional test include chest x-rays, CT scans, MRI scan, and laryngoscopy, where the surgeon uses a thin, lighted tube to examine the larynx via the throat.

Treatment

Treatment will depend on the stage of the cancer and may include surgery to partially remove parts of the larynx or complete removal of the larynx, radiation, or chemotherapy in various combinations or on their own.

Prognosis or Outcome

The outcome for small laryngeal cancers that have not spread to the lymph nodes is very good, depending on the site, size, grade, and extent of the tumor. Other factors influencing outcome are age, gender, and general health. Locally advanced or intermediate lesions are less well controlled by therapies. Recurrences after treatment usually occur within five years but are rare after that.

Prevention

The best method for avoiding this condition is to avoid smoking and excessive alcohol usage. Protecting yourself from occupational or air pollutants may also be helpful.

Choosing a healthy diet and protecting yourself from sexually transmitted infection human papillomavirus may be helpful.

Ray Marks

See also: Cancer; Swallowing Disorders; Throat Disorders

Further Reading

American Academy of Otolaryngology—Head and Neck Surgery. (2015). Laryngeal (voice box) cancer. Retrieved from http://www.entnet.org/HealthInformation/laryngealCancer.cfm.

American Cancer Society. (2015). Laryngeal and hypopharyngeal cancer. Retrieved from http://www.cancer.org/cancer/laryngealandhypopharyngealcancer/.

American Speech-Language-Hearing Association. (2015). Laryngeal cancer. Retrieved from http://www.asha.org/public/speech/disorders/LaryngealCancer.htm.

Mayo Clinic. (2015, October 1). Throat cancer. Retrieved from http://www.mayoclinic.org/diseases-conditions/oral-and-throat-cancer/basics/definition/con-20042850.

National Cancer Institute. (2015, May 19). Laryngeal cancer treatment. Retrieved from http://www.cancer.gov/cancertopics/pdq/treatment/laryngeal/Patient/page1.

LEAD POISONING

Lead poisoning, first reported in children in Australia in the late 19th century, refers to the buildup in the body of lead over a prolonged period of time. An unhealthy condition, it is especially harmful to young children, ages six and younger, who can be affected very detrimentally by excess lead in the body. If these levels are too high, they may result in death. Even if less severe, they can cause problems with both mental and physical development. In fact, adults with mildly high levels of lead can usually recover, but children, especially younger children, may not (MedlinePlus 2016).

Most commonly, lead is found in paint and older buildings that may be lead contaminated. The other sources are water, soil, and air.

Adults may also be exposed to lead if they work in auto repair shops, on home renovations, or with batteries.

It is the most important chronic environmental illness in children today, and according to the Centers for Disease Control and Prevention (CDC), there are approximately half a million U.S. children ages one to five with blood lead levels above five micrograms per deciliter, which is the level at which the CDC recommends public health actions be taken (CDC 2016). Lead poisoning varies with age, socioeconomic status, location, race, and age of the home.

In 2015, Flint, Michigan, a city of nearly 100,000, with a high number of residents who are economically disadvantaged due to the closing of industrial and auto-related factories, was found to have unacceptably high levels of lead in the city's water supply after people had complained for nearly two years about the color and taste of the water. State environmental managers denied that there were problems and also had not enforced regulations that could have prevented corrosion in the pipes. Flint residents believed that they were ignored because they were, for the most part, poor. There are many other parts of the country in which lead poisoning has been identified as a problem, including parts of Baltimore, and they are usually in low-income areas. Experts believe that, due to aging infrastructure in many locations across the country, exposure to lead is more prevalent than realized.

Signs, Symptoms, and Complications

Lead poisoning may not be easy to detect, until large amounts of lead have accumulated. In babies exposed to lead before they are born, there may be evidence of delayed growth and learning. Children suffering from lead poisoning may experience abdominal pain, constipation, fatigue and sluggishness, learning difficulties, irritability, loss of appetite, weight loss, and vomiting. Adult symptoms include abdominal pain, headaches, high blood pressure, declines in mental function, muscle weakness, pain, tingling or numbness of the extremities, mood disorders, and memory loss.

Causes and Risk Factors

Manufacturing, mining, burning fossil fuels, and related human activities can produce excess levels of lead. Some forms of paint and lead in pipes conveying tap water can release lead. Lead can be found in certain tinned products and medicines and occurs naturally in the soil, household dust, pottery, toys, and certain cosmetics.

Key risk factors are age, living in an older home, carrying out certain hobbies, and living in certain countries.

Diagnosis

Diagnosis is most commonly made through blood lead tests but may also include bone marrow biopsies and x-rays, among other tests.

Treatment

Treatment can include chelation therapy, where medication removes lead excreted in the urine, and other medications. A sudden ingestion of lead may be treated by bowel irrigation or flushing the stomach.

Prognosis or Outcome

High levels of lead can damage the kidneys and nervous systems of both adults and children. Excessively high levels may cause seizures or unconsciousness. Children can be permanently impaired, especially through mental abilities.

Prevention

Lead poisoning is preventable, to a certain extent, by carefully examining the environment and making sure that pregnant women and especially children are not exposed to any lead in paint, including on walls, furniture, and toys that were painted before 1978 when lead was finally banned in paint in the United States. Sources of water should be free of lead, and if not, filtered water should be used. Dirt, especially near construction sites, and even dust can carry lead. The Environmental Protection Agency has a website (http://www.epa.gov/lead) with information about preventing and removing lead from the home and workplace.

Ray Marks

See also: Centers for Disease Control; Environment; Failure to Thrive; Legionnaires' Disease

Further Reading

Centers for Disease Control and Prevention. (2016, January 29). Lead. Retrieved from http://www.cdc.gov/nceh/lead/.

Ganim, S., & Tran, L. (2016, January 13). How tap water became toxic in Flint, Michigan. CNN. Retrieved from http://www.cnn.com/2016/01/11/health/toxic-tap-water-flint-michigan/.

KidsHealth. (2015). Lead poisoning. Retrieved from http://kidshealth.org/parent/medical/brain/lead_poisoning.html.

Mayo Clinic. (2014, June 10). Lead poisoning. Retrieved from http://www.mayoclinic.org/diseases-conditions/lead-poisoning/basics/definition/con-20035487.

MedlinePlus. (2016). Lead Poisoning. Retrieved from https://www.nlm.nih.gov/medlineplus/leadpoisoning.html.

U.S. Environmental Protection Agency (EPA). (2016). Lead. Retrieved from http://www.epa.gov/lead.

LEGG-CALVE-PERTHES DISEASE

Legg-Calve-Perthes disease is an orthopedic disorder that affects the growing end of bones, especially in young people, and primarily firstborn children 4 to 10 years old. The bone most commonly affected is the thigh bone or femur, and the condition commonly occurs on one side only, although it can occur on both sides in about 12 percent of cases. While quite rare, affecting about 1 in 1,200 children, boys are more affected than girls, and those who are Asian, Caucasian, or Eskimo; active and very athletic; or exposed to secondhand smoke are at greatest risk. Because bone death occurs in this condition, the ball of the hip tends to fracture. As the bone fragments are slowly resorbed by the body, they are replaced by new bone and tissue. Legg-Calve-Perthes disease was discovered by Legg, Perthes, and Waldestrom in 1910. It is also termed *avascular necrosis, coxa plana, ischaemic necrosis, osteonecrosis of the hip, osteochondritis*, and *Perthes disease.*

Symptoms

Common symptoms involve limping with or without hip, knee, thigh, or groin aching or pain, especially after activity; muscle spasm; delayed bone development; possible shortness of height; leg shortness on the affected side; and limited hip joint motion or hip joint stiffness.

Causes

It is believed the condition arises as a result of unexplained loss of blood supply to the top or head of the femur, resulting in degeneration and deformity of the thigh bone, and well as growth deficiencies. Over time, the bone may break or fragment. Possible causes are infection, trauma, and inflammatory processes. The condition sometimes occurs in families.

Treatment

Treatment commonly centers around protecting the affected hip(s) from stress and injury and keeping the thigh bone's round, ball-like end in the hip socket of the pelvis. Other forms of treatment include medications for pain and swelling, physical therapy, exercises, heat or cold treatments for pain and swelling, crutches, bed rest, bracing, leg casting, and traction, where a pulling force is applied to the affected leg. Surgery known as tenotomy or contracture release may be performed if the groin muscle has shortened as a result of limping, to replace the hip ball within the socket of the pelvis, or to reposition the socket. In some children, the femur is re-angled if the head does not line up with the socket, known as osteotomy surgery.

Diagnosis

After conducting a physical exam and a review of the child's medical history and current activity, the doctor may perform x-rays, bone scans, MRI tests, or blood tests. Sometimes, bone fragments need to be removed to enable hip mobility, and sometimes the hip may need to be fixated internally by screws, wires, or plates if casting does not hold the ball and socket of the thigh together.

Prevention

There are no known ways to prevent the disease, but excess activity and high-impact activities should be avoided in affected children.

Prognosis and Outcome

The disease may be self-limiting if a new blood supply arises and allows health bone development in the area. Most people do well into their 40s and 50s if treated adequately, but thereafter, they may be at increased risk for osteoarthritis and require hip replacement surgery. The outcome may depend on the extent of the problem and its location.

Future

Studies of Legg-Calve-Perthes disease are continuing to help minimize its effects and to provide the best long-term results to the patient.

Ray Marks

See also: Bone Diseases; Secondhand Smoke

Further Reading

American Academy of Orthopaedic Surgeons. (2015, May). Perthes disease. Retrieved from http://orthoinfo.aaos.org/topic.cfm?topic=a00070.

Boston Children's Hospital. (2015). Legg-Calve-Perthes disease in children. Retrieved from http://www.childrenshospital.org/conditions-and-treatments/conditions/legg-calve-perthes-disease.

Mayo Clinic. (2014). Legg-Calve-Perthes disease. Retrieved from http://www.mayoclinic.org/diseases-conditions/legg-calve-perthes-disease/basics/definition/con-20035572.

Mount Sinai Hospital. (2015). Legg-Calve-Perthes disease. Retrieved from http://www.mountsinai.org/patient-care/health-library/diseases-and-conditions/legg-calve-perthes-disease.

National Osteonecrosis Foundation. (2014). Legg-Calve-Perthes disease. Retrieved from http://nonf.org/perthesbrochure/perthes-brochure.htm.

LEGIONNAIRES' DISEASE

Legionnaires' disease also termed *Legionellosis*, is a rare infectious disease of the lung, similar to, but more severe than, pneumonia or lung inflammation. Caused by the Legionella pneumopilia bacterium, the disease can prove fatal or, on occasion, can cause infections in wounds and other body parts in addition to the lungs, such as the heart. Most cases today occur as single isolated incidents, most commonly in the summer or early fall, although they may occur at any time. Each year, about 8,000 to 18,000 people, more men than women, are hospitalized in the United States with Legionnaires' disease. This number may be higher because the disease can be very mild and undetectable.

History

The disease emerged in 1976 when an outbreak of pneumonia occurred among members of the American Legion attending a convention. The following year, the bacterium was identified and named Legionella.

Symptoms

The symptoms can include having a high fever, chills, coughing, headaches, shortness of breath, chest pain, and muscle aches. The symptoms are very similar to pneumonia and appear three to six days after infection. The extent of the symptoms may vary and can include vomiting, nausea, diarrhea, and extremely reduced appetite. It has been reported that almost half the patients who become infected may experience confusion and altered mental states.

Key Causes and Risk Factors

Because the Legionella bacterium can be found in rivers, lakes, and other water sources and may enter artificial water supplies, it may prevail in air conditioners or in industrial cooling systems and other areas where artificial water is used. It is possible to be infected with the disease by inhaling small drops or droplets of tainted water, but the disease is not infectious as far as catching this from other people or transmitting it to others. Risk factors include having a smoking and/or drinking history, being older than 50 years of age, having a history of diabetes or cancer, and having an impaired immune system, as well as the lung condition chronic obstructive airways disease and working in air conditioning systems or cooling towers. The infection can also be transmitted if tainted liquids enter lungs directly or through contaminated soil.

Diagnosis

Diagnostic approaches include a detailed medical history, lung x-rays, blood tests, imaging scans of the chest, urine tests, or lumbar puncture tests to examine if the bacterium has traveled to the brain.

Treatment

Treatment involves a course of intravenous antibiotics and other medications to reduce the disease symptoms. Patients experiencing breathing difficulty may receive oxygen.

Prognosis

Some forms of the bacteria cause a low-grade fever called Pontiac fever, which recovers without treatment. About 10 to 15 percent of those who develop Legionnaires' and are otherwise healthy might die from the condition. The number of deaths is likely greater in those with poor health. Complications of Legionnaires' disease include respiratory failure, kidney failure, and septic shock.

Prevention

If water systems are kept at low temperatures (i.e., below 20°C) or at high temperatures (i.e., 60°C), disease outbreaks can be prevented. Water should be free of impurities and not allowed to stagnate.

Ray Marks

See also: Kidney Failure; Lung Diseases; Pneumonia; Respiratory Diseases

Further Reading

Bupa. (2015). Legionnaires' disease. Retrieved from http://www.bupa.co.uk/individuals/health-information/directory/l/legionnaires-disease.

Centers for Disease Control and Prevention. (2015, October 28). Legionella (Legionnaires' disease and Pontiac fever). Retrieved from http://www.cdc.gov/legionella/about/index.html.

Legionella.org. (2012). About the disease. Retrieved from http://legionella.org/about-the-disease/what-is-legionnaires-disease/.

Mayo Clinic. (2014, January 2). Legionnaires' disease. Retrieved from http://www.mayoclinic.com/health/legionnaires-disease/DS00853.

LEUKEMIA

Leukemia is cancer of the white blood cells, which are produced in the bone marrow. A person with leukemia has an excessive number of these cells, which grow faster and divide more chaotically than normal, accumulating and crowding the bone marrow. Because they are defective, these white blood cells cannot protect the body against disease, which is their normal function. As leukemia progresses, the production of other blood cell types, including red blood cells and platelets, also become abnormal, resulting in anemia, bleeding problems, and an increased risk of infection.

Every year, more than 54,000 cases of leukemia are reported annually in the United States, and about 24,000 people die from it; it is the seventh leading cause of cancer death. However, when compared to others, this cancer is relatively rare: About 1.5 percent of men and women will be diagnosed at some point during their lifetime; it is slightly more common in adults older than 55, especially men. It is one of the most common childhood cancers, affecting about 3,000 American children in a year, usually those younger than 15.

The main types of leukemia are acute lymphocytic leukemia, chronic lymphocytic leukemia, acute myelogenous leukemia, and chronic myelogenous leukemia.

Acute leukemias grow fast and usually worsen quickly, while chronic leukemias are slower-growing types that get worse over time. A further division of leukemia types is based on the type of blood cell affected. Lymphocytic leukemia occurs in the marrow that produces lymphocytes, a type of white blood cell inside the vertebrae immune system. Myelogenous leukemia takes place in the marrow cells that produce red blood cells, other types of white cells, and platelets. Other rare types of leukemia also exist.

Treatments depend on whether the leukemia is acute or chronic and on the type of blood cell affected. Some types can be cured, but many treatment options can help control the disease and its symptoms, even when cure is not possible. Typical treatments include chemotherapy, radiation, and stem cell transplantation. Even if symptoms disappear, therapy often continues to prevent a relapse.

Symptoms

People with chronic types of leukemia may not have any symptoms, or they may notice enlarged lymph nodes in the neck, armpit, or groin. Symptoms common to acute leukemia types are poor blood clotting (including bruising and bleeding easily), slow healing, and the development of minor hemorrhages on the body; a compromised or malfunctioning immune system, evidenced by frequent infections and an attack on beneficial cells; and anemia, which may lead to labored breathing and pale skin as good red blood cells grow in short supply.

Other symptoms may include bone or joint pain, limping, unexplained bruises, swollen lymph glands, swelling or discomfort in the abdomen, unexplained weight loss, poor appetite, fever, chills, night sweats, and fatigue. Children may have headaches, seizures, balance problems, or abnormal vision. They may also experience interference with blood flow to and from the heart, as well as breathing problems.

Causes and Risk Factors

What precisely causes leukemia is unknown, and different types are thought to have different causes. Suspected or known causes include a predisposition to genetic disorders or certain procedures for genetic health conditions; other cancers and chemotherapy and radiation treatment; exposure to chemicals, including benzene, some petrochemicals, and hair dyes; certain viruses; and exposure to environmental and artificial radiation. People with Down syndrome, who have a specific chromosomal abnormality, have been found to be at increased risk for acute myelogenous leukemia.

Diagnosis

Diagnosis will involve a physical examination and a medical history; a blood tests with a complete blood count aid in diagnosing leukemia. Bone marrow aspiration and biopsy often confirm a diagnosis and identify the leukemia cell type, and a lymph node biopsy looks for abnormal cells. With a lumbar puncture, or spinal tap, a sample of spinal fluid shows if the disease has spread to the central nervous system. X-rays, ultrasounds, CT scans, and MRIs are imaging studies that detect the location of abnormal cells, as well as if they have spread. Cell evaluations may be done to distinguish between specific types of leukemia and features of their cells.

Treatments

Of the various options, the treatment a person receives depends on the type of leukemia, age, overall health, and if the disease has spread to other parts of the body. The most common treatment is chemotherapy, which should start immediately after a diagnosis of acute leukemia; its purpose is to kill leukemia cells. Biological therapy helps the immune system recognize and attack leukemia cells, and drugs used in targeted therapy attack specific weak points within the cells. Also common is radiation therapy, in which x-rays and other high-energy beams damage leukemia cells in precise places in the body and stop them from growing. A stem cell replaces the diseased bone marrow with healthy bone marrow. Chemotherapy is often continued to prevent relapse, even if remission occurs.

Prevention

No effective way exists to prevent most types of leukemia because they develop from noninherited genetic mutations of randomly and unpredictably growing blood cells. Pregnant women can reduce the risk of prenatal radiation exposure as a trigger for leukemia by informing health care providers before having x-rays or other medical tests using radiation.

Prognosis or Outcome

The prognosis for leukemia depends on the type of blood cell affected and whether the leukemia is acute or chronic, but medical advances allow many people to live in remission with a good quality of life for at least five years after treatment ends. With appropriate treatment, most children and teens diagnosed with leukemia can look forward to very high remission rates.

Future

Many scientists are studying ways to improve treatments and patient outcomes for all types of leukemia. One example is the discovery of avocatin B, an avocado compound that targets and destroys leukemia stem cells and leaves healthy cells alone. Clinical trials in humans are many years away, but the findings suggest the possibility of a safe reliable drug that could be used in the future (Medical News Today 2015).

Ray Marks

See also: Blood Cancers; Brain Cancer; Cancer Survivorship; Childhood Cancer; Hodgkin Disease; Lymphoma; Non-Hodgkin Lymphoma

Further Reading

Kids Health. (2015). About leukemia. Retrieved from http://kidshealth.org/parent/medical/cancer/cancer_leukemia.html.

Leukemia & Lymphoma Society. (2015). Leukemia. Retrieved from http://www.lls.org/leukemia.

Mayo Clinic Staff. (2015, March 26). Leukemia. Retrieved from http://www.mayoclinic.org/diseases-conditions/leukemia/basics/definition/CON-20024914?p=1.

Medical News Today. (2015, June 16). Avocado compound holds promise for treating leukemia. Retrieved from http://www.medicalnewstoday.com/articles/295427.php.

National Cancer Institute. (2015). Leukemia. Retrieved from http://www.cancer.gov/cancertopics/types/leukemia.

News-Medical.net. (2013, October 13). What is leukemia? Retrieved from http://www.news-medical.net/health/What-is-Leukemia.aspx.

LIVER CANCER

Liver cancer is the uncontrolled, malignant growth of masses of abnormal cells in the liver. If the cancer originates in the liver cells themselves, the condition is called hepatocellular carcinoma. If the cancer originates within the ducts of the liver, the condition is called cholangiocarcinoma. Liver cancer can spread to other parts of the body, and cancer from other parts of the body (including the bladder, breast, colon, kidneys, lungs, ovaries, pancreas, stomach, and uterus) can spread to the liver.

Prevalence and Mortality

Approximately 33,000 cases of liver cancer are newly diagnosed in the United States each year, with about 23,000 annual deaths. Liver cancer has a high mortality rate. It is a serious disease that often occurs with another serious disease—cirrhosis. The average five-year survival rate for individuals with liver cancer is about 16 percent. If the cancer is diagnosed when it remains localized in the liver, the five-year survival rate is about 29 percent. If the cancer has metastasized to distant parts of the body, the five-year survival rate is only about 3 percent.

Risk Factors

The risk of liver cancer is substantially increased in people who have other chronic liver problems, especially the tissue scarring that characterizes cirrhosis. Cirrhosis, in turn, can be the result of alcohol abuse, hepatitis C infection, fatty liver disease, or hemochromatosis (excessive iron in the blood). Alcohol abuse causes most cases of cirrhosis in the United States.

Not all liver cancer cases result from cirrhosis. Some cases are believed to be related to long-term exposure to certain chemical compounds in the environment or in food. However, little is known about these associations. One possible chemical cause is aflatoxin, a toxic chemical produced by certain food molds.

Liver cancer is more common in men than women. It is also more common in older people (age 55 and over), people who are obese, and individuals of Asian or Hispanic ethnicity.

Symptoms and Diagnosis

Symptoms of liver cancer include pain on the right side of the abdomen, a full feeling when eating even small portions, decreased appetite, weight loss, abdominal swelling, foot swelling, and jaundice (yellowing of the eyes and skin). Many of these symptoms are identical to those of cirrhosis, which often precedes or coincides with liver cancer. Not all people with liver cancer have obvious symptoms, especially early in the course of the disease.

Because of the association of cirrhosis with liver cancer, many physicians recommend that individuals with cirrhosis get an ultrasound examination of the liver every six months to check for the development of tumors. These examinations may also be recommended for other people considered to be at risk for liver cancer. If the ultrasound examination yields positive results (showing possible signs of cancer), follow-up diagnostic tests are conducted. Such tests include other forms of imaging, blood analysis, and biopsy.

Computed tomography (CT) imaging and magnetic resonance imaging (MRI) are two important diagnostic tests for liver cancer. They can reveal locations in the liver in which blood appears to be supplying tumors. Blood test results that are positive for liver cancer include elevated levels of two proteins—alpha-fetoprotein (AFP) and des-gamma-carboxy prothrombin (DCP).

Although imaging and blood tests may reveal strong indications of liver cancer, a definitive diagnosis can be made only with a tissue biopsy. To obtain the tissue sample, a physician inserts a needle into the patient's liver. This can be done either in an office visit or during a surgical procedure. Microscopic examination of the tissue will show if the cells are malignant or benign.

Treatment

If liver cancer is diagnosed, the patient's particular treatment depends on the cancer's stage of development. Moderately advanced stages of liver cancer often involve some form of surgery. In some cases, surgeons are able to remove only part of the liver, thereby preserving some liver function in the patient. However, if the cancer has spread throughout the liver, the entire organ will need to be removed and replaced in a liver transplant. A healthy liver from a deceased donor is used for this procedure—the same procedure used to replace livers lost to cirrhosis. Patients undergoing liver transplants need to take antirejection drugs for the rest of their lives.

Some patients have cancer that is so far advanced and so widely metastasized that surgery would be useless. These patients are usually offered some form of palliative care to slow the further spread of the cancer, prolong life, and minimize symptoms. For example, ablation therapy involves the use of heat, lasers, or injections of special acids or alcohols to kill liver cancer cells. Embolization is an injection technique that blocks the blood vessels that feed the malignant cells.

Radiation therapy and chemotherapy are incorporated into the treatment regimens of many patients with liver cancer.

A. J. Smuskiewicz

See also: Hemochromatosis; Hepatitis; Liver Diseases

Further Reading

American Cancer Society. (2015). What is liver cancer? Retrieved from http://www.cancer.org/cancer/livercancer/overviewguide/liver-cancer-overview-what-is-liver-cancer.

Centers for Disease Control and Prevention. (2015). Liver cancer. Retrieved from http://www.cdc.gov/cancer/liver/.

Ghassan, K. A.-A. (2011). *100 Questions & Answers About Liver Cancer*. Burlington, MA: Jones & Bartlett Learning.

Mayo Clinic. (2015). Liver cancer. Retrieved from http://www.mayoclinic.org/diseases-conditions/liver-cancer/basics/definition/con-20025222.

National Cancer Institute. (2015). What you need to know about liver cancer. Retrieved from http://www.cancer.gov/publications/patient-education/wyntk-liver-cancer.

Surveillance, Epidemiology, and End Results Program, at the National Cancer Institute. (2016). SEER Stat Fact Sheets: Liver and Intrahepatic Bile Duct Cancer. Retrieved from http://seer.cancer.gov/statfacts/html/livibd.html.

LIVER DISEASES

Liver disease refers to any disease that alters the cells, tissues, structure, or function of the liver negatively. Various diseases can affect the liver. *Cirrhosis of the liver* refers to the late stage of liver disease, and liver disease can be divided into alcoholic liver disease and nonalcoholic liver disease based on the causes of the condition. Liver diseases may be acquired or congenital. Problems can occur suddenly or develop slowly over a long period of time. Men are twice as likely as women to have liver disease, and the severity of the disease can range from mild to severe.

Signs and Symptoms

Signs and symptom may vary depending on the type, cause, and severity of the problem and may include weight loss, nausea, pain, abdominal swelling, vomiting, weakness and fatigue, easy bruising, itching, confusion, appetite loss, dark colored urine, low blood sugar, muscle aches and pains, and yellow discoloration of the skin (jaundice) and eyes.

Causes and Risk Factors

The liver can be damaged by chemicals and minerals, it can be injured directly, it can be infiltrated by abnormal cells, or it can have its blood supply altered. Abuse of alcohol is the most common cause of liver disease. Taking excess amounts of certain medications or herbal remedies may increase the risk of liver disease. Hepatitis A, B, C, and D and other infectious agents and parasites can cause liver disease. Nonalcoholic fatty liver disease, Wilson's disease, metabolic cancers, heart disease, inherited diseases, and congenital birth defects can cause disease of the liver as well. Injecting drugs with other people's needles, tattoos, exposure to the blood of others, and unprotected sex might be other risk factors.

Diagnostic Procedures

A physical exam and history, plus laboratory tests, and scans may be helpful in the diagnosis. Liver function tests and liver biopsies may be performed.

Treatment

The treatment of liver disease depends on the cause. Medications, diet, fluid removal, and surgery may be performed. Immunization against hepatitis B and C may be helpful. Chemotherapy may be used to treat liver cancer. Liver transplants may be performed.

Prognosis or Outcome

Liver disease can progress to liver cirrhosis and death due to liver failure. It can also lead to gastrointestinal bleeding. Liver disease may be of short duration, but acute liver disease can develop into chronic liver disease. The overall outcome will depend on the cause of the disease as well as the treatment involved and when it began.

Prevention

Alcohol-related liver disease can be prevented by avoiding toxic substances and by reducing or eliminating alcohol usage. Screening for hepatitis C and treating fatty liver disease through a careful diet may prevent excess liver damage. Avoiding the sharing of needles is also recommended.

Ray Marks

See also: Abdominal Diseases; Alcoholism; Hemochromatosis; Hepatitis; Liver Cancer; Substance Abuse; Wilson's Disease

Further Reading

American Liver Foundation. (2015, July 2). The progression of liver disease. Retrieved from http://www.liverfoundation.org/abouttheliver/info/progression/.

Mayo Clinic. (2014, July 15). Liver disease. Retrieved from http://www.mayoclinic.org/diseases-conditions/liver-problems/basics/definition/con-20025300?footprints=mine.

News Medical. (2012, May 29). What is liver disease? Retrieved from http://www.news-medical.net/health/What-is-liver-disease.aspx.

Talk Medical. (2015). Liver disease. Retrieved from http://www.talkmedical.org/diseases
-disorders/590/liver-disease.

LUNG CANCER

Lung cancer is a type of cancer that begins in the lungs. An overwhelming number of people in the United States are diagnosed with lung cancer each year, and the incidence is increasing in developing countries (Jemal et al. 2010). The National Cancer Institute (NCI) and the *International Statistical Classification of Diseases*, 10th revision (ICD-10) (WHO 2010), define *lung cancer* as a significantly uncontrollable spread of abnormal cells within the bronchial airways and tissue of the lungs. According to the American Cancer Society (ACS), in the United States, cancer accounts for nearly one of every four deaths (ACS 2016). Lung cancer is the second most common cancer with the highest mortality rate among both men and women (ACS 2016; Jemal et al. 2010). In 2012, the Centers for Disease Control and Prevention (CDC) reported that 210,828 people in the United States were diagnosed with lung cancer and 157,423 died from lung cancer (CDC 2016). Lung cancer reportedly kills an average of 437 people per day (Xu et al. 2010). Although, the incidence rates of cancer are alarming, the deaths from lung cancer can be reduced through education and preventive steps taken to avoid potential mechanisms that may contribute to the development of lung cancer and by empowering individuals to take control of their health and that of others from by limiting exposure to eliminating passive exposure to tobacco smoke. A greater understanding of the underlying causes of lung cancer can provide an efficient vehicle for preventable efforts and reducing premature deaths due to lung cancer. This is especially the case with environmental causes of cancer, though in many cases, the built environments and sociopolitical factors present major obstacles.

Although lung cancer is almost certainly environmentally induced, family history has the potential to intensify the problem because genetic susceptibility also has a contributing role in the development of lung cancer, especially in those who develop the disease at a young age. It is important for individuals to know their family history of familial lung cancer because having a parent or sibling with lung cancer increases the risk of developing lung cancer (Bailey-Wilson et al. 2004). Tobacco smoking is a well-known risk factor for lung cancer development and accounts for about 87 percent of lung cancer deaths in men and women (ACS 2016). Smoking tobacco is the most preventable cause of lung cancers, and approximately 171,600 cancer deaths are the direct result of tobacco use (ACS 2016; CDC 2008). According to the CDC, each year smoking kills more people than AIDS, cocaine, heroin, alcohol, car accidents, homicide, and suicide combined (CDC 2016). The ninth edition report on known human carcinogens by the National Institutes of Health (NIH) reported on the increased risk of lung cancer in nonsmoking women living with smoking husbands or working with smoking coworkers (NIH 2011).

Children exposed to secondhand smoke can have lifelong respiratory health consequences including asthma, with increased risk for lung cancer. According to the

U.S. Environmental Protection Agency (EPA), children are particularly vulnerable to the effects of secondhand smoke because they are still developing physically, have higher breathing rates than adults, and run the greatest relative risk of experiencing long-term health effects. The health effects to nonsmokers from secondhand smoke are responsible for approximately 3,000 lung cancer deaths annually in the United States (EPA 2010).

Prevention and Treatment

Smoking cessation interventions help individuals reduce their personal health risks and that of others from secondhand exposure. Effective treatment strategies may include behavioral counseling and evidence-based smoking cessation aids. Although most lung cancers are associated with cigarette smoking, not all lung cancers are attributable to cigarette smoking because nonsmokers are also at risk for second-hand exposure to tobacco smoke. Currently, however, there are no generally accepted screening tests for lung cancer. Symptoms vary across individuals and are not often recognized early enough in the most treatable stage and may include chest pain, persistent cough and blood in sputum, voice change, and recurrent pneumonia or bronchitis, which is a very important dimension that influences later health outcomes.

Early detection is the best defense against any cancer. However, screening for lung cancers is not part of a typical medical evaluation or annual physicals. Lung cancer types are primarily based on a combination of factors, including imaging and biopsy analysis and the extent of disease when diagnosed. Treatments for lung cancer vary based on the tumor location, stages and cell type, and classification as small-cell or non-small-cell lung cancer. The severity of lung cancers is typed to the extent it has spread within the lungs and nearby organs and staged (i.e., I, II, III, or IV). Most will involve aggressive treatments to prevent the further spread. Early detection is critical for proper treatment and prevents more aggressive treatment regimens.

Lung Cancer Types

More people are diagnosed with non-small-cell lung cancer (NSCLC) than small-cell lung cancer (SCLC). Non-small-cell lung cancer is the most common type of lung cancer and accounts for about one out of every five new cases (ACS 2016). In addition, NSCLC is consistently diagnosed at advanced stages and has poorer prognosis than SCLC because NSCLC spreads more slowly and often goes undetected till later stages. The most common subtype of lung cancer is adenocarcinoma, with more representation among both smokers and nonsmokers compared to squamous cell carcinoma and small cell carcinoma (Kenfield et al. 2008). Primary lung cancers are when the cancer originated in the lungs. If the cancer metastasized to the lungs from elsewhere in the body it is called secondary lung cancer. Once diagnosed, the doctor may prescribe any combination of surgery, chemotherapy, and radiation therapy.

Prognosis

Survivorship from lung cancer is also lower than other cancers because, when diagnosed, the patients is often at advanced stages. The five-year survival rate for lung cancer is only 15 percent (Altekruse et al. 2010). Such a high mortality, plus the lung cancer survivor's unique health challenges that may affect their health-related quality of life, are very challenging health issues.

In the Surgeon General's Report on Health Promotion and Disease Prevention on Health Promotion and Disease Prevention, cigarette smoking was described as the single most preventable cause of death (U.S. Public Health Service 1979). Because the effect of the environment on human health is so great, the U.S. Department of Health and Human Service (HHS) continued to implement Healthy People to further reduce the health effects of tobacco use in the United States (2004). Several environmental regulations have been enforced, particularly to reduce exposure to secondhand smoke from indoor workplaces, public places, and air quality that contribute to premature death and long-term damage to the lungs and cardiovascular systems. The central problem of air pollution and the threat to human health from this is illuminated by the millions of tons of toxic air pollutants released into the air each year, primarily from transportation sources (EPA 2010b). In 2008, approximately 127 million people lived in U.S. counties that exceeded national air quality standards (EPA 2010a).

Adverse health effects have been consistently associated with exposure to particulate air pollution. National environmental laws and policies—including the U.S. National Ambient Air Quality Standards (NAAQS), National Emissions Standards for Hazardous Air Pollutants (NESHAP), and the Clean Air Act of 1990—were established by the EPA to help monitor sources of particle pollution produced by combustion sources such as power plants, vehicle exhaust, and air quality and to prevent resulting cancers from long-term exposures to air pollution. Chronic exposure to particles contributes to the risk of developing cardiovascular and respiratory diseases, as well as of lung cancer. Other policies involve reducing direct pathological effects from occupational exposures to toxic metals, asbestos, and fine particles from urban aerosol sources that are less than 2.5 microns in diameter. Workplace particles that contain asbestos—particularly quartz, crystalline and crystabolite, which are very potent lung irritants that are generated during sandblasting and similar occupational activities—can cause permanent lung disease or lung cancer.

Local and national governments strongly support the Healthy People 2020 objectives and the development of EPA policies toward air pollution reduction, clean air neighborhoods, limited construction of schools and parks near highways, and elevated smog locations in the community. Children are adversely affected because they spend more time outside during periods when air pollution is at its highest and exert themselves harder than adults; children may take in 20 to 50 percent more air pollution when exercising or playing ball with their friends (Kleinman 2000). Children not only inhale more air than adults, but they also extract more ozone from the air they breathe (EWG 2005; Kleinman 2000). Many California schools are located near freeways and other high traffic streets. Children from lower socioeconomic homes, particularly African Americans and Hispanics, are more likely to attend schools exposed to severe forms of traffic pollution (Green et al. 2004). According to a report by the Environmental Working Group (EWG 2005), the state of California, where the smog problem is severe, advises schools to keep children from playing outdoors when smog levels peak to unhealthy levels. Incentives for low- to zero-emission vehicles have also emerged and are gaining acceptance in mainstream automotive markets. Additionally, the National Cancer Institute (2011) suggests that while lung cancer death rates have been steadily declining since 1990, this is occurring more slowly among women, which could possibly be the result of inadequate knowledge of risks from secondhand tobacco smoke and the lack of standard screenings for earlier detection of lung cancers. At the same time, socioeconomic vulnerabilities and occupational factors are linked with higher lung cancer risks from elevated smog locations in the community. Clearly, focusing on issues related to timely screening, early detection, and quality treatment services and vulnerabilities among high-risk populations—such as women, youth, minorities, and workers exposed to occupational hazards—is an integral part of preventing late-stage lung cancer.

James A. Martinez

See also: Emphysema; Environment; Lung Diseases; Pneumonia; Pollution; Secondhand Smoke; Tobacco Addiction

Further Reading

Altekruse, S. F., Kosary, C. L., Krapcho, M., Neyman, N., Aminou, R., Waldron, W., & Edwards, B. K. (2010). SEER Cancer Statistics Review, 1975–2007, National Cancer Institute. Bethesda, MD. Retrieved from http://seer.cancer.gov/csr/1975_2007/.

American Cancer Society. (2016). Learn about cancer. Retrieved from http://www.cancer.org/cancer/index.

American Cancer Society. (2016). Lung cancer. Retrieved from http://www.cancer.org/cancer/lungcancer/.

Bailey-Wilson, J. E., Amos, C. I., Pinney, S. M., Petersen, G. M., de Andrade, M., Wiest, J. S., Fain, P., Schwartz, A. G., You, M., Franklin, W., Klein, C., Gazdar, A., Rothschild, H., Mandal, D., Coons, T., Slusser, J., Lee, J., Gaba, C., Kupert, E., Perez, A., Zhou, X., Zeng, D., Liu, Q., Zhang, Q., Seminara, D., Minna, J., & Anderson, M. (2004). A major lung cancer susceptibility locus maps to chromosome 623–625. *American Journal of Human Genetics*, 75, 460–474.

Centers for Disease Control and Prevention. (2016). Lung Cancer Statistics. Retrieved from https://www.cdc.gov/cancer/lung/statistics/index.htm.

Centers for Disease Control and Prevention. (2008). Cigarette smoking among adults and trends in smoking cessation—United States, 2008. *Monthly Morbidity Weekly Report*, 58(44), 1227–1232.

Environmental Working Group (EWG). (2005). Smoggy schools. Retrieved from http://www.ewg.org/reports/caschoolsozone.

Green, R. S., Smorodinsky, S., Kim, J. J., McLaughlin, R., & Ostro, B. (2004). Proximity of California public schools to busy roads. *Environmental Health Perspectives*, 112(1), 61–66.

Jemal, A., Siegel, R., Xu, J., & Ward, E. (2010). Cancer statistics, 2010. *CA: A Cancer Journal for Clinicians, 60*(5), 277–300.

Kenfield, S., Wei, E. K., Stampfer, M. J., Rosner, B. J., & Colditz, G. A. (2008). Comparison of aspects of smoking among four histologic types of lung cancer. *Tobacco Control, 17*(3), 198–204.

Kleinman, M. (2000). The health effects of air pollution on children. South Coast Air Quality Management District. Retrieved from http://www.aqmd.gov/forstudents/health_effects_on_children.html.

U.S. Department of Health and Human Services, Office of Disease Prevention and Health Promotion. (2010). *Healthy People 2020*. Washington, DC. Retrieved from http://www.healthypeople.gov.

U.S. Department of Health and Human Services (HHS), Public Health Service, Office of the Surgeon General. (2004). The health consequences of smoking: A report of the Surgeon General. Rockville, MD: HHS. Retrieved from http://www.cdc.gov/tobacco/data_statistics/sgr/2004/index.htm.

U.S. Environmental Protection Agency (EPA), Office of Air Quality Planning and Standards. (2010). *Our Nation's Air: Status and Trends through 2008*. Washington: EPA.

U.S. Environmental Protection Agency (EPA). (2010). History of the Clean Air Act. Retrieved from http://epa.gov/oar/caa/caa_history.html.

U.S. Public Health Service (USPHS). (2020). *Healthy People: The Surgeon General's Report on Health Promotion and Disease Prevention*.

Centers for Disease Control and Prevention. (2010). U.S. cancer statistics: 1999–2007 incidence and mortality web-based report. Atlanta, GA: Department of Health and Human Services. Retrieved from http://www.cdc.gov/uscs.

National Cancer Institute. (2011). U.S. cancer statistics: 1999–2007 incidence and mortality web-based report. Retrieved from http://www.cdc.gov/uscs.

World Health Organization (WHO). (2010). *International Statistical Classification of Disease and Related Health Problems,* 10th Revision (ICD-10R).

Xu, J. Q., Kochanek, K. D., Murphy, S. L., & Tejada-Vera, B. (2010). Deaths: Final data for 2007. *National Vital Statistics Reports, 58*(19), web release. Hyattsville, MD: National Center for Health Statistics.

LUNG DISEASES

The lungs are part of the respiratory system and assist us with breathing. However, if the lungs become diseased, the function of the lungs may become impaired and problems, with breathing can occur as a result. Respiratory diseases affect all ages—children, teens, adults, and seniors. Most of these diseases are chronic in nature, and all have a major impact not only on the individual with the disease, but on the family, the community, and the health care system. Chronic lung diseases or disorders are among the most common medical conditions worldwide. Tens of millions of people in the United States suffer from lung diseases. Some of the most common lung diseases include asthma, chronic obstructive airways disease, pulmonary fibrosis, cystic fibrosis, occupational lung disease, chronic bronchitis, tuberculosis, pneumoconiosis or a category of conditions caused by inhalation of substances that injure the lungs, and infections of the lung. Others include cancer of the lungs, pulmonary hypertension, and pulmonary embolism. Obstructive sleep apnea syndrome is a clinical disorder marked by frequent pauses in breathing during sleep, usually accompanied by loud snoring. These pauses cut off the oxygen supply to your body for a few seconds and halt the removal of carbon dioxide. As a result of this, your brain briefly wakes you up, reopens the airways and restarts breathing. This can occur many times during the night and makes proper sleep impossible. One or more of these lung diseases can affect the thin lining around the lungs, the blood vessels in the lungs, or the lung airways or air sacs, or chest wall, as well as the nerves controlling the respiratory muscles. Lung diseases can affect all ages-children, teens, adults and seniors. Most of these diseases are chronic in nature and all have a major impact not only on the individual with the disease, but on the family, the community, and the health care system.

Signs, Symptoms, and Complications

With almost all of the long-standing or chronic lung diseases, there may be a persistent or chronic cough, breathlessness, wheezing, chest pain, gasping, or coughing up of blood or mucus; due to lack of oxygen, some patents may exhibit a bluish skin color around the mouth, inside of the lips, or on the fingernails. The color of the skin may also appear pale or gray. Others may develop an enlargement of the fingertips and experience abnormal fingernail growth, chronic chest pain, nose flaring (the openings of the nose spread because the person is working harder to breathe), and sweating if the breathing rate is very fast. Problems may occur both with inhaling and exhaling, depending on the health condition and its severity, and a grunting sound may be heard each time the person exhales.

Causes and Risk Factors

Smoking, infections, and genetic explanations are the most common reasons for lung conditions. Asbestos dust, allergens, and other air pollutants may damage the lung tissues. Premature babies can incur lung injury that leads to chronic lung disease. The two most important risk factors for chronic respiratory diseases are tobacco smoke (through personal smoking and exposure to secondhand smoke) and indoor and outdoor air quality.

Diagnosis

Diagnostic testing for lung disease can include evaluation of blood gas composition or lung or pulmonary function tests, such as spirometry, to measure the amount and rate of air exhalation and evaluation of air flow with a peak flow meter to measure the exhalation rate, lung volume, or quantity of air a person takes into his or her lungs and how much is left after exhalation. Chest x-rays or CT scans may help to examine lung structure, as may MRI, ultrasound scans, nuclear lung scans, and PET scans. Additional tests may include cystic fibrosis tests, tests for specific infections, and tests for autoantibodies to help determine if an autoimmune disorder is affecting the lungs. Other tests may include a lung biopsy to examine the lung for cancer or tissue damage, sputum tests, drug screening tests because overdoses can cause respiratory distress, and electrocardiograms to examine heart rhythm to determine whether the heart may be affecting breathing.

Treatment

The goal of treatment is to prevent the disease, treat infections and prevent their spread to other areas, reduce inflammation, and stop or slow the progression of any lung damage. Other treatment goals are to relieve symptoms, ease breathing, minimize the side effects associated with some forms of treatment, and ensure the person is taking in enough oxygen. Surgery might be carried out and may include removal of a lung. Radiation and chemotherapy may be used to treat lung cancer. Physical therapy and respiratory therapy, as well as ventilators, are also commonly used to assist breathing and to clear the airway passages. Antibiotic medications, steroids, bronchodilators, anti-inflammatory medications, or cough remedies may be needed. Exercise, too, might be helpful for improving lung function, and avoiding toxic environments may be indicated as well—for example, those that are polluted.

Prognosis or Outcome

The prognosis depends on the condition and whether early treatment, as well as ongoing treatment, is sought.

Prevention

Avoiding smoking, secondhand smoke, and working in environments where the air is filled with irritants or allergens may be helpful.

Ray Marks

See also: COPD (Chronis Obstructive Pulmonary Disease); Cor Pulmonale; Emphysema; Legionnaires' Disease; Lung Cancer; Pneumonia; Pollution; Respiratory Diseases; Secondhand Smoke; Sleep Disturbances and Sleep Disorders; Tobacco Addiction; Tuberculosis

Further Reading

American Lung Association. (2015). Warning signs of lung disease. Retrieved from http://www.lung.org/lung-health-and-diseases/warning-signs-of-lung-disease/.

National Heart Lung and Blood Institute. (2012, July 17). Lung diseases and conditions. Retrieved from http://www.nhlbi.nih.gov/health/health-topics/topics/hlw/condition.

Stanford Children's Health. (2015). Chronic lung disease. Retrieved from http://www.stanfordchildrens.org/en/topic/default?id=chronic-lung-disease-90-P02348&sid=.

Womenshealth.gov. (2012, July 16). Lung disease fact sheet. Retrieved from http://womenshealth.gov/publications/our-publications/fact-sheet/lung-disease.html.

LUPUS

Lupus is a chronic autoimmune disease that can damage the joints, skin, kidneys, blood cells, nervous system, or any other organ; its most common type is known as *systemic lupus erythematosus*. Other types are those affecting the skin, a side effect of medications, and the rare form that affects newborns. Lupus occurs when the body's immune system attacks its own healthy tissues and cells, which causes inflammation. Symptoms can range from mild to life-threatening; they commonly include joint pain or swelling, muscle pain, fatigue, fever, and a red butterfly-shaped facial rash, and symptoms often flare up and go into remission intermittently. An estimated 1.5 million adults in the United States have lupus, with about 16,000 new cases every year. Anyone can get lupus, which usually develops between the ages of 15 and 44. Women are 10 times more at risk, and African American, Hispanic, and Asian women are more likely to develop the disease. There is no cure, but medications can relieve symptoms, prevent flare-ups, and protect against damage to organs. Most people have a normal life span with appropriate medical care.

Symptoms

A wide range of symptoms are possible because lupus can affect any part of the body. They vary among individuals, and they may come and go, develop slowly or rapidly, be mild or severe, or be temporary or permanent; new symptoms may appear during the course of the disease. Common symptoms include joint pain or swelling; muscle pain; fatigue; fever without a known cause; a red, butterfly-shaped rash across the bridge of the nose; chest pain with deep breathing; hair loss; sensitivity to sunlight; headaches; swelling of the feet, legs, hands, or around the eyes; mouth or nasal ulcers; swollen glands; anemia; abnormal blood clotting; and fingers turning pale or purple due to cold.

Causes and Risk Factors

The specific cause of lupus is unknown, but it may develop as a response to the combination of hormones, especially estrogen; genetics and family history; and environmental agents. Those with a genetic predisposition may develop lupus when they come into contact with something that can trigger it. Those commonly cited include ultraviolet light from the sun and fluorescent light bulbs, infections, exposure to silica dust in agricultural or industrial settings, drugs that increase sensitivity to the sun, exposure to cold or a virus, exhaustion, injury, and emotional or physical stress. Risk factors that increase the likelihood of developing lupus include being female; being between the ages of 15 and 44; and being African American, Hispanic, or Asian.

Diagnosis

No single test can diagnose systemic lupus, and symptoms vary significantly among people, as well as over time for an individual, and they often overlap with other disorders. In addition to the symptoms, a diagnosis is based on medical history, physical symptoms, and blood and urine tests.

A list of diagnostic criteria has been established to distinguish lupus from other immune system disorders. A person with four of the following criteria, which may be experienced at the same time or separately over time, is classified as having lupus: butterfly rash; discoid rash on the face, arms, neck, or torso; skin rashes resulting from photosensitivity; mouth or nasal ulcers; swelling, stiffness, or pain in two or more joints; inflammation of the membranes around the lungs or heart; urine with increased protein or clumps of red blood cells or kidney cells; seizures or psychosis, without a known cause; anemia or reduced numbers of platelets or white blood cells; lab tests indicating increased antibodies attacking normal tissue; and a positive antinuclear antibody (ANA) test, which is a blood test that checks for specific antibodies.

Treatments

There is no cure for lupus, and treatment depends on the symptoms and their severity. The goals are to relieve symptoms, including preventing flare-ups and treating them as they appear, and to reduce or protect against organ damage.

A variety of medications may be prescribed separately or in combination to treat mild to moderate lupus: nonsteroidal anti-inflammatory drugs to diminish joint swelling and pain, as well as fever; antimalarial drugs to reduce fatigue, joint pain, skin rashes, or mouth sores and help prevent abnormal blood clotting; corticosteroids and immune suppressants for serious or life-threatening complications, including kidney inflammation, lung or heart involvement, and central nervous system symptoms; and biologics, which are proteins derived from human genes designed to inhibit specific parts of the immune system.

Prevention

Because the cause of lupus is unknown, it is not possible to prevent it. Avoiding exposure to the sun and using sunscreen may prevent flare-ups. Adequate rest and sleep can help relieve lupus-related fatigue, exercise can help maintain joint flexibility and may prevent heart disease and strokes, and lowering other risk factors for heart disease and kidney disease can prevent complications.

Prognosis or Outcomes

The prognosis for those with lupus has improved over the past few decades due to more accurate monitoring tests and treatments. The disease has no predictable outcome, but with appropriate medical care and a healthy lifestyle, most people can lead a full life and expect to have a normal lifespan. But life expectancy and quality of life can vary depending the disease's severity. Those with lupus face a slightly increased risk for developing infections, cancer, kidney disease, heart disease, and, for women, pregnancy complications.

Future

Research studies are ongoing to discover and identify genes associated with susceptibility or that play a role in the development of lupus; biomarkers found in cells or tissues that predict lupus flare-ups or the disease process itself; how lupus affects different organs, including how it behaves in its early stages; and new treatments, such as the medication rituximab, which lowers the number of white blood cells that produce antibodies.

Ray Marks

See also: Immune System Disorders; Musculoskeletal Disorders

Further Reading

American College of Rheumatology. (2015, June). Lupus. Retrieved from http://www
    .rheumatology.org/I-Am-A/Patient-Caregiver/Diseases-Conditions/Lupus.
Lupus Foundation of America. (2015). What is lupus? Retrieved from http://www.lupus
    .org/answers/entry/what-is-lupus.
Mayo Clinic. (2011). Lupus. Retrieved from http://www.mayoclinic.org/diseases-conditions
    /lupus/basics/definition/con-20019676.
National Institute of Arthritis and Musculoskeletal and Skin Diseases. (2014, November).
    What is lupus? Fast facts: An easy-to-read series of publications for the public. Retrieved
    from http://www.niams.nih.gov/Health_Info/Lupus/lupus_ff.asp.
Thomas, D. E., Jr. (2014). *The Lupus Encyclopedia: A Comprehensive Guide for Patients and
    Families.* Baltimore, MD: Johns Hopkins University Press.

LYME DISEASE

Lyme disease is transmitted to humans by the bite of a deer tick and is a bacterial infection. In its early stages, it can resemble the flu and sometimes involves a red-colored, bull's-eye rash called *erythema migrans.* The Centers for Disease Control and Prevention (CDC) defines this rash as a skin lesion that typically begins as a red spot and expands over a period of days to weeks to form a large round lesion, at least five centimeters (about two inches) across. A red circular spot that begins within hours and is smaller is usually a reaction to the tick bite. Left untreated, symptoms of the primary illness usually go away on their own within a few weeks, although the rash may reoccur. Late-stage cases are harder to treat and can involve the heart, brain, and entire body.

Lyme disease was first recognized in 1975, after researchers investigated why unusually large numbers of children were being diagnosed with juvenile rheumatoid arthritis in Lyme, Connecticut, and two neighboring towns.

Ticks carry the Lyme bacterium in their stomachs. They can transmit the bacterium to humans with a tick bite. The number of cases of the disease in an area depends on the number of ticks present and how often the ticks are infected with the bacteria.

The number of reported cases of Lyme disease, as well as the number of geographic areas where Lyme disease occurs, is increasing. It has been found in nearly all states in America, although most cases are located in the coastal northeast, Mid-Atlantic States, Wisconsin, Minnesota, and northern California. Lyme disease is also found in large areas of Asia and Europe, as well as South America. It is the most common tick-borne illness in North America and Europe. Lyme disease can occur more than once in the same individual if he or she is bitten by another tick and re-infected by the Lyme disease bacterium known as *Borrelia burgdorferi*.

Signs, Symptoms, and Complications

Lyme disease can initially occur with no symptoms or very mild symptoms. The disease often, however, causes a rash with symptoms of arthritis, fatigue, muscle aches, joint pain, especially in the knees. It can cause symptoms of flu such as chills, fever, and swollen lymph glands. It can also cause symptoms of eye inflammation; heart problems, such as an irregular, slow heart beat; liver inflammation; and brain disease. There may also be neurological symptoms such as a stiff neck, severe headaches, temporary paralysis of the facial muscles, numbness, pain, severe fatigue, or weakness. In later disease stages, there may be evidence of motor and sensory nerve damage and brain inflammation as well as memory loss, difficulty with concentration, and mood changes or sleeping habits, although these symptoms may be reversible with appropriate treatment.

Causes and Risk Factors

Exposure to deer ticks and being bitten by a deer tick are the main causes and risk factors of Lyme disease.

Diagnosis

Lyme disease may be difficult to diagnose and is based largely on physical findings because some of its symptoms are similar to those of other disorders. A medical history may reveal if a tick bite has occurred, but many patients may not remember being bitten by a tick or have no idea ticks can transmit disease. The easiest way for a doctor to diagnose Lyme disease is if a bull's-eye rash is present on the skin. If there is no visible rash, the doctor might order a blood test three to four weeks after the onset of the suspected infection to look for antibodies against the bacteria. These blood tests include an:

- *Enzyme-linked immunosorbent assay or ELISA test*—a blood test that measures the levels of antibodies or molecules that fight infection such as that produced by the Lyme disease bacteria present in the body.
- *Western blot*—a blood test that identifies antibodies directed against certain proteins found on the Lyme bacteria; it may be ordered if the ELISA test result is unclear.
- *Polymerase chain reaction test or PCR*—a test that helps detect bacterial DNA in fluid drawn from an infected joint.

A spinal tap may be ordered at some point if there are neurological symptoms.

Treatment

Lyme disease can be effectively treated within a few weeks with antibiotics orally or intravenously in its early phases.

Prevention

- Protect yourself, if outdoors, and while biking, hiking, and gardening in tick infested areas.
- Avoid areas with lots of ticks.
- Use insect repellent.
- Keep ticks off of the skin.
- Remove ticks properly. According to the Lyme Awareness of Cape Cod website, you should grasp the tick with fine tweezers, as near the skin as you can, and gently pull it straight out. Be careful not to squeeze the tick when removing it, which could result in more bacteria being injected. Don't try to remove the tick with your fingers or with lighted cigarettes, matches, nail polish, or Vaseline.
- Educate yourself about Lyme disease and how it is transmitted.

Pregnant women should avoid exposure to ticks in Lyme disease areas because the infection can be transferred to the unborn child and make the woman more likely to miscarry.

Prognosis

Lyme disease in its initial stage is often easily treatable; however, if the diagnosis is delayed or the treatment is inadequate, serious brain, heart, or joint problems can arise. Many people who suffer from Lyme disease experience symptoms that fluctuate over time. Continued symptoms or the development of new symptoms after being treated may indicate the presence of a persistent infection or a new infection.

Ray Marks

See also: Brain Diseases; Neurological Diseases

Further Reading

Centers for Disease Control and Prevention. (2016, May 27). Lyme disease. Retrieved from http://www.cdc.gov/lyme/index.html.

Horowitz, R. (2013). *Why Can't I Get Better? Solving the Mystery of Lyme and Chronic Disease.* New York: St. Martin's Press.

Mayo Clinic. (2015, August 27). Lyme disease. Retrieved from http://www.mayoclinic.org/diseases-conditions/lyme-disease/basics/definition/con-20019701.

National Institute of Allergy and Infectious Diseases. (2015, September 4). Lyme disease. Retrieved from http://www.niaid.nih.gov/topics/lymedisease/Pages/lymeDisease.aspx.

LYMPHATIC DISORDERS

The lymphatic system is the body's drainage network. Its purpose is to fight infections and keep fluid levels balanced throughout the body by ridding it of toxins, waste, and other unwanted materials. It is comprised of lymphatic vessels that transport *lymph*, a clear watery fluid of water, white blood cells, proteins, and fats. Lymph passes through the lymph nodes, hundreds of small organs along the network of lymph vessels that contain *lymphocytes*, the white blood cells that fight infection. The lymph nodes also filter out cancer and damaged cells and foreign particles. Bone marrow, the spleen, and thymus also have lymph with high white blood cells.

When the lymphatic system fails to function properly, fluids may build up in tissues and lymph nodes may become swollen or enlarged. This can occur with an excessive amount of fluid or when lymphatic vessels or nodes are damaged or removed in surgery, become blocked by a tumor, or become inflamed. The most common lymphatic disorders are *lymphadenopathy*, or enlarged lymph nodes, and *lymphedema*, which occurs when lymphatic fluid accumulates and causes swelling, most often in the arms or legs. It may be caused by a birth defect or damage to the lymphatic system. Lymphatic diseases affect as many 10 million Americans, including children, and hundreds of millions around the world.

Less common lymphatic disorders include Castleman disease, a group of inflammatory disorders that enlarge lymph nodes and can cause many organs to malfunction; lymphangiomatosis, or cysts or lesions formed from lymphatic vessels; Klippel-Trenaunay syndrome, a birth defect of blood or lymph vessels that form improperly and may appear as port wine stains, varicose veins, and enlarged bones and soft tissue; lymphangioma, or defects that usually develop during fetal growth but may also develop due to trauma; lymphangioleiomyomatosis (LAM), in which abnormal smooth muscle cells (LAM) grow out of control in the lungs, lymph nodes, and kidneys, eventually destroying normal lung tissue; lymphatic filariasis, a parasitic disease caused by microscopic worms that live in the human lymph system; mesenteric lymphadenitis, inflammation of the lymph nodes in the membrane that attaches the intestine to the mesentery, or abdominal wall, usually from an intestinal infection; lymphangiectasia, improperly formed intestinal lymph vessels or blockage of lymph flow from the intestines; and lymphoma, or cancer of the lymph nodes.

Symptoms

Common symptoms of many lymphatic disorders include swelling of an arm, leg, or the groin and weight loss, fever, and night sweats. Lymphedema is characterized by a full or heavy sensation in a limb; skin or tissue tightness; decreased flexibility or difficulty fitting into clothing in an affected area; tightness associated with otherwise normal wearing of a ring, wristwatch, or bracelet; and noticeable swelling.

Causes and Risk Factors

Enlarged lymph nodes, known as lymphadenopathy, are most often caused by strep throat, infected skin wounds, or other bacterial infections, as well as by upper respiratory viral infections or mononucleosis. Lupus, rheumatoid arthritis, and other immune system disorders may also cause enlargement. More dangerous causes are cancer, HIV, and tuberculosis, but less than 1 percent of those with enlarged lymph nodes have cancer.

The most common cause of lymphedema is the removal of or damage to lymph nodes, which blocks lymph fluid from draining properly, which leads to a buildup and swelling, as in surgery and radiation therapy for cancer. It often takes place in women who have had breast cancer surgery that involves removing lymph nodes in the armpit. Those receiving treatment for melanoma, as well as head, neck, prostate, and ovarian cancer, are also at high risk. Physical trauma, as seen in wounded combat veterans, can also lead to the development of lymphedema. Primary lymphedema, caused by developmental problems of lymph vessels, is a rare inherited condition.

Diagnosis

The diagnosis of lymphadenopathy is based on a physical examination to check for other signs of infection or lumps and a medical history. If an infection can't be identified, blood tests, a CT scan, or a chest x-ray may be taken as well as possible tests for tuberculosis, HIV, lupus, mononucleosis and, occasionally, toxoplasmosis and syphilis. A lymph node biopsy is performed if cancer or lymphoma is suspected or if swelling continues for several weeks.

Diagnosis of lymphedema is based on symptoms, particularly if symptoms appear after surgery that included removal of lymph nodes. Otherwise, diagnostic tools may include ultrasound; MRI and CT scans; and a lymphoscintigraphy, in which a radioactive dye is ingested and images show the dye moving through the lymph vessels and highlighting areas of lymph blockage.

Treatments

Lymphadenopathy, or enlarged lymph nodes, are not treated directly; treatment is focused on appropriate treatment of the underlying illness or infection.

Lymphedema has no cure, but compression and pneumatic garments on the legs or arms can reduce swelling and lessen pain. Other treatments to manage symptoms include elevation of the affected limbs, exercise, and manual lymph drainage—a specialized type of massage that promotes the flow of lymph fluid away from an arm or leg.

Prevention

Facing surgery or lymph node removal, it may be possible to reduce the risks of developing lymphedema. For the affected limb, recommendations include elevation;

avoiding injuries and infections; and avoiding heat and cold applications, as well as constricting clothing. Following surgery, exercise and stretching may reduce the risk.

Prognosis

Swollen lymph nodes, the result of many factors, cannot be prevented. Although there is no cure for lymphedema, it can be managed with early diagnosis and treatment, which minimizes symptoms and may improve the outcome.

The risk of developing lymphedema falls within the first year following surgery and radiation therapy, and nearly all cases develop within three years. If it has not developed by then, the risk remains but is very small.

Ray Marks

See also: Cancer; Lymphoma; Non-Hodgkin Lymphoma; Tuberculosis

Further Reading

Mayo Clinic. (2014, October 23). Lymphedema. Retrieved from http://www.mayoclinic.org /diseases-conditions/lymphedema/basics/symptoms/con-20025603.

Mayo Clinic. (2014, January 2). Swollen lymph nodes. Retrieved from http://www .mayoclinic.org/diseases-conditions/swollen-lymph-nodes/basics/definition/con -20029652.

Merck Manual. (2015). Overview of the lymphatic system. Retrieved from http://www .merckmanuals.com/home/heart-and-blood-vessel-disorders/lymphatic-disorders /overview-of-the-lymphatic-system.

National Lymphedema Network. (2015). What is lymphedema? Retrieved from http://www .lymphnet.org/le-faqs/what-is-lymphedema.

LYMPHOMA

Lymphoma is a cancer that originates in cells of the immune system called lymphocytes. It involves rapid uncontrolled multiplication of the lymphocyte cells. Lymphocytes are white blood cells that move throughout the body within a network of lymph channels to form part of the immune system. The lymphocytes are designed to fight and destroy infectious agents. There are two types, B-cells and T-cells. Lymphoma occurs when these B- and T-cells start to divide uncontrollably. These cells may collect in lymph nodes or lymph tissues and can also form solid tumors or cell masses in areas of the body such as the spleen, thymus, tonsils, adenoids, and bone marrow, as well as the channels (called lymphatics or lymph vessels) that connect them. The abnormal cells can metastasize or travel from an affected lymph node to another lymph node to the lymph system and related organs. Lymphomas are the most common form of blood cancer in the United States, affecting more than 50,000 cases each year, including about 1,700 young people.

Types

There are two main types of lymphoma, Hodgkin lymphoma, which develops from B lymphocytes and non-Hodgkin lymphoma, which involves B and T lymphocytes. Both can occur in the same tissues but differ when viewed microscopically.

Symptoms

Symptoms are frequently minor or nonexistent in the early stages and may mimic symptoms of common, nonthreatening diseases. The first signs of lymphoma may be the presence of swelling in the regions of the neck, armpits, or groin. The swollen lymph glands may be tender and painful to some degree or simply swell and become firm, with no symptoms of pain in non-Hodgkin disease. If the tumors start to grow and press on nerves and blood vessels, or the stomach, the person can experience tingling and numbness, have swollen arms or legs, or feel full as though they have eaten. There may also be chest pain, lower back pain, fever, weight loss, fatigue or lack of energy, breathlessness due to swelling in the region of the chest, night sweating, itching of the skin, skin rashes that may appear red or skin with the appearance of purple lumps, and chills.

The symptoms will vary depending on how far the cancer has spread and the size of the tumors.

Causes

The cause of lymphoma is not known. Lymphoma may be linked genetically to a family predisposition for having this disease. Older age, which may predispose to genetic mutations, or the presence of other health conditions may increase the risk of acquiring lymphoma. These conditions include HIV and autoimmune diseases that are being treated such as Lupus.

Treatment

Treatment depends on the extent of the problem and the type of lymphoma that is present and may include radiation therapy, chemotherapy, or biological therapy. The ultimate goal is to clear the cancer and prevent any return of this, known as remission.

Diagnosis

Physical exams, a careful medical history, and blood tests may be helpful in diagnosing lymphoma. Also useful are kidney and liver performance tests, as well as imaging tests such as:

- X-rays
- Computerized tomography (CT) scans
- Magnetic resonance imaging (MRI)

- Lymphangiogram
- Gallium scan
- Positron emission tomography (PET) scans

Other tests are bone marrow tests and biopsies or removal of small pieces of tissue that can be examined microscopically in a laboratory. The tissue samples can then be used to stage the lymphoma as follows. Both Hodgkin lymphoma and non-Hodgkin lymphoma use a similar staging system to describe the extent of the disease:

- Stage I or early disease is said to occur when lymphoma is found in a single lymph node region or in a single organ outside the lymph node.
- Stage II or locally advanced disease is said to occur when two or more lymph node regions on the same side of the diaphragm or one lymph node region and a nearby tissue or organ carries lymphoma.
- Stage III or advanced disease is said to occur when two or more lymph nodes or a lymph node and an organ on the opposite side of the body are affected by lymphoma.
- Stage IV or widespread, disseminated disease is said to occur when the lymphoma has spread to the spleen, bone marrow, bone, or central nervous system.

According to Crosta (2009), both types of lymphoma may receive an A classification, indicating no symptoms like fever and weight loss are present, a B classification indicating such symptoms are occurring, or an E classification indicating that the tumor has spread directly from a lymph node to an organ.

Prevention

There is no way at present to prevent lymphoma.

Prognosis and Outcome

Lymphoma is treatable and curable depending on the type, stage, and extent of the condition. Crosta (2009) notes that, after therapy, the patient may see improvement (i.e., the lymphoma may shrink), attain a stable disease state (where the lymphoma is the same size as before therapy), see progression of the condition (where the lymphoma worsens), or enter a refractory disease state (where the lymphoma resists treatment).

Ray Marks

See also: Brain Cancer; Breast Cancer; Cancer Survivorship; Childhood Cancer; Hodgkin Disease; Leukemia; Lymphatic Disorders; Non-Hodgkin Lymphoma

Further Reading

American Cancer Society. (2015). Lymphoma. Retrieved from http://www.cancer.org/cancer /lymphoma/index.

Leukemia and Lymphoma Society. (2015). Lymphoma. Retrieved from http://www.lls.org /lymphoma.

Lymphomainfo.net. (2015). Lymphoma symptoms. Retrieved from http://www.lympho mainfo.net/lymphoma/symptoms.html.

Mayo Clinic. (2015, January 23). Non-Hodgkin's lymphoma. Retrieved from http://www .mayoclinic.org/diseases-conditions/non-hodgkins-lymphoma/basics/definition/con -20027792.

Medical News Today. (2016, January 8). Lymphoma: Causes, symptoms and research. Retrieved from http://www.medicalnewstoday.com/articles/146136.php.

MedlinePlus. (2016, June 16). Lymphoma. Retrieved from https://www.nlm.nih.gov /medlineplus/lymphoma.html.

National Cancer Institute. (2015). Lymphoma for patients. Retrieved from http://www.cancer .gov/types/lymphoma.

MACULAR DEGENERATION

There are two types of macular degeneration: dry macular degeneration and wet macular degeneration. Dry or atrophic macular degeneration, or non-neovascular macular degeneration, is more common and is a chronic health condition that causes vision loss owing to the deterioration of the light-sensitive cells of the macula, located in the center of the layer of tissue lining the back wall of the eyeball called the retina. This condition causes blurring of central vision that is needed for everyday tasks such as reading, driving, and recognizing faces. The condition can occur in one or both eyes, may cause severe vision loss, and is characterized by the presence of small yellow deposits in the macula, called drusen.

Dry macular degeneration can progress to wet macular degeneration and rapid vision loss.

Wet macular degeneration, or exudative or neovascular macular degeneration, is the more advanced and damaging form of eye disease caused by the abnormal growth of blood vessels that are located under the retina the leak blood and fluid. The leakage causes permanent damage to light-sensitive retinal cells, which die and create blind spots centrally in about 10 percent of people with macular degeneration. All people with wet macular degeneration first had dry macular degeneration.

Macular degeneration is also termed *age-related macular degeneration* (AMD or ARMD).

Signs and Symptoms

The symptoms of dry macular degeneration occur slowly, and as these occur, painless changes in vision may arise such as blurriness of printed material, distorted vision, changed color perception, and difficulty recognizing faces. Objects may not be as bright as they used to be, and in advanced stages, hallucinations of geometric shapes or people may occur.

Drusen are an early sign of age-related macular degeneration and are yellow deposits under the retina of small or large size that can be seen with a dilated eye exam test. Drusens do not cause loss of vision, but people who have large drusens are at risk for more severe age-related macular degeneration that commonly results in severe losses of vision.

Causes

The causes of dry macular degeneration are not known but are probably age related. Family history, genetic changes leading to oxidative stress, race (especially being Caucasian and female), and having a lighter eye color, smoking, sleep apnea, having an overactive immune system, exposure to sunlight, some forms of medication, and obesity increase the chances of macular degeneration and/or its progression. Other factors include an unhealthy diet, cardiovascular disease, and having elevated levels of cholesterol.

Age-related macular degeneration is common among people age 50 and older and is the leading cause of vision loss in older adults.

Diagnosis

A medical history and comprehensive routine eye examination may be used to confirm the diagnosis of macular degeneration. The degree of dry macular degeneration can be categorized into early, intermediate, and advanced stages. The tests used are visual acuity tests, visual field tests, dilated eye exams, Amsler grid tests (a chart of black lines), optical coherence tomography or photography, microperimetry using a scanning laser opthalmoscope or regular opthalmoscope, fluorescein angiograms using dye to highlight blood vessels of the retina, or indocyanine green angiography procedures.

Treatment

Treatment can slow the disease progression even if it cannot reverse it. Certain vitamins and supplements may help to reduce the risk of progression, complications, and extent of the problem. Lifestyle changes such as eating healthier foods and stopping smoking may be helpful. In wet macular degeneration, injections to slow its progression may be used. Another method involves photodynamic therapy using a laser. Both these methods try to deliver drugs or anti-angiogenesis agents into the eye. Laser surgery, designed to destroy new blood vessels, and submacular surgery to remove abnormal blood vessels or blood in the eyes or retinal translocation surgery may be used as well.

For selected patients, implanting a telescopic lens in one eye may improve both distance and close vision in persons with damage to both eyes.

In cases of vision loss, low vision aids and rehabilitation may be desirable.

Prognosis or Outcome

People with age-related macular degeneration rarely lose complete vision, but this can occur if both eyes are affected by the wet form.

Even after treatment, the wet type can reoccur. Successful and timely treatment will, however, slow the rate of vision loss and improve vision.

Prevention

Prevention strategies include having regular routine eye examinations; controlling the presence of high blood pressure and cholesterol; stopping smoking; and including a nutritious diet, nutritional supplements, and exercise routine into your life.

Future

Researchers are continuing to study the effects of omega-3-fatty acids and lutein in persons with macular degeneration.

Ray Marks

See also: Cholesterol; Colorblindness; Diabetes, Type 1; Eye Diseases; Glaucoma; Hyperopia; Myopia; Sjögren's Syndrome

Further Reading

American Macular Degeneration Foundation. (2015). What is macular degeneration? Retrieved from https://www.macular.org/what-macular-degeneration.
Mayo Clinic. (2015, September 19). Dry macular degeneration. Retrieved from http://www.mayoclinic.org/diseases-conditions/macular-degeneration/basics/definition/con-20075882.
Mayo Clinic. (2015, September 19). Wet macular degeneration. Retrieved from http://www.mayoclinic.org/diseases-conditions/wet-macular-degeneration/basics/definition/con-20043518.
National Eye Institute. (2015). Facts about age-related macular degeneration. Retrieved from https://nei.nih.gov/health/maculardegen/armd_facts.

MALARIA

Malaria is a serious, often fatal, disease commonly caused by a microscopic parasite (known as plasmodium) that feeds on a certain mosquito (called Anopheles mosquitoes), which then feeds on or bites humans, mainly between dusk and dawn. It can also be transmitted on occasion directly from a mother to an unborn child, through blood transfusions, or sharing needles to inject drugs, and once in the body, one of the five types of parasites that affect humans multiply in the liver and then infect and destroy red blood cells. Occurring mostly in hot, tropical countries, there are about 1,500 cases reported each year in the United States, mainly from those who have traveled to affected areas of Africa. Malaria can be classified as uncomplicated or severe, and in 2010, an estimated 660,000 deaths occurred from malaria, mostly among African children. In areas with high malaria, it is a chronic disease: Increased efforts toward malaria prevention and control are reducing the malaria burden in areas where it is prevalent.

People with malaria can be very sick and exhibit:

Fever
Shaking or chills
Flu
Sweating
Nausea
Headaches, dizziness, and blurred vision
Vomiting

Body aches, intense muscle pain, and malaise between 10 and 15 days after receiving a mosquito bite, or within seven days after being bitten, are other symptoms; symptoms can lie dormant in the body for months or even years.

Physical signs such as respiratory distress, an abnormally enlarged spleen, convulsions, cerebral malaria causing brain damage, kidney problems, dehydration, low blood sugar, and severe anemia may occur in children or adults with severe disease.

The same pattern of symptoms can be repeated at intervals of two to three days, depending on the particular species of malaria parasite causing the infection.

Causes and Risk Factors

People living in infested areas, young children, people with HIV/AIDS, and those who are pregnant and exposed to the mosquito are especially vulnerable. Nonimmune travelers from malaria-free areas are very vulnerable to the disease if infected. Certain climactic conditions that affect mosquito number and survival and areas where people have little to no immunity against malaria can influence the risk of acquiring malaria.

Diagnosis

The World Health Organization (WHO) recommends all suspected cases be tested using a parasite-based diagnostic test before administering treatment. This can be done by taking a blood sample.

Treatment

Antimalarial drugs by mouth or injection for treatment or prevention of malaria by travelers is indicated, although the WHO reports the parasites have developed resistance to a variety of malarial medicines. Treatment depends on the type of malaria parasite, the severity of the symptoms, a person's age, and whether a woman is pregnant or not.

Prognosis or Outcome

The outcome will depend on the severity of the condition and is curable if diagnosed early on and treated promptly and appropriately with artemisinin-based combined therapies, insecticide-treated mosquito nets, window screens, and indoor residual spraying with insecticide. If untreated, malaria can become life-threatening because it can disrupt the blood supply to vital organs. Some varieties of the malaria parasite—usually those causing milder disease—can persist for years and cause relapses of the condition.

Prevention

Malaria can be prevented by simple measures such as by using clothes that cover or protect the body and by using mosquito repellents, spraying the home, and sleeping under a net. Use air conditioning and electric fans and stay indoors after dark in infected areas. Research is under way to test a vaccine for preventing malaria.

Ray Marks

See also: Environment; World Health Organization

Further Reading

Centers for Disease Control and Prevention. (2015, October 21). Malaria. Retrieved from http://www.cdc.gov/malaria/.

KidsHealth.org. (2015). Malaria. Retrieved from http://kidshealth.org/parent/infections /parasitic/malaria.html.

Mayo Clinic. (2015, June 20). Malaria. Retrieved from http://www.mayoclinic.org/diseases -conditions/malaria/basics/definition/con-20013734.

National Institute of Allergy and Infectious Diseases. (2015, November 2). Malaria. Retrieved from http://www.niaid.nih.gov/topics/malaria/Pages/default.aspx.

MALE BREAST CANCER

Although it is rare, breast cancer can affect men. It makes up less than 1 percent of all breast cancers and it is 100 times more common in women than in men; the lifetime risk of developing breast cancer for a man is about 1 in 1,000. Men of any age can contract the disease, but it is most often detected between the ages 60 and 70, and it is rare under age 35. Just like female breast cancer, male breast cancer is the growth of malignant cells in breast tissue. The most common type of male breast cancer is infiltrating ductal carcinoma, which spreads into the surrounding tissue. Lumps, skin changes, and nipple discharge are symptoms to breast cancer in women. Age, family history, a high level of estrogen, and exposure to radiation are primary risk factors for male breast cancer. Treatments include surgery and chemotherapy, as well as radiation and hormone therapy. As with breast cancer in women, the prognosis improves with early detection and treatment.

Symptoms

The most common sign of male breast cancer is a painless lump or thickening found in the breast tissue. Other symptoms include dimpling, puckering, redness, or scaling in the skin over the breast; nipple retraction (turning inward), redness, or scaling; and discharge from the nipple that can be opaque or bloody.

Causes and Risk Factors

The exact causes of male breast cancer are unknown, but environmental and genetic factors play a role; one factor may be the level of sex hormones in the body. Risk factors that increase the likelihood of a man contracting breast cancer include exposure to radiation, especially in the chest; age, with the average diagnosis around 68; high levels of estrogen, which can be due to hormone medications, cirrhosis of the liver (as a result of excessive alcohol consumption), obesity, environmental estrogens (as in beef or pesticides), or the rare genetic disorder Klinefelter syndrome; family history, including female relatives with breast cancer and inherited gene mutations; and testicle disease or surgery.

Diagnosis

Men with breast cancer are often diagnosed at advance stages of the disease because they ignore breast lumps until they've grown very large.

A doctor diagnoses breast cancer in men based on a physical examination, including the breasts, and medical history. Diagnostic tools may include a mammogram, ultrasound, or MRI scan, which provide different types of pictures of breast tissues; blood tests; and a biopsy, which checks for cancer cells. These tests also detect the spread of cancer cells elsewhere in the body.

Treatments

Treatment depends upon the size and location of a tumor and the man's overall physical health. Standard treatment includes surgery, which most often is a mastectomy, or removing the breast, lymph nodes under the arm, chest muscle lining, and part of the chest wall muscles. If appropriate, a partial mastectomy or lumpectomy may be performed to remove cancerous cells and some surrounding tissue but leave the breast. Other standard treatments include chemotherapy, or medications to stop the growth and division of cancer cells; hormone therapy, which removes or blocks hormones from growing; radiation therapy, or high-energy x-rays that kill or stop the growth of cancer cells; and targeted therapy, which is the use of medications to attack cancer cells without harming normal cells.

Prevention

The cause or causes of most cancers, including male breast cancer, are unknown, so prevention is not possible. But some risk factors can be modified, including maintaining a healthy body weight and lowering alcohol consumption. Early detection and treatment have been shown to reduce the number of deaths from male breast cancer.

Prognosis

The size, extent, and type of breast cancer in men influence prognosis. It is more common for breast cancers in men to have spread once they are diagnosed, which indicates a more advanced stage of the disease that may be less likely to be cured.

Future

Scientists are examining common gene variations that could affect breast cancer risk. One study of male breast cancer identified several genetic variations, showing that the effect of these variations on risk for men and women differs, as does the biology of breast cancer in men and women.

Ray Marks

See also: Breast Cancer; Cancer; Men's Health

Further Reading

American Cancer Society. (2014, October 10). What is breast cancer in men? Retrieved from http://www.cancer.org/cancer/breastcancerinmen/detailedguide/breast-cancer-in-men-what-is-breast-cancer-in-men.

Breastcancer.Org. (2013). Symptoms of male breast cancer. Retrieved from http://www.breastcancer.org/symptoms/types/male_bc/symptoms.

Mayo Clinic. (2015, February 17). Male breast cancer. Retrieved from http://www.mayoclinic.org/diseases-conditions/male-breast-cancer/basics/definition/con-20025972.

National Cancer Institute. (2015, August 12). Male breast cancer treatment. Retrieved from http://www.cancer.gov/cancertopics/pdq/treatment/malebreast/Patient/page1.

MELANOMA

Melanoma is a type of skin cancer that develops from malignant *melanocytes*—melanin-producing cells—that form on the skin and sometimes the eyes and internal organs such as the intestines. It is the most common cancer for people 25 to 29 years old, although the risk of developing melanoma increases with age. If treated early, melanoma is curable. However, the longer the melanomas are able to develop, the greater the chance that the cancer will spread to other parts of the body, making it more difficult to treat and potentially fatal. While melanoma is not the most common form of skin cancer, it is the deadliest.

Melanoma is caused by DNA damage to new melanocytes, the cells that give skin its pigment. When skin cells experience DNA damage, they can grow into cancerous masses known as melanomas. There are several factors that can cause DNA damage to the skin. One of the most common causes is exposure to UVA and UVB rays from the sun or tanning booths, which can result in sunburns or other damage to the skin. Individuals with lighter complexions, light-colored eyes, and blond or red hair are most at risk for sun damage, though people of all skin complexions can develop melanoma. A weakened immune system can also increase the risk of DNA damage to the skin. Heredity is another major contributing factor to melanoma. Individuals with a first-degree relative who has had the disease have a 50 percent greater chance of developing melanoma than someone who has not had the disease in the family. Individuals with more than 50 moles or atypical moles, known as *dysplastic nevi*, have an increased risk of developing melanoma, especially when combined with long periods of sun exposure or a family history of the disease.

The main symptom of the disease is the appearance of a melanoma, or several, on the skin. Melanomas typically develop out of already existing moles or as entirely new growths. While the majority of moles are harmless, they do have the potential to become cancerous. Melanomas can appear anywhere on the body, though they are most likely to be found on areas exposed to the sun such as the face, legs, arms, or back. Melanomas that appear on areas that do not receive much sun such as the soles of the feet or palms are more common in individuals with darker skin complexions or a family history of the disease. Moles that have become melanomas typically have an asymmetrical shape, irregular border, and a change in color, and they have grown larger. The mole may also become itchy or begin to bleed or ooze fluid. While melanomas are generally brown or black in color, they can also be pink, red, blue, purple, or white. If left untreated, melanomas will spread deeper into the skin and to other parts of the body.

In order to diagnose melanoma, a health care professional will begin by examining the skin from head to toe in order to detect any potential melanomas. If a potential melanoma is found, a biopsy will be conducted in order to make sure that it is cancerous. The three biopsy procedures used to diagnose melanoma are punch biopsies, excisional biopsies, and incisional biopsies. While punch and incisional biopsies only remove a portion of the mole, excisional biopsies remove the entire growth. The sample will then be analyzed to determine if the growth is cancerous. If it is found to be cancerous, the doctor will attempt to determine the stage of the cancer by examining the thickness of the melanoma. There are four stages of the disease, which are differentiated by how thick the melanoma is and how far it has spread through the skin and body. In order to determine if the cancer has spread, the doctor will conduct a sentinel node biopsy, in which dye is injected into the melanoma and travels into the lymph nodes. The first lymph nodes stained by the dye are then biopsied and tested. It they are cancer free, then it is unlikely the cancer has spread beyond the initial melanoma.

There are several treatments available for melanoma depending on the severity of the cancer. Early stages of the disease are generally treated by removing the melanoma or removing the normal skin surrounding the growth as well as tissue underneath. If the cancer has not spread beyond the initial growth, this may be all the treatment necessary. If the cancer has spread, surgery may be required in order to remove the disease from the affected areas. Radiation therapy, which uses high-energy radiation to kill cancer cells, is typically used after surgery if the cancer is contained to one area. If surgery is unsuccessful or not an option, chemotherapy may be used to kill the cancer cells by injecting powerful drugs into the site of the melanoma. Biological therapy, in which drugs such as interferon or interleukin-2 are used to boost the immune system, is another treatment option. In order to prevent melanoma, individuals are encouraged to limit their exposure to the sun; wear sunscreen of at least SPF 15, as well as protective clothing, while in the sun; and avoid tanning beds. Regular examinations of the skin for any new growths or unusual changes to moles are also recommended in order to catch the disease early. The survival rate for melanoma ranges from a five-year rate of 97 percent for stage I to a five-year rate of 15 to 20 percent for stage IV.

The first account of melanoma is believed to have come from the Greek physician Hippocrates in the 5th century BCE. In 1787, Scottish surgeon John Hunter became the first to successfully operate on a melanoma patient, though he did not know the growth he was removing was melanoma at the time. The melanoma was sent to the Hunterian Museum of the Royal College of Surgeons of England for preservation after it was removed. Melanoma was first described as a distinct disease in 1804 by French physician René Laennec, who called the condition "melanose." In 1820, English general practitioner William Norris became the first to recognize a link between heredity and melanoma. By 1857, Norris had found a link between melanoma and moles and a possible relationship between the disease and environmental factors; he determined that it could spread to other parts of the body. The first case of melanoma in North America was reported in 1837 by Isaac Parish. In 1838, the word *melanoma* was officially coined by Sir Robert Carswell to describe the disease. After treating a woman with the disease in 1905, the findings of Scottish physician William Handley would contribute significantly to the surgical treatment of melanoma for the next 50 years. In 1966, Wallace Clark created a scale to help doctors and patients determine the chances of surviving the disease. The scale, known as Clark's levels, consisted of five levels, with each based on how far the melanoma had spread into the skin. Expanding on Clark's work, in 1970 pathologist Alexander Breslow reported that the degree to which the melanoma had spread into the skin was a major factor in patient prognosis.

Today, instances of melanoma in the United States are increasing. Around 120,000 new cases of the disease are diagnosed each year. Men are generally at greater risk for developing melanoma than women. The average age for developing melanoma is 61, though rates among individuals under 30 have been increasing. Among racial groups, whites have a 2 percent risk of developing the disease, while Latinos have a 0.5 percent risk, and African Americans have a 0.1 percent risk.

Renee Dubie

See also: Basal Cell Carcinoma; Skin Cancer; Skin Conditions; Squamous Cell Carcinoma

Further Reading

American Academy of Dermatology. (2015). Melanoma: Overview. Retrieved from https://www.aad.org/public/diseases/skin-cancer/melanoma.

American Cancer Society. (2015). What is melanoma skin cancer? Retrieved from http://www.cancer.org/cancer/skincancer-melanoma/detailedguide/melanoma-skin-cancer-what-is-melanoma.

Kwabi-Addo, B., & Laura, T. (2011). *Cancer Causes and Controversies: Understanding Risk Reduction and Prevention.* Santa Barbara, CA: Praeger.

MacMillan, A. (May 10, 2013). The ABCDE's of melanoma: 5 letters that can save your life. *Self.* Retrieved from http://www.self.com/flash/health-blog/2013/05/health-abcdes-melanoma/.

Mayo Clinic. (2016). Melanoma. Retrieved from http://www.mayoclinic.org/diseases-conditions/melanoma/basics/definition/con-20026009.

National Cancer Institute. (2015). What does melanoma look like? Retrieved from http://www.cancer.gov/types/skin/melanoma-photos.

Skin Cancer Foundation. (2015). Melanoma warning signs and images. Retrieved from http://www.skincancer.org/skin-cancer-information/melanoma/melanoma-warning-signs-and-images.

MENIERE'S DISEASE

Also called *endolymphatic hydrops*, Meniere's disease is a chronic inner ear condition that affects balance and hearing. Although the condition generally affects only one ear at first, over time approximately 50 percent of all patients will develop the problem in both ears. Less than 1 percent of the worldwide population is thought to have Meniere's disease, and only around 45,000 new cases are diagnosed in the United States each year. Although anybody can have the condition, it is most often initially detected in adults between the ages of 40 and 60.

Although the exact cause of Meniere's disease is not yet fully understood, the disorder is usually connected to an overabundance of fluid in the inner ear. Head injuries, viral infections in the middle or inner ear, allergies, and migraine headaches are among the risk factors associated with the condition. The condition usually presents with four major symptoms: ringing in the ear (tinnitus), fluctuating hearing loss, increased pressure in the ear, and reoccurring bouts of dizziness (vertigo). Such issues as diarrhea, vomiting, loss of vision or blurred vision, and chest pain may also be symptoms of Meniere's disease. A person with Meniere's disease will typically suffer from a cluster of episodes or attacks in which their symptoms are acute, followed by lengthy stretches of time without symptoms. Such periodic attacks often occur without warning and may be as short as 20 minutes or as long as several hours. In extreme cases, an attack may extend for a full 24-hour period. The intensity, frequency, and length of a Meniere's disease attack varies from person to person and from episode to episode.

In order to be diagnosed with Meniere's disease, a patient must have experienced at least two separate, spontaneous dizzy spells of at least 20 minutes in length and have had verified hearing loss at some point in time because hearing loss may come and go, depending on whether a person is in the throes of an episode or not. To diagnose the disease, a medical practitioner will conduct a physical exam along with a hearing test and some type of balance assessment. Such tests as magnetic resonance imaging (MRI) of the brain and a caloric stimulation test may also be used to rule out the possibility of other ailments. Although there is currently no cure for Meniere's disease, medications to treat vertigo and to reduce fluid retention may be prescribed. In circumstances where attacks are consistently severe, surgery may be performed to help regulate fluid levels in the inner ear and correct problems with vertigo and balance. A reduced-sodium diet is also recommended for those with Meniere's disease, and at times, the condition will reverse on its own without any medical interference at all.

Meniere's disease is a relatively new condition, having been officially defined by the American Academy of Otolaryngology in 1995; however, the origins of information about the condition can be traced back to the 1860s, when French physician Prosper Meniere developed his theory that vertigo and hearing loss were associated with inner ear issues rather than problems with the brain as scientists believed at the time. Meniere's theory was debated for many years before being accepted by the medical community in the mid-20th century. As medical advances were made, his broad ideas about the inner ear (along with others that followed) were synthesized, and a list of criteria used to diagnose Meniere's disease was eventually developed in the early 1970s. Wording of the criteria was changed in the mid-1980s and again in the 1990s to allow for degree of debilitation and other more recently discovered factors.

Throughout history, several notable people have been diagnosed with Meniere's disease, including American astronaut Alan Shepard and iconic actress Marilyn Monroe. While there is still no cure or known cause for the disease, in 2013 researchers at the University of Colorado School of Medicine theorized that the condition may be caused by a combination of a malformation in the inner ear and vascular disease, which decreases the flow of blood in the brain and the ear. Recent studies have also shown that the application of anti-inflammatory steroid medication behind the eardrum successfully controlled symptoms of the disorder in some 90 percent of patients tested.

Tamar Burris

See also: Allergies; Ear Diseases; Tinnitus; Vestibular Diseases

Further Reading

Crane, R. (2011). *Overcoming Meniere's Disease: A Practical Guide.* Bogotá, Colombia: Mejorando Endeavors.

Dalebout, S. (2008). *The Praeger Guide to Hearing and Hearing Loss: Assessment, Treatment, and Prevention.* Westport, CT: Praeger.

Haybach, P. J., & Underwood, J. (1998). *Meniere's Disease: What You Need to Know.* Portland, OR: Vestibular Disorders Assoc.

Mayo Clinic. (2015). Meniere's disease. Retrieved from http://www.mayoclinic.org/diseases-conditions/menieres-disease/basics/definition/con-20028251.

Vestibular Disorders Association. (2015). Meniere's disease. Retrieved from http://vestibular.org/menieres-disease.

MENINGITIS

Basics

Meningitis is classified as an inflammatory disease. The inflammation that occurs in meningitis is localized to the protective membranes covering the brain and spinal cord, called *meninges*, hence the term, *meningitis*. Most cases of meningitis are caused by bacteria or viruses, but some cases are may be causes by the presence of certain medications and/or illnesses. People of any age can get meningitis, but because it can be easily spread among those living in close quarters, teens, college students, and students in boarding schools are at higher risk for infection.

The two forms of meningitis that can occur are acute meningitis and chronic meningitis. Acute meningitis strikes suddenly, while chronic meningitis develops over two weeks or more when slow-growing organisms invade the membranes and fluid surrounding the infected person's brain. The signs and symptoms of chronic meningitis, such as headaches, fever, vomiting, and mental cloudiness, are similar, however, to those of acute meningitis.

Types of Meningitis

There are five types of meningitis:

Bacterial meningitis, which is serious and contagious when transmitted by oral contact, such as kissing, can also occur when bacteria directly invade the meninges—for example, as a result of sinus and ear infections, a fracture of the skill, of after some types of surgery—but this is rare. It hurts those with weakened immune systems the most.

The most common bacterial strains include:

Streptococcus pneumonia (pneumococcus), the most common cause of bacterial meningitis in infants, young children, and adults in the United States.

Neisseria meningitidis (meningococcus), causing meningococcal meningitis that is highly contagious, and mostly affects teenagers and young adults. It may cause local epidemics in college dormitories, boarding schools, and military bases.

Haemophilus influenzae (haemophilus), now greatly reduced in prevalence due to the availability of a vaccine against this strain.

Listeria monocytogenes (listeria), a strain that may affect pregnant women, newborns, older adults, and people with weakened immune systems.

Fungal meningitis is caused by inhaling fungal spores from the environment.

Noninfectious meningitis can be caused by cancers, Systemic Lupus Erythematosus (lupus), certain drugs, or head injury, or brain surgery, rather than being spread from person to person.

Parasitic meningitis, caused by *Naegleria fowleri,* infects people by entering the body through the nose. This typically occurs when people go swimming or diving in warm freshwater places, like lakes and rivers. The *Naegleria fowleri* ameba travels up the nose to the brain where it destroys the brain tissue.

Viral meningitis is spread through contact with a variety of enteroviruses, which tend to reside in the digestive tract. Most cases of meningitis in the United States are caused by a viral infection, but bacterial and fungal infections also can lead to meningitis.

Symptoms

Meningitis often triggers characteristic or classic signs and symptoms, including headaches, fever and a stiff neck.

Other signs and symptoms that may occur in anyone older than age of two include:

Vomiting or nausea with headache
Confusion or concentration difficulty
Seizures
Sleepiness or difficulty waking up
Sensitivity to light
Lack of appetite
Less common symptoms
Localized weakness or loss of strength or sensation, especially in the face

Joint swelling and pain in one or more joints
A new skin rash that often looks like a bruise

The severity of illness and the treatment for meningitis differ depending on the cause. Thus, it is important to know the specific cause of meningitis.

Key Causes and Risk Factors

Many of the bacteria and viruses that cause meningitis are fairly common and are associated with other illnesses. In some cases of bacterial meningitis, the bacteria spread to the meninges from a severe head trauma or a severe local infection, such as a serious ear or nasal sinus infection.

Meningitis may develop in response to physical injury, cancer or certain drugs. Risk factors for meningitis include:

Skipping vaccinations in children
Age—younger than age 5 or under age 20, especially if living in community settings
Pregnancy
Having a compromised immune system

Diagnosis

A doctor will diagnose meningitis by physical exams, lab tests (possibly including samples of spinal fluid), as well as medical history. An initial diagnosis of the type of meningitis known as meningococcal is made by clinical examination followed by a lumbar puncture to extract infected spinal fluid. The bacteria can sometimes be seen in microscopic examinations of the spinal fluid. The diagnosis is supported or confirmed by growing the bacteria from specimens of spinal fluid or blood, by agglutination tests, or by polymerase chain reaction (PCR) amplification (a test to check for antibodies against certain viruses to check for the specific causes of meningitis).

An at-risk child or adult may hence undergo the following diagnostic tests:

Blood cultures. Here, blood is drawn from a vein and sent to a laboratory and examined under a microscope for bacteria.
Imaging. X-rays and computerized tomography (CT) scans of the head, chest, or sinuses may be used to reveal swelling or inflammation.
Spinal tap (lumbar puncture). This procedure includes an analysis of the suspected victim's cerebrospinal fluid.

Treatments

Treatments are based on the type of meningitis: In acute meningitis prompt treatment is essential.

Bacterial meningitis: A course of treatment with intravenous antibiotics and cortisone medications is used to bring down swelling in the body.

Viral meningitis: Because it is a viral disease, viral meningitis cannot be cured by antibiotics. Instead, bed rest, fluids, and over-the-counter pain medications are usually enough for a person to be cured, with the exception being infants and those with weakened immune systems.

Other kinds of meningitis: Fungal meningitis is treated with intravenous antifungal medications in a hospital. Chronic meningitis is treated based on the underlying cause, which is often fungal.

Noninfectious meningitis due to allergic reactions or autoimmune disease may be treated with cortisone or may require no treatment, and resolve on their own. Meningitis related to cancer will be treated based on the type of cancer.

Prognosis

Viral meningitis may improve without treatment, but bacterial meningitis is serious and requires immediate antibiotic treatment to improve the chances of a recovery and to prevent the risk of permanent brain damage or death, which can occur in a matter of days.

There's no way to know what kind of meningitis a person has without seeing the doctor and undergoing spinal fluid testing.

This should be done quickly, if necessary, because the complications of meningitis can be severe, and the longer one has the disease without treatment, the greater the risk of seizures and permanent neurological damage, including:

Hearing loss
Memory difficulty
Learning disabilities
Brain damage
Gait problems
Seizures
Kidney failure
Shock
Death

Prevention

Anyone at risk, or suspected to have the condition should seek medical care immediately to prevent serious complications.

These steps can help prevent meningitis:

Washing hands. Careful hand-washing is important to avoid exposure to infectious agents, and it's a good idea to keep unwashed hands away from the nose, eyes, and mouth.
Practicing good hygiene. Food, drinks, toothbrushes, lip balms, etc., should not be shared.
Staying healthy. Keeping the immune system healthy by a good diet, regular exercise, and enough sleep will prevent many diseases.
Covering the mouth. When coughing or sneezing, cover the mouth or nose, preferably with the inside of the elbow.
If pregnant, take care with food. Make sure that meat is cooked properly and avoid unpasteurized milk, including soft cheeses made from it. Check labels to make sure that the milk has been pasteurized.

Immunizations

Some forms of bacterial meningitis are preventable with the following vaccinations:

Haemophilus influenzae type b (Hib) vaccine
Pneumococcal conjugate vaccine (PCV7)
Haemophilus influenzae type b and Neisseria meningitidis serogroups C and Y vaccine (Hib-MenCY)
Pneumococcal polysaccharide vaccine (PPSV)
Meningococcal conjugate vaccine (MCV4)

To prevent meningitis, routine vaccinations are important, as are knowing the signs of meningitis.

Future

In December 2010, a new meningococcal vaccine was introduced nationwide in Burkina Faso, and in selected regions of Mali and Niger, with a total of 20 million persons 1 to 29 years of age vaccinated. In 2011, the lowest number of confirmed meningitis A cases ever recorded during an epidemic season was reported. Other African countries are hence pursuing similar nationwide campaigns.

It is hoped that all 26 countries in the African meningitis belt will have introduced this vaccine by 2016. High coverage of the target age group of 1 to 29 years is expected to eliminate meningococcal A epidemics from this region of Africa.

Ray Marks

See also: Brain Diseases; Inflammation; Nasal Disorders; Vaccines

Further Reading

Abramovitz, M. (2014). *Meningitis (Diseases and Disorders)*. Farmington Hills, MI: Greenhaven Press.
Centers for Disease Control and Prevention. (2015, October 1). Meningitis. Retrieved from http://www.cdc.gov/meningitis/index.html.
Mayo Clinic. (2015, September 15). Meningitis. Retrieved from http://www.mayoclinic.org/diseases-conditions/meningitis/basics/definition/con-20019713.
National Meningitis Association. (2015). Disease prevention and information. Retrieved from http://www.nmaus.org/disease-prevention-information/.
National Institute of Neurological Disorders and Stroke. (2015, April 30). Meningitis and encephalitis fact sheet. Retrieved from http://www.ninds.nih.gov/disorders/encephalitis_meningitis/detail_encephalitis_meningitis.htm.
World Health Organization. (2015, November). Meningococcal meningitis. Retrieved from http://www.who.int/mediacentre/factsheets/fs141/en/.

MEN'S HEALTH

Like women, men face gender-related health issues, in addition to general health issues shared by both genders. Threats to the health of men are found to specifically arise with respect to three health issues—heart disease, cancer, and unintentional injury. Fortunately, these three health threats are largely preventable and depend on healthy lifestyle choices, such as eating a healthy diet and including physical activity in one's daily routine. It is also important for men to manage their risky behaviors, such as drinking too much and engaging in casual sex, among other more general types of safety, such as wearing a seat belt.

As men get older, their health concerns are likely to change and the percentage of men 18 years and over in fair or poor health is about 12.5 percent. In addition, the percentage who are 20 years and over who are obese is about 33.9 percent (2007–2010). This is important because obese men were more likely to have precancerous lesions detected in their benign prostate biopsies, compared with non-obese men, and were at a greater risk for subsequently developing prostate cancer, according to data published in *Cancer Epidemiology, Biomarkers & Prevention*, a journal of the American Association for Cancer Research.

Health Risk Factors

The failure to get enough exercise is an important risk factor for men, and data show that of men 18 years and over, only 52.3 percent met the 2008 federal physical activity guidelines for aerobic activity through leisure-time aerobic activity. However, as reported in *Science News*, a new study suggests that exercise may reduce Caucasian men's risk of developing prostate cancer. And among Caucasian men who *do* have prostate cancer, exercise may reduce their risk of having more serious forms of the disease. Unfortunately, the benefits do not seem to apply to African American men. In addition, the percentage of men 18 years and over who currently smoke is about 21.5 percent. The percentage of men 18 years and over who had five or more drinks in one day at least once in the past year is about 31.2 percent.

Leading Causes of Death among Men

Heart disease
Cancer
Accidents (unintentional injuries)

Research

Research shows men with prostate cancer who take cholesterol-lowering drugs called statins are significantly less likely to die from their cancer than men who don't take such medication, according to a 2013 study (Geybels et al. 2013). The study followed about 1,000 Seattle-area prostate cancer patients. Approximately 30 percent of the study participants reported using statin drugs to control their cholesterol. After a mean follow-up of almost eight years, the researchers found that the risk of death from prostate cancer among statin users was 1 percent as compared to 5 percent for nonusers.

Prevention

Eating healthy foods; staying at a normal weight; being smoke free; getting annual check-ups and screening; avoiding drinking; managing stress; being safe at work, home, and play; and knowing one's health risks may be helpful.

Ray Marks

See also: Alcoholism; Cancer; Diet and Nutrition; Heart Disease; Male Breast Cancer; Physical Activity; Pneumothorax; Prostate Cancer; Testicular Cancer; Women's Health

Further Reading

Agency for Healthcare Research and Quality. (March 2014). Men: Stay healthy at any age. Retrieved from http://www.ahrq.gov/patients-consumers/patient-involvement/healthy -men/healthy-men.html.

Centers for Disease Control and Prevention. (2015, November 4). Men's health. Retrieved from http://www.cdc.gov/men/.

Geybels, M. S., Wright, J. L., Holt, S. K., Kolb, S., Feng, Z., & Stanford, J. L. (2013). Statin use in relation to prostate cancer outcomes in a population-based patient cohort study. *The Prostate*, 73(11), 1214–1222.

Mayo Clinic. (2014, April 4). Men's health. Retrieved from http://www.mayoclinic.org /healthy-lifestyle/mens-health/basics/mens-health/hlv-20049438.

Men's Health Network. (2015). A-Z—Men's health. Retrieved from http://menshealthnetwork .org/azmenshealth.

Rundle, A., Jankowski, M., Kryvenko, O. N., Tang, D., & Rybicki, B. A. (2013). Obesity and future prostate cancer risk among men after an initial benign biopsy of the prostate. *Cancer Epidemiology, Biomarkers & Prevention, 22*(5), 898–904.

Womenshealth.gov. (2011, January 10). Men's health. Retrieved from http://womenshealth .gov/mens-health/tips-for-men-for-a-healthly-life/index.html.

MENTAL HEALTH DISORDERS

Mental health can be defined as a state that is represented by successful performance of mental functions, the engagement in productive activities, fulfilling relationships with other people, and the ability to adapt to change and to cope with challenges. Mental health is essential to personal well-being, family and interpersonal relationships, and the ability to contribute to community or society.

Mental disorders, in contrast, are health conditions characterized by alterations in thinking, mood, and/or behavior that are associated with distress and/or impaired functioning. Mental disorders contribute to a wide variety of associated health problems, including disability, pain, drug addictions, criminal behavior, or premature death.

Mental illness is the term applied to collectively represent all diagnosable mental disorders, which comprise a wide array of problems, with different symptoms and presentation. However, they are generally characterized by some combination of abnormal thoughts, emotions, behaviors, and relationships with others. Examples are schizophrenia, depression, mental retardation, and disorders due to drug abuse.

Mental disorders are among the most common causes of disability, and the resulting disease burden is among the highest of all diseases. According to the National

Institute of Mental Health (NIMH 2016), in any given year, an estimated 13 million American adults (approximately 1 in 17) are found to have a seriously debilitating mental illness. Mental health disorders are also shown to account for 25 percent of all years of life lost to disability and premature mortality in the United States. Moreover, suicide is the 11th leading cause of death in the United States, accounting for the deaths of approximately 30,000 Americans each year.

Importantly, mental health and physical health are closely connected, and good mental health greatly influences a person's ability to maintain good physical health. Conversely, mental illnesses, such as depression and anxiety, can affect people's ability to participate in health-promoting behaviors, and thus their physical health may be compromised. In turn, problems with physical health, such as chronic diseases, can have a serious impact on mental health and diminish a person's ability to participate in treatment and recovery.

Other Key Facts

- More than 450 million people worldwide suffer from mental disorders, and many more have mental problems.
- Mental health is an integral part of health; indeed, there is no health without mental health.
- Strategies and interventions exist to promote mental health and most mental health disorders can be successfully treated.

According to the World Health Organization (WHO 2013): "Health is a state of complete physical, mental and social well-being and not merely the absence of disease or infirmity." An important consequence of this definition is that mental health is described as more than the absence of mental disorders or disabilities.

Consequently, an individual who is mentally healthy is possibly able to realize his or her own goals, can cope with the normal stresses of life, can work productively, and is able to make a contribution to his or her community. In this positive sense, mental health appears to serve as the foundation for individual well-being and the effective functioning of a community.

Determinants of Mental Health

Multiple social, psychological, and biological factors determine the level of mental health of a person at any point in time. For example, persistent socioeconomic pressures are recognized risks to mental health for individuals and communities. The clearest evidence is associated with indicators of poverty, including low levels of education.

Poor mental health is also associated with rapid social change, stressful work conditions, gender discrimination, social exclusion, unhealthy lifestyle, risks of violence and physical ill health, and human rights violations.

There are specific psychological and personality factors that make people vulnerable to mental disorders. There are also certain biological causes of mental disorders, including genetic factors and chemical imbalances in the brain.

Types of Mental Health Disorders

- *Anxiety disorders:* Anxiety disorders include generalized anxiety disorder, panic disorder and panic attacks, agoraphobia, social anxiety disorder, selective mutism, separation anxiety, and specific phobias. Obsessive-compulsive disorder and posttraumatic stress disorder are closely related to anxiety disorders.
- *Mood disorders:* These disorders, also called affective disorders, involve persistent feelings of sadness or periods of feeling overly happy or fluctuations from extreme happiness to extreme sadness. The most common mood disorders are depression and bipolar disorder.
- *Psychotic disorders:* Psychotic disorders involve distorted awareness and thinking. Two of the most common symptoms of psychotic disorders are hallucinations—the experience of images or sounds that are not real, such as hearing voices—and delusions—false beliefs that the ill person accepts as true, despite evidence to the contrary. Schizophrenia is an example of a psychotic disorder.
- *Eating disorders:* Eating disorders involve extreme emotions, attitudes, and behaviors involving weight and food. Anorexia nervosa, bulimia nervosa, and binge eating disorder are the most common eating disorders.
- *Impulse control and substance use disorders:* People with impulse control disorders are unable to resist urges, or impulses, to perform acts that could be harmful to themselves or others. Pyromania (starting fires), kleptomania (stealing), and compulsive gambling are examples of impulse control disorders. Alcohol and drugs are common objects of addictions. Often, people with these disorders become so involved with the objects of their addiction that they begin to ignore responsibilities and relationships.
- *Personality disorders:* People with personality disorders have extreme and inflexible personality traits that are distressing to the person and/or cause problems in work, school, or social relationships. In addition, the person's patterns of thinking and behavior significantly differ from the expectations of society and are so rigid that they interfere with the person's normal functioning. Examples include antisocial personality disorder, obsessive-compulsive personality disorder, and paranoid personality disorder.

Strategies and Interventions

Mental health promotion involves actions to create living conditions and environments that support mental health and allow people to adopt and maintain healthy lifestyles. These strategies include a range of actions to increase the chances of more people experiencing better mental health.

This may include strategies to promote a climate that respects and protects basic civil, political, socioeconomic, and cultural rights, which is fundamental to mental health promotion because without the security and freedom provided by these rights, it is very difficult to maintain a high level of mental health.

Specific ways to promote mental health include but are not limited to:

- The provision of early childhood interventions, such as home visits for pregnant women; combined nutritional and psychosocial help for disadvantaged populations
- Support to children by offering skills building programs and child and youth development programs
- The socioeconomic empowerment of women

- The provision of social support for elderly populations
- Programs targeted at vulnerable groups, including minorities, indigenous people, migrants, and people affected by conflicts and disasters
- Mental health promotional activities in schools and worksites
- Housing improvements
- Violence prevention programs
- Community development programs

Diagnosis methods include clinical and medical examination, psychological examination, and neuroimaging. The prognosis depends on condition and when it is diagnosed. Prevention includes mental health screening and dealing with stress as effectively as possible when indicated.

Future

Emerging issues in mental health include challenges by veterans who have experienced physical and mental trauma; people in communities with large-scale psychological trauma caused by natural disasters; older adults, as the understanding and treatment of dementia and mood disorders continues to improve; and the availability of guns for mentally ill people.

Ray Marks

See also: Alzheimer's Disease; Anxiety Disorders; Bipolar Disorder; Brain Disorders; Dementia; Depression; Fetal Alcohol Syndrome; Men's Health; Psychotic Disorders; PTSD (Post-Traumatic Stress Disorder); Schizophrenia; Season Affective Disorder; Social Health; Women's Health

Further Reading

Anxiety and Depression Association of America (ADAA). (2016). Understand the facts. Retrieved from http://www.adaa.org/understanding-anxiety.

Diagnostic and Statistical Manual of Mental Disorders, 5th ed. (DSM-5). (2013). Washington, DC: American Psychiatric Association.

Healthy People.gov. (2013). Mental health and mental health disorders. Retrieved from http://www.healthypeople.gov/2020/topicsobjectives2020/overview.aspx?topicId=28.

MedlinePlus. (2013). Mental disorders. U.S. National Library of Medicine. National Institutes of Health. Retrieved from http://www.nlm.nih.gov/medlineplus/mentaldisorders.html.

National Institute of Mental Health (NIMH). (2016). Health and education. Retrieved from https://www.nimh.nih.gov/health/index.shtml.

WebMD. Mental Health Center. (2013). Mental health. Retrieved from http://www.webmd.com/mental-health/default.htm.

World Health Organization. (2013). Mental disorders. Retrieved from http://www.who.int/topics/mental_disorders/en/.

METABOLIC DISORDERS

Metabolism refers to the complex sets of chemical processes and reactions that occur in the body in association with the breakdown of foods—namely, protein, fats, and carbohydrates. Disorders of metabolism affect the ability of the body to convert food into fuel or energy. It is also termed *in-born errors of metabolism*. Metabolism is affected by age and gender, and many conditions affecting metabolism are inherited or genetic in origin. They can also be acquired due to the presence of endocrine organ disease or failure of a metabolically important organ such as the liver or due to respiratory failure, cancer, or end-stage chronic obstructive pulmonary disease and HIV/AIDS. Most people with inherited metabolic disorders appear to have a genetic defect that affects one of their enzyme levels or its function. There are several hundred types of genetic metabolic disorders, and their symptoms, treatments, and prognoses vary widely. Inherited metabolic disorders fall into different categories, depending on the specific substance affected and whether this builds up in harmful amounts because it can't be broken down, is too low, or missing.

Types of Metabolic Disorders

The most common types of metabolic diseases or disorders are Addison's disease, cystic fibrosis, Tay-Sachs disease, Gaucher disease, Hurler disease, galactosemia, Friedrich's disease, hyperthyroidism, hypothyroidism, phenylketonuria, and Type I diabetes, among others.

Symptoms

Metabolic disorders result in different symptoms, depending on the particular disorder. The symptoms can vary in intensity among individuals from mild to severe and can be life-threatening.

Some symptoms of inherited metabolic disorders include:

Abdominal pain
Abnormal odor of urine, breath, sweat, or saliva
Coma
Developmental delay
Failure to gain weight or thrive
Jaundice
Lethargy
Loss of vision or changes in vision
Muscle twitching, spasms, or seizures
Muscle weakness
Paralysis
Poor appetite
Seizures
Vomiting
Weight loss

The symptoms may come on suddenly or progress slowly. Symptoms may be brought on by foods, medications, dehydration, minor illnesses, or other factors. Symptoms appear within a few weeks after birth in many conditions. Other inherited metabolic disorders may take years for symptoms to develop.

Key Causes and Risk Factors

In genetically inherited metabolic disorders, either one enzyme is not adequately produced or, if produced, does not function adequately.

Metabolic disorders can be due to other factors, such as a combination of inherited and environmental factors. Other examples of conditions that can cause metabolic disorders include: alcohol abuse; diabetes; diuretic abuse; gout; ingestion of poison or toxins, including excessive aspirin, bicarbonate, alkali, ethylene glycol, or methanol; and sepsis (life-threatening bacterial blood infection).

Factors increasing the risk of developing metabolic disorders include:

- The presence of certain chronic medical conditions, such as lung or kidney disease (includes any type of kidney problem, such as kidney stones, kidney failure, and kidney anomalies)
- Having a family history of genetic metabolic disorder
- HIV/AIDS

Diagnosis

Inherited metabolic disorders are present at birth, and some are detected by routine screening.

If an inherited metabolic disorder is not detected at birth, it is often not diagnosed until symptoms appear.

Once symptoms develop, specific blood or DNA tests are available to diagnose most genetic metabolic disorders, and referral to a specialized center increases the chances of a correct diagnosis.

Treatment

Limited treatments are available for inherited metabolic disorders. The essential genetic defect causing the condition can't be corrected with current technology. Instead, treatments try to minimize problems that occur due to impaired metabolism.

Common general treatment principles include:

- Reducing or eliminating intake of any food or drug that can't be metabolized properly
- Replacing the enzyme or other chemical that is missing or inactive
- Removing the toxic products of metabolism that accumulate due to the metabolic disorder

Treatment may include such measures as:

- Special diets that eliminate certain nutrients
- Taking enzyme replacements or other supplements that support metabolism
- Treating the blood with chemicals to detoxify dangerous metabolic by-products

Whenever possible, treatment for metabolic disorders should begin by seeking medical care from a qualified health care provider. The treatment approach for metabolic disorders depends on the specific disorder. Inborn errors of metabolism (inherited metabolic disorders) are often treated with nutritional counseling and support; periodic assessment; physical therapy; and other supportive care options, including bone marrow transplantation, medications to reduce symptoms (such as pain or low blood sugar), mineral supplementation, surgery to relieve pain or symptoms, and vitamin supplementation.

Acquired metabolic disorder treatment will include normalizing the metabolic balance by both reversing the cause and administering medications.

A person with an inherited metabolic disorder should receive care at a medical center with experience with these rare conditions.

Children and adults with inherited metabolic disorders can become quite ill, requiring hospitalization and sometimes life support. Treatment during these episodes will usually focus on emergency care and improving organ function.

Prognosis

Complications of untreated metabolic disorders can be serious and even life-threatening in some cases. You can help minimize your risk of serious complications by following the treatment plan you and your health care professional design specifically for you. Complications of metabolic disorders include:

- Organ failure or dysfunction
- Seizures and tremors
- Unconsciousness and coma

Future

Scientists are studying many aspects of this problem and are trying to examine the role of gene therapy, but there is no cure for any condition currently.

Ray Marks

See also: Addison's Disease; Cystic Fibrosis; Diabetes, Type 1; Hyperthyroidism; Hypothyroidism; Phenylketonuria; Sugar Diabetes; Tay-Sachs Disease; Thyroid Disease

Further Reading

KidsHealth.org. (2015, June). Metabolic disorders. Retrieved from http://kidshealth.org /parent/general/body_basics/metabolism.html#.

Mayo Clinic. (2015, March 31). Inherited metabolic disorders. Retrieved from http://www .mayoclinic.org/diseases-conditions/inherited-metabolic-disorders/basics/definition /con-20036708.

MedlinePlus. (2016, May 25). Metabolic disorders. Retrieved from http://www.nlm.nih.gov /medlineplus/metabolicdisorders.html.

METABOLIC SYNDROME

Identified risk factors that exist together are termed *metabolic syndrome.* The presence of these risk factors raises the incidence for medical disorders such as coronary artery disease, stroke, and Type 2 diabetes. A plethora of names are associated with metabolic syndrome: metabolic syndrome X, cardiometabolic syndrome, syndrome X, insulin resistance syndrome, and Reaven's syndrome. The combination of any risk factors that increase or produce the development of medical disorders is typically classified under one of these associated names.

Symptoms

Many government and public health organizations have reached a consensus that three or more of the following signs present represents individuals with metabolic syndrome. Individuals with increased blood pressure, fasting blood glucose, large waist circumference, cholesterol, and triglycerides are symptoms associated with metabolic syndrome. Individuals with one of these factors likely have others. The more factors individuals have, the greater the risk of serious diseases and diminished quality of life. If individuals are unsure or notice an apple-shape body, they may want to inquire with their physician about metabolic syndrome testing.

Causes

The exact cause of metabolic syndrome remains a mystery. Researchers believe a multitude of causes rather than a single cause may explain the high incidence across the United States. However, a majority of the research indicates obesity is a likely culprit of metabolic syndrome.

The main components suggested are classified as extra pounds around the abdominal section, described as "apple-shaped," and insulin resistance. Other important factors are aging, genetic predisposition, changes associated with hormones, and physical inactivity. After the development of metabolic syndrome, many patients develop intensive blood clots and increased signs of inflammation.

Diagnosis

A constellation of cardiovascular diseases risk factors comprise metabolic syndrome. Several national organizations, such as the National Cholesterol Education Program (NCEP) and the American Heart Association (AHA), have created criteria for diagnosis based on large waist circumferences, triglyceride level, reduced HDL, increased blood pressure, and elevated fasting blood sugar. Individuals with three or more of these traits are diagnosed with metabolic syndrome.

Treatment

The primary objective of treatment is to reduce heart disease and diabetes. General prescription consists of lifestyle changes or pharmacological agents to reduce blood pressure and blood glucose.

Four primary areas are targeted by health care professionals to affect metabolic syndrome. The first task is to lose weight by reduced caloric intake per day (500 to

1,000 calories). Second, increase moderate physical activity to at least 30 minutes between five and seven days a week. Third, control cholesterol by either losing weight or using medication to decrease cholesterol. Finally, maintain blood pressure through increased physical activity, weight reduction, or medication. More importantly, individuals who smoke must quit immediately. Also, over-the-counter aspirin may help provide an added benefit for some individuals.

Prevention

Lifestyle changes are paramount for individuals with one, two, or three components of metabolic syndrome. The acceptance of change through commitment toward a healthy diet, regular physical activity, and scheduled checkups will reduce the risk of cardiovascular diseases such as heart attack, diabetes, and stroke. Home remedies for individuals to embrace lifestyle changes by using ELSE model of success: Exercise, Lose weight, Stop smoking, and Eat fiber-rich foods. Implementation of the ELSE model curbs bad habits by adding new habits that reduce symptoms associated with metabolic syndrome.

Prognosis and Outcomes

Metabolic syndrome increases the long-term risk for developing many chronic diseases (cardiovascular and kidney disease) and impedes blood circulation in lower extremities.

Future

Prevention and treatment of metabolic syndrome requires individuals to address several risk factors together. The improvement of quality of life begins with eating better, getting active, and taking medications if prescribed. The adoption of more fruit and vegetable consumption, coupled with at least 150 minutes a week of physical activity, leads toward positive body weight reduction. In order for change to occur, individuals will need a balance between healthy eating and attainable exercise goals that gets their heart rate up.

Ray Marks

See also: Coronary Artery Disease; Diabetes, Type 2; Stroke

Further Reading

American College of Sports Medicine. (2009). *ACSM's Guidelines for Exercise Testing and Prescription. Volume 220*, 8th ed. Philadelphia: Lippincott Williams & Wilkins.

American Heart Association. (2014). Metabolic syndrome. Retrieved from http://www.heart .org/HEARTORG/Conditions/More/MetabolicSyndrome/Metabolic-Syndrome_UCM _002080_SubHomePage.jsp.

International Diabetes Foundation. (2007). The IDF consensus world-wide definition of the metabolic syndrome. Retrieved from https://www.idf.org/webdata/docs/MetS_def _update2006.pdf.

Knowler, W. C., Barrett-Connor, E., Fowler, S. E., Hamman, R. F., Lachin, J. M., Walker, E. A., & Nathan, D. M. (2002). Reduction in the incidence of type 2 diabetes with lifestyle intervention or metformin. *New England Journal of Medicine, 346*, 393–403.

Mayo Clinic. (2014). Metabolic syndrome. Retrieved from http://www.mayoclinic.com /health/metabolic%20syndrome/DS00522.

National Heart, Lung, and Blood Institute. (2015). What is metabolic syndrome? Retrieved from http://www.nhlbi.nih.gov/health/health-topics/topics/ms/.

MINORITY, CHRONIC DISEASE

In the United States, minority groups—including African Americans, Hispanics, Asians, and American Indians, among others, who now make up approximately 25 percent of the population—often suffer disparities or inequalities in health services and health outcomes such as life expectancy and infant mortality rates, as well as higher rates of disability and deaths from chronic diseases. This has led to a movement focused on narrowing the inequality gap.

Key causes of the health disparity gap between minorities and the mainstream are lack of education, language issues, lack of job opportunities, hazardous environments, poor housing, discrimination, exclusion, lack of access to high-quality health care, and risky behaviors, among other factors.

Among the most frequent minority health issues in New York are heart disease (or cardiovascular disease), diabetes, obesity (or overweight and obesity), hypertension (or high blood pressure), and HIV/AIDS. According to the U.S. Department of Health and Human Service Office of Minority Health and other health literature sources, African Americans, Hispanics/Latinos, American Indians and Alaska Natives, Asian Americans, Native Hawaiians, and Pacific Islanders have higher rates of infant mortality, cardiovascular disease, diabetes, HIV/AIDS, and cancer, and lower rates of immunizations and cancer screening, in general.

Instead of reliable, consistent access to health care, they have poorer access to health monitoring and are less likely to receive screenings, timely diagnoses, and appropriate treatment for chronic diseases and conditions. In addition, racial and ethnic minorities are more likely than whites to be underinsured or to lack health insurance coverage altogether. For example, although racial and ethnic minorities constitute one-third of the total U.S. population, they comprise more than one-half (52 percent) of the uninsured population. In fact, in 2003, 23 million of the 45 million uninsured were racial and ethnic minority Americans. It is not surprising, therefore, that racial and ethnic minorities are more likely than whites to have higher illness rates and to experience higher rates of premature death and suffer worse health outcomes. Young people from racial and ethnic minority groups in the United States suffer disproportionately from chronic health conditions, which may continue into adulthood, so much more needs to be done to achieve health equity.

Because the factors contributing to poor racial/ethnic minority health—and to racial/ethnic health disparities—are many and complex, they have been organized into three categories or levels, including individual-level factors, environmental-/community-level factors, and systems-level factors.

Each of these factors, along with research to better understand the factors influencing minority health are needed to achieve the nation's health equity goals.

Ray Marks

See also: AIDS; Diabetes, Type 1; Environment; Heart Disease; Hypertension; Lead Poisoning; Obesity

Further Reading

American Cancer Society. (2013). Cancer facts & figures for African Americans 2013–2014. Retrieved from http://www.cancer.org/research/cancerfactsfigures/cancerfactsfiguresfor africanamericans/cancer-facts-figures-african-americans-2013-2014.

American Heart Association. (2015.) African Americans and heart disease, stroke. Retrieved from http://www.heart.org/HEARTORG/Conditions/More/MyHeartandStrokeNews /African-Americans-and-Heart-Disease-Stroke_UCM_444863_Article.jsp#.V2Q _gzVPjKE.

Centers for Disease Control and Prevention. (2014.) National diabetes statistics report: Estimates of diabetes and its burden in the United States. Atlanta GA: U.S. Department of Health and Human Services, 2014. Retrieved from www.cdc.gov/diabetes/pubs /statsreport14/national-diabetes-report-web.pdf.

Centers for Disease Control and Prevention. (2014). Factors that contribute to health disparities in cancer. Retrieved from http://www.cdc.gov/cancer/healthdisparities/basic _info/challenges.htm.

Families USA. (2014). Health equity. Retrieved from http://familiesusa.org/issues/health -equity.

Health Power for Minorities. (2015). Racial & ethnic channels. Retrieved from http:// healthpowerforminorities.com/special-channels/racial-ethnic/.

Kochanek, K., Arias, E., & Anderson, R. N. (2013). How did cause of death contribute to racial differences in life expectancies in the U.S. in 2010? *National Center for Health Statistics Data Brief,* No. 125. Hyattsville MD: National Center for Health Statistics.

Shonkoff, J., & Garner, A. (2012). Life-long effects of early childhood adversity and toxic stress. *Pediatrics, 129,* 2011–2663.

National Heart, Lung, and Blood Institute. (2012, February 29). The Heart Truth® for African American Women: An Action Plan. Retrieved from http://www.nhlbi.nih.gov /health/educational/hearttruth/downloads/html/factsheet-actionplan-aa.htm.

Office of Disease Prevention and Health Promotion. (2014). *Healthy People 2020.* Social determinants of health. Retrieved from http://www.healthypeople.gov/2020/topics -objectives/topic/social-determinants-health

Office of Minority Health. (2014, June 13). Profile: Blacks/African Americans. Retrieved from http://minorityhealth.hhs.gov/omh/browse.aspx?lvl=3&lvlid=61.

MULTIPLE MYELOMA

Overview

Multiple myeloma is a very debilitating condition affecting the white blood cells or plasma cells located in the bone marrow, which begin to multiply. Abnormal but related problems caused by multiple myeloma are bone problems, immune system problems, kidney-related problems, and red blood cell count problems. It is also termed *myeloma.*

As the condition progresses, the cancerous plasma cells begin to emerge from the bone marrow and can be deposited elsewhere in the body, where they cause further organ damage. Inside the bone marrow, multiple myeloma plasma cells release chemicals that stimulate the body to dissolve areas of bone. This can create weak bone areas, called *lytic lesions.*

First described in 1848, multiple myeloma is characterized by the excessive growth of malignant plasma cells and a subsequent overabundance of a substance known as *monoclonal paraprotein* (M protein).

In 2009, the American Cancer Society estimated that about 20,580 new cases would be diagnosed and that the five-year relative survival rate for the condition would be around 35 percent. The American Cancer Society estimates that 24,000 new cases of multiple myeloma will be diagnosed in 2014, suggesting that the number of cases is rising.

Signs and Symptoms

The signs and symptoms of myeloma may vary and include a high level of calcium in the blood, kidney failure, anemia related to fatigue, and bone damage or bone fractures.

Bone pain, bleeding, spinal cord compression, feeling weak, experiencing frequent infections and fevers, feeling thirsty, weight loss, nausea, constipation, or frequent urination are also common symptoms of the condition.

Less common are shortness of breath, chest pain, confusion, and numbness in the fingers and toes during cold weather.

Key Causes and Risk Factors

The cause of multiple myeloma is unknown.

Older age and being male, black, and obese, with a history of monoclonal gammopathy of undetermined significance (MGUS), increases the risk of developing the condition.

Exposure to radiation and workplace petrochemicals and having a family history of multiple myeloma are also potential risk factors. Exposure to herbicides, insecticides, heavy metals, plastics, and various dusts (including asbestos) may be risk factors for the disease, yet none of these associations is strong, and in most cases, multiple myeloma develops in individuals with no known risk factors.

Diagnosis

Diagnostic procedures may include one or more of the following: blood and urine tests, diagnostic imaging tests (including x-rays and bone scans), kidney function tests, bone biopsy, and bone marrow biopsy examinations and may help with the diagnosis of the condition.

The tests may result in one of four categories of disease: smoldering multiple myeloma or early disease with no symptoms, Stage I disease, Stage II disease, and Stage III disease—where the stage takes into account the severity of the cancer as far as if it is causing bone or kidney damage. Early disease with symptoms such as bone damage is found in Stage I. In Stages II or III, the disease is more advanced, and more cancer cells are found in the body.

Treatments

Treatment approaches for multiple myeloma will depend on the stage of the disease and may include chemotherapy, steroids and other drugs, radiation therapy, stem cell therapy, targeted therapy to block the growth of the cancerous cells, bone marrow transplants, or simply observation if the disease or condition is mild.

As well, lifestyle modifications and reducing stress may be advantageous. Survival may range from 1 to 10 years or more but depends on a number of factors.

Future

Researchers are studying the DNA of plasma cells to try to understand what changes cause these cells to become cancerous. To date, it appears most people with multiple myeloma have genetic abnormalities in their plasma cells though they haven't yet discovered the cause of these changes.

Ray Marks

See also: Bone Diseases; Immune System Disorders; Kidney Diseases

Further Reading

American Cancer Society. (2015). Multiple myeloma. Retrieved from http://www.cancer .org/cancer/multiplemyeloma/detailedguide/multiple-myeloma-what-is-multiple -myeloma.

International Myeloma Foundation. (2013). Newly diagnosed? Retrieved from http:// myeloma.org/Main.action.

Mayo Clinic. (2015). Multiple myeloma. Retrieved from http://www.mayoclinic.com/health /multiple-myeloma/DS00415.

Multiple Myeloma Research Foundation. (2015). Multiple myeloma. Retrieved from http:// www.themmrf.org/living-with-multiple-myeloma/newly-diagnosed-patients/what-is -multiple-myeloma/.

PubMed Health. (2015). Multiple myeloma. Retrieved from http://www.ncbi.nlm.nih.gov /pubmedhealth/PMH0001609/.

MULTIPLE SCLEROSIS

Multiple sclerosis, commonly called MS, is a progressive disease of the central nervous system. The immune system attacks and damages the *myelin sheath*, or the protective covering of the nerve cells. The disease slows down, disrupts, or blocks the flow of messages from the brain and spinal cord to other parts of the body and may eventually create areas of thick scar tissue along the permanently damaged myelin. This scar tissue gives the disease its name—*multiple* refers to many and *sclerosis* to scars. The symptoms of MS, which can be debilitating, may include muscle weakness, stiffness, or spasms; trouble with balance or coordination; problems with bladder, bowel, or sexual function; memory or concentration difficulties; blurred vision; depression or anxiety; and numbness, tingling, or prickling sensations, depending on which nerves are affected. MS is usually mild, but some people experience severe symptoms such as losing the ability to write, speak, or walk. About 400,000 adults in the United States have MS, and some 2.5 million worldwide. It affects women more often than men, and most people are diagnosed between the ages of 15 and 50. Because there is no cure for MS, treatment involves delaying its progression and managing the symptoms; those with mild symptoms may not need treatment.

Symptoms

The symptoms of MS vary widely among individuals, and they depend on which nerves are affected and the amount of damage. Severe symptoms may result in the inability to walk or paralysis, while mild symptoms may enter long periods of remission. Common initial symptoms are often blurred or double vision, red or green color distortion, or blindness in one eye. Other typical symptoms may include one or more of the following that progress for several days: muscle weakness and difficulty with coordination, balance, or walking; clumsiness; tingling, numbness, or prickling sensations; sexual dysfunction; pain; slurred speech; tremors; dizziness; fatigue; depression; bladder or bowel problems; trouble swallowing; or hearing loss. About half of those with MS have mild difficulties with concentration, attention, memory, and poor judgment.

Causes and Risk Factors

MS is considered an autoimmune disorder in which the immune system attacks and destroys its own myelin. But its causes are not known, and it is also not clear why some people develop the disease, although genetics and environmental factors may play a small role. Women face about twice the risk. Other risk factors that increase the chance of developing the disease include age (between 15 and 50); family history, especially a parent or sibling; other autoimmune disorders (thyroid disease, Type 1 diabetes, and inflammatory bowel disease); Caucasians; and possibly Epstein-Barr virus or a vitamin D deficiency. Previously, those who live in temperate climates far from the equator (in Canada, the northern United States, Europe, New Zealand, and southeastern Australia) were thought to be at risk, but in past decades, more cases have been diagnosed in Latin America and other more temperate regions. Diet, exercise, and smoking tobacco are not considered risk factors.

Diagnosis

There is no single test for MS, but a diagnosis can be made after a person has experienced several episodes of symptoms. Most people have MS confirmed with an MRI scan, a detailed image of the brain and spinal cord that can reveal damaged myelin MRI. Doctors also take a medical history and perform a physical exam and may conduct other tests to confirm a diagnosis, including a neurological examination to test coordination, balance, reflexes, vision, speech, and sensation; lumbar puncture, also called a spinal tap, which analyzes spinal fluid; evoked potentials test to monitor the brain's responses to visual and auditory stimulation and show how well nerve transmission is occurring; and blood tests to check for any other causes of symptoms.

Treatments

There is no cure for MS, but medications are prescribed to slow down and manage symptoms, help speed recovery from attacks, and reduce the length and severity of relapses. Physical or occupational therapy, psychotherapy, support groups, or social work interventions are often recommended to help reduce symptoms, prevent greater disability, and improve overall quality of life.

Prevention

No preventive measures for MS have been identified. For those living with the disease, living healthfully and reducing stress may prevent its rapid progression.

Prognosis and Outcomes

Once diagnosed, most people who receive appropriate treatment for MS can expect a normal life expectancy; most have mild symptoms or occasional flare-ups, and some remain stable with no progression following an initial attack. The disease can go into remission spontaneously. If untreated, MS can become severe, limiting mobility and causing pneumonia and other serious complications.

Future

Researchers are working on naturally occurring interferons, or naturally occurring antiviral proteins; beta interferon has been shown to reduce the number of attacks and may slow the progression of physical disability. Others are examining genetic factors that may help diagnose and predict a person's response to treatment options; evaluating drugs that show promise in eliminating or preventing new scarring from forming; and stem cell therapy, which may help the immune system prevent scars from forming. Treatments are also being developed that would protect the myelin from additional damage, help repair it, and possibly help those with MS regain lost function.

Ray Marks

See also: Color Blindness; Environment; Genetics and Genomics; Immune System Disorders

Further Reading

Furney, K. O. F. (2009). *When the Diagnosis Is Multiple Sclerosis: Help, Hope, and Insights from an Affected Physician.* Baltimore, MD: Johns Hopkins University Press.

Mayo Clinic. (2015). Multiple sclerosis. Retrieved from http://www.mayoclinic.org/diseases -conditions/multiple-sclerosis/home/ovc-20131882.

Multiple Sclerosis Association of America. (2015, September 9). MS overview. Retrieved from http://mymsaa.org/about-ms/overview/.

National Institute of Neurological Disorders and Stroke. (2015, July 17). Multiple sclerosis information page. Retrieved from http://www.ninds.nih.gov/disorders/multiple_sclerosis /multiple_sclerosis.htm.

National Multiple Sclerosis Society. (2015). What is MS? Retrieved from http://www .nationalmssociety.org/What-is-MS.

MUSCLE CRAMPS

Muscle cramps are the sudden and involuntary tightening of a muscle or group of muscles. Although the most commonly affected muscles are in the legs, muscle cramps can also affect the arms, hands, abdomen, and feet. When a cramp occurs, a hard bulge may be felt in the affected muscle, accompanied by intense pain. Although most cramps last only a few seconds, they usually render the affected muscles useless for the duration, followed by a feeling of tenderness, similar to how a sore muscle feels after working out too hard.

There are a variety of causes of muscle cramps. The three most frequent causes are overuse of a muscle, dehydration, and mineral depletion. An intense workout or frequent overuse of a muscle can lead to oxygen depletion in the muscle tissue. This leads to muscle fatigue, and the muscle may cramp for lack of oxygen. Dehydration may occur when a person fails to drink enough fluids while working out or simply doing normal activity in a dry, hot climate. The lack of water in the body causes nerve endings to compress together more tightly, leading to involuntary discharges that cause muscle twitches. These twitches can develop into cramps if the fluid level is not replenished. Mineral depletion may be caused either by inadequate dietary intake or as a side effect of dehydration. Diets lacking in potassium, calcium, or magnesium may lead to increased risk of muscle cramps. A person may lose too much of these minerals during an intense workout, in which the minerals are expelled from the body through large amounts of sweat.

Other, less frequent, causes of muscle cramps include medical or nutritional reasons. Cramps are fairly common in pregnant women. It can also be a symptom of kidney failure, diabetes, liver problems, or hypothyroidism, a condition in which the thyroid gland is underactive. Alcoholism also may cause muscle cramps because dehydration may accompany high alcohol levels in the body. Leg cramps are sometimes caused by narrowing of the arteries that supply blood to the legs and are usually brought on by exercising because the blood flow cannot keep up with the demand for oxygen to the muscles. The compression of spinal nerves may cause cramping while walking. Finally, people gradually lose muscle mass with advancing age, which may cause muscles to become fatigued more quickly.

Most of the time, muscle cramps can be self-treated and will disappear on their own. Two of the most effective ways to treat muscle cramps are stretching and applying heat or cold. Because most cramps occur in the back of the calf (charley horse) or the front or back of the thigh, knowing how to stretch the leg during a cramp can be helpful. Pulling the top of the foot toward the head while keeping the leg straight and massaging the bulging area of the muscle will help to make the cramp subside. Alternately, a warm towel or heating pad can be applied to the affected muscle until the cramp is gone. Massaging the muscle with ice after the cramp disappears may help alleviate pain.

However, there are some cases in which muscle cramps do indicate the need for professional care. It is best to consult with a doctor if the cramps occur very frequently and last an unusually long time or cause severe pain. In addition, if the skin around the affected muscle swells or develops a rash, or if the muscle seems weak after cramping occurs, medical care should be sought.

The best way to avoid muscle cramps is to ensure the consumption of plenty of fluids and to always stretch before and after any physical activity.

Christina M. Girod

See also: Diabetes, Type 1; Hypothyroidism; Kidney Diseases; Liver Diseases

Further Reading

Allen, R. E., & Kirby, K. A. (2012, August 15). Nocturnal leg cramps. American Academy of Family Physicians. Retrieved from http://www.aafp.org/afp/2012/0815/p350.html.

American Cancer Society. (2015). Leg cramps. Retrieved from http://www.cancer.org/treatment/treatmentsandsideeffects/physicalsideeffects/dealingwithsymptomsathome/caring-for-the-patient-with-cancer-at-home-leg-cramps.

Cleveland Clinic. (2015, October 28). Health essentials: Don't let foot cramps and charley horses slow you down. Retrieved from http://health.clevelandclinic.org/2015/10/dont-let-foot-cramps-charley-horses-slow/.

Mayo Clinic. (2016). Muscle cramp. Retrieved from http://www.mayoclinic.org/diseases-conditions/muscle-cramp/basics/definition/con-20014594.

Tobias, A. J. (2015, June 10). Here's what you need to know about cramps: The condition that felled Matthew Dellavedova. Cleveland Clinic. Retrieved from http://www.cleveland.com/metro/index.ssf/2015/06/heres_what_you_need_to_know_ab.html.

MUSCULOSKELETAL DISORDERS

Comprised of muscles, bones, cartilage, tendons, ligaments, joints, and other connective tissue that support and join tissues and organs, the musculoskeletal system gives the body shape and stability, protects its vital organs, and allows it to move. Musculoskeletal disorders are injuries to these areas in the body. Among of the most common health problems and sources of chronic disability, they can affect people of all ages. About one-third of adults in the United States have symptoms of musculoskeletal disorders, and the prevalence tends to increases with age: Most people over age 75 have arthritis or some type of musculoskeletal disorder.

Often the result of sudden exertion or repetitive movement, musculoskeletal disorders range from lower back pain (the most common) to rheumatoid arthritis, as well as different types of arthritis. The term *soft-tissue rheumatism* describes conditions that cause pain, swelling, or inflammation in the tendons, muscles, bursas, and ligaments—the soft tissues around the joints—such as bursitis and tendinitis.

Most disorders cause pain; the muscles are the most commonly affected, along with spinal discs in the lower back, tendons and nerves in the neck and the upper limbs, and osteoarthritis in the lower limbs, but the disorders can affect all areas of the body. Of the many musculoskeletal disorders, these are among the most common: types of arthritis, carpal tunnel syndrome, tendinitis, muscle or tendon strain, ligament sprain, tension neck syndrome, rotator cuff tendinitis, lateral epicondylitis (tennis elbow), trigger finger, plantar fasciitis, degenerative disc disease, and ruptured or herniated discs. Less common are gout, fibromyalgia, and rheumatoid arthritis. Medications for pain relief and inflammation and physical therapy are effective treatments.

Symptoms

Pain is the most common symptom of most musculoskeletal disorders—ranging from mild to severe, from acute and short-lived to chronic or recurrent, and from localized to throughout the body. Other common symptoms include joint ache and stiffness; swelling; fatigue; muscle burning, twitching, or the feeling of being pulled; dull aches and discomfort; weakness; and reduced mobility.

Causes and Risk Factors

The largest category of workplace injuries, musculoskeletal disorders can also be caused or worsened by recreational and daily activities that include sudden or forceful exertion and long-term exposure to repetitive motions, force, vibrations, or awkward postures. Diseases and unexpected movements; automobile accidents; falls; fractures; sprains; dislocations; overuse, underuse, or lack of stretching; poor posture; and long periods of immobilization can injure the muscles, bones, and connective tissues.

Anyone of any age can experience a musculoskeletal disorder, but risk factors that increase the likelihood include aging, level and frequency of regular activity, lifestyle, and occupation. Job-related risk factors include activities that require repetitive heavy lifting, bending and twisting, uncomfortable sitting or standing positions, and working without a break for long periods or in environments that are too cold or hot.

Diagnosis

Diagnostic tools include a medical history and a physical examination to locate the origin of the pain. Laboratory tests may include x-rays for images of bones, including arthrography, which shows torn ligaments or fragmented cartilage in a joint; DXA scans for bone density; CT scans for more detailed images of bones; MRI scans for abnormalities in muscles, ligaments, tendons, and other soft tissues; ultrasounds to identify inflammation in and around joints and tears or inflammation of tendons; bone scans; and tests that can determine if the nerves supplying the muscles are functioning properly. Blood tests can confirm a disorder such as rheumatoid arthritis and lupus. For swollen joints, a doctor may test the joint fluid for bacterial infection or crystals that can cause gout.

Treatments

The treatment of a musculoskeletal disorder depends on its severity and cause and the location of the pain. Prescription medications may be required to reduce inflammation and pain; occasional pain may be alleviated with nonprescription pain relievers. Physical or occupational therapy teaches pain-management techniques.

Depending on the underlying cause, the application of heat or cold or immobilizing a joint with a splint can relieve musculoskeletal pain. Other treatments may include reducing workload and increasing rest periods; relaxation and biofeedback techniques to reduce stress; acupuncture or acupressure; stretching exercises and those to strengthen and condition muscles; chiropractic care; therapeutic massage; and osteopathic manipulation, which evaluates and treats illness or injury to restore normal functioning.

Prevention

Preventive measures include avoiding overuse or injury during daily activities, adding regular strengthening and stretching exercises, maintaining good posture, and taking care when lifting or moving heavy objects.

Prognosis and Outcomes

Depending on the cause and severity of a musculoskeletal disorder, many can be treated effectively to improve or restore mobility and normal functioning. Although these disorders tend to increase with age because muscles, bones, and joints naturally break down, some risk factors may be reduced by adherence to preventive measures.

Ray Marks

See also: Arthritis; Bursitis; Carpal Tunnel Syndrome; Fibromyalgia; Gout; Joint Disorders; Lupus; Osteoarthritis; Rheumatoid Arthritis

Further Reading

Cleveland Clinic. (2014, November 14). Musculoskeletal pain. Retrieved from https://my .clevelandclinic.org/health/diseases_conditions/hic_musculoskeletal_pain.

HealthLine. (2013, June 18). Musculoskeletal disorders. Retrieved from http://www
.healthline.com/galecontent/musculoskeletal-disorders.

Merck Manual. (2015). Musculoskeletal pain. Retrieved from http://www.merckmanuals
.com/home/bone-joint-and-muscle-disorders/symptoms-of-musculoskeletal-disorders
/musculoskeletal-pain.

MYOPATHIES

The term *myopathy* is a basic one describing any form of neuromuscular disease
that affects a muscle but not its nerve. It is a skeletal muscle disorder that is usually
chronic and that progresses slowly. In these infrequently occurring disorders, the
muscle commonly undergoes structural changes and often degenerates, atrophies,
or wastes, thus becoming thinner, and/or the affected muscles often become weak,
thus having an effect on movements of everyday living. In other areas, the muscles
may be conspicuously enlarged or exhibit metabolic dysfunction, muscle spasm,
or rigidity. Weakness of the muscles, or muscle strength imbalances, can transfer
forces unequally to the joints and can cause restrictions of mobility and resultant
joint deformity. This may affect the limbs as well as the spinal joints. The degree of
disability and mortality associated with the condition vary. In those with severe
weakness, there may be respiratory failure and death. Prevalence is higher in males
for muscular dystrophy and higher for women for inflammatory myopathies.

Types

The main types of myopathy are congenital myopathy, inflammatory myopathy,
muscular dystrophies, endocrine-related myopathies, and drug-induced myopathy.

Congenital myopathy is the term describing muscle disorders that are present at
birth; it is classified as one of four types: central core disease, nemaline rod disease, centronuclear or myotubular myopathy, and multicore myopathy.

Muscular dystrophy refers to a group of genetic diseases that are progressive and
can cause progressive weakness and muscle degeneration and movement control
problems. Major forms include Duchenne, myotonic, and limb-girdle, among others.

Inflammatory myopathies involve inflammation and degeneration of the muscle
over time and appear associated with autoimmune system disorders. Examples include polymyositis and dermatomyositis.

Endocrine-related myopathies can be caused by poorly functioning endocrine
systems—for example, thyroid gland problems—or from excess intake of corticosteroid drugs.

Drug-induced myopathies are those caused by toxic substances that destroy the
muscle and can occur generally or locally.

Signs and Symptoms

Muscles affected by myopathy may exhibit poor tone, muscle weakness, and wasting, especially among those muscles closest to the center of the body, such as the

thigh and shoulder muscles. More rarely, the muscles of hands and feet may be involved. This condition can thus affect the ability of the child or adult to carry out certain motor skills, such as walking or grasping. Other symptoms associated with myopathies are muscle cramps, pain, stiffness, spasm, or an inability to relax the muscle, called *myotonia*. In certain myopathies, there may be acute flare-ups and breakdown of muscle fibers that are released into the blood as a red pigment or myoglobin.

In most cases, the symptoms are consistent and do not fluctuate from day to day, although in some rare forms, the weakness may appear in acute forms, while the patient is well at other times.

Key Causes and Risk Factors

Myopathies can be inherited conditions that are acquired at birth or occur later in life. They can also occur in association with metabolic disorders, infection or inflammation of the muscle, endocrine disorders, drugs, genetic mutations, or exposure to infectious agents.

Diagnosis

Clinical tests as well as genetic and laboratory tests may be used to diagnose the presence of a myopathy. Other tests involve muscle and/or nerve biopsies, blood tests, or electromyogram that record the electrical activity of the muscle. Early diagnosis can allow for the best chances of the best possible care.

Treatments

Treatments for myopathy depend on the disease or the condition and its specific causes, but no cure exists for any myopathy. Supportive and symptomatic treatment may be the only available and/or needed interventions. Others may require drug therapy intervention, physical therapy, bracing, splinting, or surgery.

Prognosis

The prognosis will vary depending on the type of myopathy. It could vary from being severely disabled and wheelchair bound to a condition that is a threat to life to a condition with little impact on longevity and function. The disease can be fatal at any age, and the risk of serious complications can be reduced by following a personalized treatment plan. No forms of prevention exist.

Future

Research is under way to better prevent, treat, or cure myopathies.

Ray Marks

See also: Musculoskeletal Disorders; Neuromuscular Disorders

Further Reading

Muthusamy, P. (2010). Myopathy. Cleveland Clinic Center for Continuing Education. Retrieved from http://www.clevelandclinicmeded.com/medicalpubs/diseasemanagement/neurology/myopathy/.

Myopathies. (2013). Patient.co.uk. Retrieved from http://www.patient.co.uk/print/1703.

National Institute of Neurological Disorders and Stroke. (2015). NINDS myopathy information page. Retrieved from http://www.ninds.nih.gov/disorders/myopathy/myopathy.htm.

Swierzewski, S. J., III. (2015). Myopathies. Health Communities.com. Retrieved from http://www.healthcommunities.com/myopathies/overview-of-myopathy.shtml.

MYOPIA

Myopia (nearsightedness) is a vision condition in which a person can see close objects with clarity but objects that are farther away are out of focus. The problem is extremely common—some 30 percent of all Americans suffer from myopia. The percentage of sufferers is particularly high in Asia, where some 80 percent of the population has myopia. Although the condition is most often seen in adults between 40 and 50 years of age, it is also found in school-aged children and the elderly. Even though symptoms may take years to appear, typically the problem begins in childhood and progresses until the eye stops growing later in life.

Myopia is created through a refractive error in the eye. In a person with normal eyesight, when light rays enter the eye, they will focus on the retina. This creates visual acuity. In a person who is nearsighted, the light rays will focus in front of the retina. This creates blurriness. This refractive error may occur because the clear surface of the eye, the cornea, is overly curved. It may also occur because the eye itself is longer than normal. The exact cause of myopia is unknown; however, nearsightedness tends to run in families—if one or both parents have myopia, there is a higher risk that their children will develop it as well. The condition also appears to occur more often in people who engage in a lot of reading or other types of close work that may cause visual stress.

In addition to having blurry vision when looking at objects that are far away, a person with myopia may experience such symptoms as headaches, excessive blinking, and a need to squint the eyes in order to see far away objects clearly. Myopia may be more acute at night or while working on the computer or doing other types of close work. The problem can usually be diagnosed through a simple eye exam. As part of the testing, a person will be asked to read letters on a chart. Using such instruments as a hand-held lighted retinoscope and several different lenses, an optometrist will also evaluate the focusing ability of the eye to determine whether a person has myopia.

Although there are currently no ways to stop myopia from occurring, there are several different treatment options for the condition. The most common is corrective eyeglasses and/or contact lenses. There are also several refractive surgical procedures that can be used to correct myopia, including LASIK surgery and a less mainstream method called intraocular lens implantation, in which a surgeon will implant a corrective lens in front of the natural lens in the eye. If a person suffers from myopia due to a problem with muscle spasms, doctors may recommend eye exercises and vision therapy to strengthen these muscles and improve the ability to focus on far away objects. Orthokeratology, or corneal refractive therapy, is another option for treating myopia. This treatment method involves slowly reshaping the cornea by wearing a series of rigid contact lenses for a limited time each day.

Physicians in ancient Rome and Greece are among those first thought to have discovered myopia, and the condition—including the possibility of it being a family problem—was greatly studied through the 19th century. As early as the late 1700s, information was being published on night myopia, or nearsighted issues that occurred mostly after dark, and by the mid-1800s, scientists had already determined that close work contributed to the vision problem. Throughout the 20th century, numerous clinical trials were conducted to try to determine the cause and best course of treatment for myopia, and treatment possibilities greatly expanded with the development of such surgical procedures as LASIK. In 2010, scientists at Duke University uncovered a new gene associated with nearsightedness. Three years later, researchers in the United Kingdom discovered several new genes that are thought to trigger the condition. In part because of growing concern over the increase of myopia around the world, the World Health Organization (WHO) has made it a goal to eradicate preventable blindness by 2020—with myopia and other refractive disorders considered part of its top five priorities.

Tamar Burris

See also: Colorblindness; Diabetes, Type 1; Eye Diseases; Glaucoma; Hyperopia; Macular Degeneration; Sjögren's Syndrome

Further Reading

American Optometric Association. (2015). Myopia (nearsightedness). Retrieved from http://www.aoa.org/patients-and-public/eye-and-vision-problems/glossary-of-eye-and-vision-conditions/myopia?sso=y.

Boyd, K. (2013, September 1). Nearsightedness: What is myopia? American Academy of Opthalmology. Retrieved from http://www.aao.org/eye-health/tips-prevention/myopia-nearsightedness.

Johns Hopkins Medicine. (2015). Nearsightedness, farsightedness and astigmatism. Retrieved from http://www.hopkinsmedicine.org/wilmer/conditions/nearsight.html.

Kitchen, C. K. (2007). *Fact and Fiction of Healthy Vision: Eye Care for Adults and Children.* Westport, CT: Praeger.

Langdell, C. C., & Langdell, T. (2010). *Coping with Vision Loss: Understanding the Psychological, Social, and Spiritual Effects.* Westport, CT: Praeger.

N

NASAL DISORDERS

The nose processes the air that enters the lungs, about 18,000 to 20,000 liters of air daily in an adult, by removing dust, germs, and other irritants and warming the air so the lungs and nasal passages do not become dry. Inside the nose are the nerve cells that aid the sense of smell. A nasal disorder can affect the entire body. Common disorders include rhinitis, which describes two types of inflammation, one of which is caused by allergies; nasal polyps, or growths in the nasal lining; nosebleeds; and nasal obstructions such as a deviated septum, when the wall between the nostrils and nasal passages is crooked. Because of its prominent position on the face, the nose is also vulnerable to fractures.

Symptoms are usually characterized by runny or stuffy nose, trouble breathing, temporary loss of smell or taste, sneezing, bleeding, sore throat, postnasal drip, and pain in the case of injuries. The causes are varied and can include viruses, infection, allergies, injuries, as well as environmental irritants such as dry air, smog, perfume and other scents, cigarette smoke, and exhaust fumes. Nasal polyps may develop as an immune system response in some people. Over-the-counter and prescription medications, as well as home remedies can treat most nasal disorders effectively. Surgery may be the preferred treatment for a badly deviated septum or a nasal fracture. Anyone at any age can develop a nasal disorder. For example, some 58 million people in the United States have allergic rhinitis, and about 19 million have nonallergic rhinitis.

Symptoms

Nasal disorders have many common symptoms, including pain or excess pressure in the forehead, face, or upper teeth; swelling; nosebleeds; difficulty breathing; runny nose; sneezing; congestion; red or itchy eyes; headache; coughing; fatigue; sore throat; postnasal drip; snoring; and the loss of smell or taste. It may be difficult to tell if a nose is fractured, particularly until the swelling subsides. A deviated septum may not present any symptoms.

Causes and Risk Factors

The causes of nasal disorders are many and varied, but they commonly include allergies, viruses, and environmental irritants or injuries. The causes of nonallergic rhinitis are unknown, but triggers associated with it include exposure to the strong odors of exhaust fumes and other pollutants, chlorine, and cleaning solutions; cigarette smoke; perfumes, hairsprays, and other scents; and dry air, laundry detergents, Latex, and the overuse of overuse decongestants. It can often take place with sudden changes in temperature and during puberty, menstruation, or pregnancy, which are periods of hormonal changes.

Allergic rhinitis, commonly known as hay fever in children and adults, is an overreaction of the immune system to tree and grass pollens, dust, mold, animal dander, or other allergens.

Nasal polyps, or fluid-filled growths, are most common in young and middle-age adults. They may develop in those who have a specific type of immune system response and chemical markers in their mucous membranes; risk factors include family history and a predisposition to asthma, allergies, and other causes of chronic inflammation in the nasal passages. Because the nose lining has so many tiny blood vessels close to its surface, they can be damaged easily and cause a nosebleed; dry air and nose picking are the most common causes, although irritants, allergies, infections, and injuries are also known causes. The primary cause of a deviated septum—the cartilage and bone between the nasal cavities—is an injury that moves it out of normal position. Most fractures are also caused by traumatic events, as in sports injuries, falls, or accidents.

Diagnosis

Nosebleed and most other nasal disorders can be diagnosed with a general physical examination where specific attention is paid to the nose and a description of the symptoms. Nonallergic rhinitis has no specific diagnostic test, but a doctor can make a diagnosis based on symptoms and by ruling out allergies. Allergic rhinitis is diagnosed with skin tests that show how the skin reacts to an allergen and a blood test to measure antibodies made by the body in response to allergens. Nasal polyps and a deviated septum are often visible with the use of lighted instruments, and a doctor can diagnose them based on appearance. A broken nose diagnosis may be confirmed by an x-ray.

Treatments

Treatment of the symptoms of chronic rhinitis may be managed with the regular use of prescription anti-inflammatory nasal sprays. Antihistamine medications can relieve sneezing, itching, and a runny nose, but they do not relieve congestion; decongestants can unclog stuffy noses; antibiotics fight infections. Desensitization injections, commonly known as allergy shots, are effective against allergic rhinitis. Usually, a deviated septum does not require treatment, or it can be managed with nasal sprays to help breathing; surgery can make repairs, if necessary. Surgery is usually considered only when other treatments cannot reduce symptoms.

Nasal disorders are incurable, but nasal polyps are commonly treated with nasal saline sprays and corticosteroid medications, as well as antibiotics in the presence of a bacterial sinus infection. In severe cases, surgery may be performed. Most nosebleeds resolve on their own, rarely needing any medical intervention. Surgery is not usually necessary for a broken nose, but procedures to realign the bones may be required.

Prevention

There is no sure way to prevent nonallergic rhinitis or allergic rhinitis, but measures to reduce symptoms include identifying and avoiding known triggers and allergens, not overusing nasal decongestants, and receiving effective treatment. Strategies to prevent nasal polyps include following instructions on taking allergy or asthma medications, avoiding breathing known airborne allergens or irritants, and using a humidifier to help moisten breathing passages and a saline nasal rinse or spray to remove allergens or irritants from the nose. Steps to prevent nosebleeds similarly focus on keeping the nasal membranes moist by using a humidifier and a saline nasal spray, as well as the application of a thin coating of petroleum jelly or antibiotic ointment inside the nose. To avoid an injury-related deviated septum or nasal fracture, precautionary measures include wearing a helmet or other sport-appropriate safety gear and using a seat belt while riding in any motor vehicle.

Prognosis and Outcomes

Most nasal disorders, including those caused by trauma, can be managed and controlled by a variety of effective treatments so normal breathing is restored.

Ray Marks

See also: Allergies; Bleeding Disorders; Meningitis; Respiratory Diseases

Further Reading

American Academy of Otolaryngology—Head and Neck Surgery. (2015). Your nose, the guardian of your lungs. Retrieved from http://www.entnet.org/?q=node/1365.

Mayo Clinic. (2014, March 8). Nasal polyps. Retrieved from http://www.mayoclinic.org /diseases-conditions/nasal-polyps/basics/definition/con-20023206.

Mayo Clinic. (2013, February 19). Nonallergic rhinitis. Retrieved from http://www.mountsinai .org/patient-care/service-areas/ent11/areas-of-care/nasal-sinus-and-allergy-disorders.

Mount Sinai Hospital. (2015). Nosebleeds/epistaxis. Retrieved from http://www.mountsinai .org/patient-care/service-areas/ent/areas-of-care/nasal-sinus-and-allergy-disorders /nosebleeds-epistaxis.

NATIONAL INSTITUTES OF HEALTH (NIH)

The National Institutes of Health (NIH) is a component of the U.S. Department of Health and Human Services. It is the largest research agency in the United States and is involved in important discoveries that improve health and save lives as outlined at its website (https://www.nih.gov/).

NIH is made up of 27 institutes and centers, each with a specific research agenda, often focusing on particular diseases or body systems. Its leadership plays an active role in shaping the agency's research planning, activities, and outlook. It is the primary federal agency for conducting and supporting basic, clinical, and translational medical research, and it investigates the causes, treatments, and cures for both common and rare diseases.

As a result of the research at NIH, Americans today are living longer and healthier lives, and their life expectancy jumped from 47 years in 1900 to 78 years as reported in 2009. Disability in people over age 65 has dropped dramatically in the past three decades, and according to the website, nationwide rates of new diagnoses and deaths from all cancers combined have fallen significantly in recent times.

Many studies at NIH have led to the significant scientific advances such as the development of MRI, understanding how viruses can cause cancer, and factors influencing cholesterol control. We have better knowledge of how our brain processes visual information, as well as research training programs and educational programs—all designed to improve the nation's health. NIH's long-term efforts to understand, treat, and prevent chronic diseases is helping to reduce the global burden of these conditions.

As a result of the efforts at NIH, it is believed that we are not only living longer, but that the American quality of life is improving. Over the last quarter century, the proportion of older people with chronic disabilities has dropped by nearly one-third. NIH also drives job creation and economic growth, and its research funding directly supports hundreds of thousands of American jobs. It also serves as a foundation for the medical innovation sector, which employs 1 million U.S. citizens (http://www.nih.gov/about/impact/index.htm).

It is not, however, without critics, including those who claim it rewards safe and mediocre, not innovative, projects for funding (Nicholson and Ioannis 2012) and both political conservatives, who believe the NIH wastes money, and liberals, who believe it is not spending enough, especially on curing diseases.

Ray Marks

See also: Centers for Disease Control (CDC); World Health Organization

Further Reading

Cook-Deegan, R. (2015, Winter). Has NIH lost its halo? *Issues in Science & Technology, 31*(2), 36–47.

National Institutes of Health. (2016). Impact of NIH Research. Retrieved from https://www.nih.gov/about-nih/what-we-do/impact-nih-research.

National Institutes of Health (NIH). (2016). Retrieved from http://www.nih.gov/.

Nicholson, J. M., & Ioannidis, J. P. A. (2012, December 6). Research grants: Conform and be funded. *Nature, 492*, 34–36.

YouTube. (2016). NIHOD (NIH Channel). Retrieved from https://www.youtube.com/user/NIHOD.

NEOPLASMS

Neoplasms are collections of abnormal cells. Also called *tumors*, they can be benign, precancerous, or premalignant, or cancerous or malignant. If a cancerous tumor is not treated, it will continue to grow and invade healthy tissues. Tumors come in different sizes and can occur anywhere in the body, including the brain. Different types of tumors are made up of different types of cells.

Symptoms

The symptoms of a tumor, if present may depend on where the tumor is situated and how large it is. If it is visible or large, it can be palpated. Weight loss, illness, feeling less than well, or having a fever might indicate the presence of a nonmalignant tumor. Swelling, nausea, easy bruising, skin changes, bowel changes, nosebleeds, night sweating, and pain are other possible symptoms. Some tumors are more common in one gender versus another or one age group versus another.

Causes and Risk Factors

According to the *New York Times* (2010), one reason a person may develop a tumor is related to a problem with the body's immune system. In addition to exposure to tobacco, toxic substances, excessive exposure to sunlight, radiation, viruses, and toxins may foster the development of a tumor. Excess alcohol intake, environmental factors, and family history may also increase the risk for developing a tumor.

Diagnostic Procedures

A biopsy is the most frequent form of test to examine if a tumor is cancerous or not. This can be done surgically or with a needle that isolates tissue that can be studied under the microscope.

Blood tests, x-rays, CT scans, or MRI exams may also be helpful.

Treatments

Chemotherapy, radiation, surgery, or a combination of these factors may be used to treat a tumor.

Outcome

If a tumor is benign, the outlook is good. If a tumor is premalignant or cancerous, treatment may be helpful in reducing the problem, depending on the form of cancer. Some are more curable than others.

Prevention

Leading a healthy lifestyle and avoiding toxic exposure to chemicals and radiation is strongly indicated for preventing neoplasms.

Ray Marks

See also: Cancer; Environment; Immune System Disorders; Neurofibromatosis

Further Reading

American Cancer Society. (2014). Signs and symptoms of cancer. Retrieved from http://www .cancer.org/cancer/cancerbasics/signs-and-symptoms-of-cancer.

New York Times. (2016). Tumor. Retrieved from http://www.nytimes.com/health/guides /disease/tumor/overview.html.

Nordqvist, C. (2015). Tumors: Benign, premalignant and malignant. *Medical News Today.* http://www.medicalnewstoday.com/articles/249141.php.

St. Jude Children's Hospital. (2016). Recognizing the symptoms: Warning signs of solid tumors. Retrieved from http://www.stjude.org/stjude/v/index.jsp?vgnextoid=090afa318 6e70110VgnVCM1000001e0215acRCRD&vgnextchannel=3b7bbfe82e118010VgnV CM1000000e2015acRCRD.

NEPHRITIS

Nephritis is any type of inflammation of the kidney that impairs its function. The kidneys, which look like two bean-shaped organs, are the body's waste-removal system. Daily, they process about 200 quarts of blood and remove two quarts of waste products and excess water. Kidneys impaired in some way may stop working completely, which is known as kidney failure. Nephritis can involve any part of the kidneys: the glomeruli (clusters of filtering capillaries), tubules (small tubes), or the tissues surrounding these parts. Acute nephritis is when the kidneys suddenly become inflamed. Chronic nephritis refers to the condition that develops without symptoms over time, usually several years, often leading to complete kidney failure. Symptoms common to nephritis are swelling, changes in urine, and fatigue. Autoimmune disorders, infections, and toxins are the most common causes of nephritis. Treatment of nephritis depends on the underlying cause.

The most common form of acute nephritis is the condition of *glomerulonephritis*, which is often referred to as nephritis without other qualification; it is inflammation of the glomeruli, or microscopic blood vessels in the kidneys with small pores through which blood is filtered. Children and teenagers are more likely than adults to be affected by glomerulonephritis. Other types of nephritis refer to specific affected areas in the kidneys, as in interstitial nephritis, or the cause, such as lupus or radiation nephritis. Pyelonephritis, or inflammation of the kidney and upper urinary tract is more common in adult women; athletic nephritis results from strenuous exercise; and hereditary nephritis is a rare condition.

Symptoms

Common symptoms for the different types of acute and chronic nephritis may include pelvic, abdominal, or back pain; frequent or painful urination, including a burning sensation; cloudy, pink-colored, or foamy or bubbly urine; swelling due to fluid retention in the face, hands, legs, and feet; shortness of breath; cough; fever; and high blood pressure. Symptoms of kidney failure include lack of appetite, fatigue, vomiting, difficulty sleeping, dry or itchy skin, and muscle cramps at night.

Causes and Risk Factors

The different types of nephritis can have distinct causes. The primary cause of acute glomerulonephritis is not known, but some known factors include lupus and other immune disorders; viral and bacterial infections such as strep throat, an abscess traveling to the kidneys, and endocarditis; and vasculitis, or blood vessel inflammation. Chronic glomerulonephritis is often the result of family history, immune system disorders, urinary tract surgery, or excess antibiotic or pain medications.

Acute interstitial nephritis is most commonly caused by an allergic reaction to a medication, including side effects of antibiotics and other medications. Other causes are autoimmune disorders (including Sjögren's syndrome, systemic lupus erythematosus, and Kawasaki disease); infections; long-term use of aspirin, nonsteroidal anti-inflammatory drugs, and other medications; too little blood potassium; and excess blood calcium or uric acid.

Most pyelonephritis infection results from the E.coli bacteria in the intestine. Other possible causes include infection following a urinary examination with a cystoscope, as well as bladder, kidney, or ureter surgery. Kidney stones, enlarged prostate, cancerous abdominal or pelvic masses, and other conditions reducing urine flow allow bacteria to travel to the kidneys. Those with diabetes or immune systems conditions are more likely to experience this type of nephritis.

Diagnosis

The diagnosis of all types of nephritis starts with the symptoms, a physical examination, and medical history.

A diagnosis of acute glomerulonephritis is further based on blood and urine tests to identify the infectious organisms or antibodies in the immune system and a biopsy to determine the cause of the disease and the amount of damage to the kidneys. A doctor tests for chronic glomerulonephritis also with a urine test, usually as part of a complete medical examination, and an ultrasound or CT scan of the kidneys. A kidney biopsy distinguishes chronic glomerulonephritis from other kidney disorders.

During a physical exam for interstitial nephritis, a doctor listens for abnormal sounds in the lungs or heart and looks for high blood pressure and fluid in the lungs; blood and urine lab tests may be conducted, as well as a kidney ultrasound and biopsy.

A diagnosis of pyelonephritis is based on urine and blood cultures, a CT scan, and kidney ultrasound. Doctors also check for kidney stones, congenital urinary tract defects, and other conditions that can make pyelonephritis more likely.

Treatments

If an underlying cause is the reason for a type of nephritis, treatment focuses on that illness or disorder.

Acute glomerulonephritis, particularly following a strep infection, usually improves without medical treatment. No specific medical treatment is prescribed for the chronic type of glomerulonephritis, but those who have been diagnosed are advised to reduce the amount of protein, salt, and potassium in their diets, as well as to take calcium supplements and diuretics to increase urination, and to control high blood pressure; steroids may be helpful. At the final or end stage of chronic nephritis, treatment may include a kidney transplant and dialysis.

Treatment of interstitial nephritis is based on its underlying cause, especially avoiding the medications that lead to the symptoms. Limiting protein, salt, and fluids can improve swelling, as well as help control high blood pressure and the buildup of waste products in the blood. Dialysis, if necessary, is usually required for a short period of time. This type of machine filters the blood as the kidneys should, and it is no longer needed when kidney function improves. Corticosteroids or other anti-inflammatory medications may be helpful.

Pyelonephritis, a serious infection, requires treatment with antibiotics and, if necessary, pain medication; most cases are acute; severe cases may require hospitalization. The chronic form of pyelonephritis is a rare condition that is usually caused by congenital kidney defects. Calcium channel blockers help control high blood pressure, and corticosteroids or other immune suppressing medications may be prescribed as needed.

Prevention

Key to preventing glomerulonephritis is to avoid strep infections, especially for children, or get immediate treatment if infected. Adults can take steps to avoid viral infections that can lead to the illness. Interstitial nephritis is difficult to prevent, but the risk can be decreased by avoiding or reducing the use of medications that can cause this condition. Those with a history of urinary tract infections can try to prevent pyelonephritis by consuming plenty of fluids, urinating frequently, and practicing good hygiene, especially after urination. Reducing the amount of the protein, salt, and potassium in the diet and taking calcium supplements and diuretics increases urination and helps control high blood pressure.

Prognosis and Outcomes

To live a healthy life, it is recommended that people with chronic glomerulonephritis restrict salt intake, lower consumption of protein and potassium, control blood sugar levels (diabetes), maintain a healthy weight, and quit smoking. Although there is no known cure, many people can live normally for many years, helped by dialysis or kidney transplantation when necessary.

Interstitial nephritis is usually short term, although rarely it may cause chronic kidney failure or other permanent damage. Its acute form is more serious and likely to lead to long-term or permanent kidney damage, particularly in older adults. After treatment with antibiotics, most people with pyelonephritis do not experience a recurrence and rarely have permanent kidney damage.

Jean Kaplan Teichroew

See also: Inflammation; Kawasaki Disease; Kidney Diseases; Kidney Failure; Sjögren's Syndrome

Further Reading

Healthline. (2015). Acute nephritis. Retrieved from http://www.healthline.com/health/acute-nephritic-syndrome#Overview1.

Medical News Today. (2019, October 14). What is glomerulonephritis? What causes glomerulonephritis? Retrieved from http://www.medicalnewstoday.com/articles/167252.php.

Merck Manual. (2015). Overview of kidney filtering disorders. Retrieved from http://www.merckmanuals.com/home/kidney-and-urinary-tract-disorders/kidney-filtering-disorders/overview-of-kidney-filtering-disorders.

National Kidney Foundation. (2015). Glomerulonephritis. Retrieved from https://www.kidney.org/atoz/content/glomerul.

NEURODEGENERATIVE DISEASES

There are more than 600 types of neurodegenerative diseases, which affect the nerve cells of the brain, known as neurons. Examples of neurodegenerative diseases are Alzheimer's disease, Parkinson's disease, and Huntington's disease. Because they are associated with progressive degeneration of the neurons, they are irreversible diseases that cause very high rates of disability, especially among older adults. Both mental and physical function may be affected adversely, and these diseases are becoming more common as populations age.

Symptoms

Headaches, nausea, dizziness, loss of balance, tremors, and memory loss are common symptoms of neurodegenerative health conditions.

Causes and Risk Factors

Neurodegenerative disorders and neuronal damage may occur due to genetic factors or gene mutations, but they may also occur spontaneously. A defect in energy metabolism or increased damage to macromolecules due to oxidative factors may be additional causes. Many of the neurodegenerative diseases are associated with the aggregation and deposition of misfolded proteins or insoluble filaments of normally soluble proteins, and those conditions where this occurs are called *disease* due to brain amyloidosis.

Diagnostic Procedures

In addition to a careful clinical and physical examination, neuroimaging examination may be helpful at arriving at a definitive diagnosis. Biopsies, and possibly biochemical analyses, may be helpful. X-rays, myelograms, arteriograms, electroencephalograms, or lumbar puncture tests may also be helpful.

Treatments

Treatments for neurodegenerative health conditions are dependent on the health problem and its severity. Medications, antibiotics, physical therapy, and occupational therapy may be helpful, depending on the problem.

Prognosis

Most neurodegenerative health conditions have a poor prognosis and are very challenging for providers as well as families.

Prevention and Future

Early detection may increase the chances for a more favorable outcome. Scientists are seeking disease-modifying drugs. Research is predicted to accelerate in the next decade or beyond.

Ray Marks

See also: Alzheimer's Disease; Dementia; Parkinson's Disease

Further Reading

Beal, M. F. (1995). Aging, energy, and oxidative stress in neurodegenerative diseases. *Annals of Neurology, 38*, 357–366.

European Commission. (2015). Major and chronic diseases—Neurodegenerative diseases. Public Health. Retrieved from http://ec.europa.eu/health/major_chronic_diseases /diseases/brain_neurological/index_en.htm.

Halliwell, B. (2001). Role of free radicals in the neurodegenerative diseases. Therapeutic implications for antioxidant treatment. *Drugs and Aging, 18*, 685–716.

JPND Research. (2014). What is neurodegenerative disease? Retrieved from http://www .neurodegenerationresearch.eu/about/what/.

Perelman School of Medicine, University of Pennsylvania. (2013). Center for Neurodegenerative Disease Research. Retrieved from http://www.med.upenn.edu/cndr/.

Skovronsky, D. M., Lee, V. M-Y., & Trojanowski, J. Q. (2006). Neurodegenerative diseases: New concepts of pathogenesis and their therapeutic implications. *Annual Review of Pathological Mechanisms of Disease, 1*, 151–170.

University of California—San Francisco. (2013). Institute for Neurodegenerative Diseases. Retrieved from http://ind.ucsf.edu/.

Young, A. B. (2009). Four decades of neurodegenerative disease research: How far have we come? *The Journal of Neuroscience, 29*, 12722–12728.

NEUROFIBROMATOSIS

Neurofibromatosis is a neurological health condition that can affect many body parts, including the brain and spinal cord, as well as the skin or other parts of the body. It can cause noncancerous tumors to develop and grow, but fortunately, these often do not pose a large threat to those who are affected, most commonly children ages 3 to 16. The tumors that characterize neurofibromatosis grow along the nerves of the body or areas of skin and become problematic if they press on vital body parts or nerves.

Categories or Subtypes

There are two types of neurofibromatosis. These are termed neurofibromatosis types 1 and 2. Type 1 is more common and is said to affect approximately 100,000 Americans. It is also known as von Recklinghausen disease or bilateral acoustic neurofibromatosis.

Type 2 occurs more rarely and is associated with benign tumors on the nerves of the ear that can cause deafness and balance problems. It occurs less frequently that type 1, or in 1 of 40,000 births. It is also termed central or vestibular neurofibromatosis. Occurrences of either type are found in all races and affect both genders to the same degree.

The tumors originate from changes that occur in nerve and skin cells; as these grow, they press on important functional areas of the body. Children with this condition may experience developmental abnormalities as well as an increased risk of acquiring a learning disability. A third rare disease form of is schwannomatosis.

According to information posted at KidsHealth (2013), the severity of both neurofibromatosis types varies greatly, and when diagnosed, it is not possible to know right away whether a case will be mild or associated later on with complications.

Symptoms

Neurofibromatosis is characterized by the presence of flat, light brown spots on the skin, arms, or groin area. They may be very small and look like freckles. There may be soft bumps under the skin, on the iris of the eye, or on bones causing bone deformities. Only 3 to 5 percent of the brown flat spots will possibly become cancerous. The symptoms the person may experience may be very mild, but they may also be severe and affect hearing, learning ability, the heart and blood vessels, and the eyes, causing vision loss.

Children with type 1 neurofibromatosis may have larger than normal heads, but they may be shorter than the average child in height. Those with type 2 may have pain, numbness, and weakness in the arms and legs, eye problems, balance problems, and muscle wasting.

Causes and Risk Factors

The condition is genetic in origin. Having a family history of the condition is the most important risk factor.

Diagnostic Procedures

A physical examination, including an eye exam and ear exam, plus a medical history can help with the diagnosis of the condition. Imaging and genetic blood test may help as well.

Treatments

The tumors or fibromas can usually be removed surgically without any ill effect. Auditory brainstem implants or cochlear implants may help with hearing loss. If a tumor becomes malignant, it will be treated using standard cancer therapy approaches of radiation, chemotherapy, and surgery.

Prognosis

Doctors find it difficult to know in advance who will have problems with the tumors and who will not.

Prevention and Future

There is no cure for neurofibromatosis, but periodic and early evaluation is likely to help prevent complications or to minimize these. Research is under way to better understand the causes of the condition and how to diagnose and treat the condition.

Ray Marks

See also: Neoplasms; Neurological Diseases

Further Reading

KidsHealth. (2013). Neurofibromatosis. Retrieved from http://kidshealth.org/parent/general /aches/nf.html.

Janus, C., & Bhogal, P. (2014, Fall). Skin warriors. *Abilities,* 14–18.

Mayo Clinic. (2015). Neurofibromatosis. Retrieved from http://www.mayoclinic.com/health /neurofibromatosis/DS01185.

National Human Genome Research Institute. (2014). Learning about neurofibromatosis. Retrieved from http://www.genome.gov/14514225.

U.S. National Library of Medicine. National Institutes of Health. (2014). Neurofibromatosis. MedlinePlus. Retrieved from http://www.nlm.nih.gov/medlineplus/neurofibromatosis .html.

NEUROLOGICAL DISEASES

Neurological diseases are those that involve the brain and spinal cord and/or the nerves that are interconnected with these structures. These diseases include amyotrophic lateral sclerosis (ALS), Parkinson's disease, Huntington's disease, stroke, brain tumors, epilepsy, multiple sclerosis (MS), muscular dystrophy, spinal cord tumors, neuropathies, brain aneurysms, encephalitis, movement disorders, speech disorders, and various forms of dementia, among other diseases. These diseases and disorders are largely irreversible but may be manageable, or prevented from worsening, by early detection and intervention. They are major causes of disability, functional limitations, and huge direct and indirect medical and social costs.

Symptoms

Symptoms of a neurological disorder will vary depending on the site of the problem, as well as on its severity.

Some common symptoms are headaches, weakness, blackouts, tingling, numbness, loss of motor ability, tremors, problems with swallowing, confusion, pain, shuffling gait, paralysis, poor coordination, loss of balance, alterations of gait, or loss of memory.

Causes and Risk Factors

Causes of neurological disorders range from genetics to environmental factors, trauma, and high-risk behaviors. High blood pressure, obesity, heart disease, infections, and diabetes are additional risk factors.

Diagnostic Procedures

Diagnosis of neurological disorders may involve a clinical examination, MRI brain scans, lumbar puncture tests, physical function tests, sensory tests, and electrophysiological or nerve condition tests to examine if nerves are functioning adequately.

X-rays, blood test, physical examination, and biopsies are other methods of diagnosing the presence of a neurological problem.

Treatments

Treatment is often very challenging and will vary depending on the cause of the problem, as well as its severity. Assistive devices, various forms of physical therapy, and occupational therapy may be helpful. Neurosurgery, medications, or specialized neurological or electrophysiological treatments may be helpful.

Healthful eating, giving up smoking, monitoring one's blood pressure, and exercise may decrease the risk of stroke. Frequent screening for aneurysms may also be helpful.

Prevention and Future

Preventing exposure to harmful substances and avoiding trauma may be helpful in reducing the burden of neurological disorders. Researchers are working to understand the various neurological diseases, their risk factors, and what is needed to prevent and treat them.

Ray Marks

See also: ALS (Amyotrophic Lateral Sclerosis); Charcot-Marie-Tooth Disorder; Lyme Disease; Neurofibromatosis; Neuromuscular Disorders; Parkinson's Disease; Peripheral Nerve Disorders; Polio and Post-Polio Syndrome

Further Reading

Disabled World. (2008). List of neurological disorders. Retrieved from http://www.disabled
    -world.com/artman/publish/neurological-disorders-list.shtml.

Mollema, N. J., & Orr, H. T. (2013, November/December). One family's search to explain
    a fatal neurological disorder. *American Scientist, 101*(6), 442–449.

Neurological Institute. (2013). How to prevent neurological disease. Retrieved from http://
    www.neurologicalinstitute.com/educational_resources/e_prevent.html.

Public Agency of Canada. (2014). Neurological conditions. Retrieved from http://www.phac
    -aspc.gc.ca/cd-mc/nc-mn/index-eng.php.

Science Daily. (2013). Researchers work to prevent neurological diseases. Retrieved from
    http://www.sciencedaily.com/releases/2010/06/100624183013.htm.

UCSF Medical Center. (2013). Neurological disorders. Retrieved from http://www.ucsfhealth
    .org/conditions/neurological_disorders/.

NEUROMUSCULAR DISORDERS

Neuromuscular diseases are fairly rare diseases that affect the muscles and nerves of the limbs and trunk and the motor cells of the spinal cord. The problem can be located either in the muscle or the nerve supplying the muscle(s). Common conditions that fall under this category are amyotrophic lateral sclerosis (ALS), carpal tunnel syndrome, myasthenia gravis, peripheral neuropathy, muscular dystrophy, and motor neuron disease. Many are progressive, and some are fatal.

Symptoms

Common symptoms of the presence of neuromuscular disease are muscle weakness and wasting or atrophy. Other symptoms include numbness, tingling, muscle twitching, paralysis, cramps in the muscles, and low endurance with prolonged activity. Other problems may include double vision, muscle pain, spasticity, swallowing, and functional and breathing problems.

Causes and Risk Factors

Most common causes are genetic. Tumors, autoimmune diseases, and exposure to toxic substances are other causes.

Diagnostic Procedures

The varied diagnostic procedures include a physical and clinical examination of the neuromuscular system and general body strength.

Depending on the problem, tests may include genetic testing; laboratory blood, biochemical, or cerebrospinal fluid tests; radiographs; or scanning tests. Other tests include electrodiagnostic testing using nerve conduction tests to test if the nerves are able to transmit impulses effectively, tests to examine the state of the autonomic nervous system, muscle function tests, tests of sensation, and examination of tissue samples of muscles or nerves.

Treatments

Depending on the problem, those affected by a neuromuscular condition may require medications or drug therapy, Botox injections, medical interventions to improve life quality, surgery, specialized care, home health aides, assistive devices, nutritional support, and counseling. They may require help from allied health professionals such as nurses, physical therapists, respiratory therapists, and social workers.

Prognosis, Prevention, and Future

Prognosis depends on the condition and its extent and severity. Sometimes, neuromuscular disorders can be fatal or long standing.

No known prevention strategies exist.

Researchers at the Mayo Clinic are studying many aspects of neuromuscular disorders. These studies have made it easier to predict who is at risk genetically for neuromuscular disease and may help to prevent or minimize disability in the future.

Ray Marks

See also: ALS (Amyotrophic Lateral Sclerosis); Carpal Tunnel Syndrome; Cor Pulmonale; Genetics and Genomics; Myopathies; Neurological Diseases; Peripheral Nerve Disorders; Polio and Post-Polio Syndrome; Polymyositis

Further Reading

Mayo Clinic. (2015). Neuromuscular disease group. Retrieved from http://www.mayoclinic.org/neurology/neuromuscgroup.html.

Cooperative International Neuromuscular Research Group. (2016). Neuromuscular disorders. Retrieved from http://www.cinrgresearch.org/aboutnd/diseases.cfm.

University of Pittsburgh. Department of Neurology. (2012). What is neuromuscular disease? Retrieved from http://www.neurology.upmc.edu/neuromuscular/patient_info/what.html.

NEUROPATHY

Overview

Neuropathy is a general term that refers to diseases or dysfunction of the nerves in any region of the body. Neuropathies are commonly classified according to the types or location of nerves affected or according to the disease causing this problem

Types

There are four types of neuropathy:

- *Peripheral neuropathy,* where the nerve problem lies outside of the brain and spinal cord, can affect the nerves of the extremities—the toes, feet, legs, fingers, hands, and arms. The term *proximal neuropathy* refers to nerve damage causing pain in the thighs, hips, or buttock regions.

- *Cranial neuropathy* occurs when any of the 12 cranial nerves that exit from the brain directly are damaged. Two specific types of cranial neuropathy are optic neuropathy and auditory neuropathy. The optic nerve transmits visual signals from the retina of the eye to the brain, and the auditory nerve carries signals from the inner ear to the brain and enables one to hear.
- *Autonomic neuropathy* refers to damage of the nerves of the involuntary nervous system, such as those that control the heart and circulation, digestion, bowel and bladder function, the sexual response, and perspiration, as well as other organs.
- *Focal neuropathy* is a condition that is restricted to one nerve or group of nerves, or one area of the body.

Symptoms

Regardless of cause, neuropathy has some characteristic symptoms, although some may not have and symptoms. The degree to which an individual is affected by a particular neuropathy varies.

In peripheral neuropathy, symptoms often begin in the feet with a gradual onset of loss of feeling, numbness, tingling, or pain that can gradually progress toward the center of the body. The arms or legs may be involved, determining joint position may be challenging, and the person may appear uncoordinated and clumsy or fall frequently. Extreme sensitivity to touch can be another symptom of peripheral neuropathy.

When damage to the motor nerves occurs, symptoms include weakness, loss of reflexes and muscle mass, cramping, and/or loss of dexterity.

Autonomic neuropathy may cause a tingling or burning sensation or sharp, jabbing, or electric-like pain.

There may be skin, hair, or nail changes; heat intolerance; bowel, bladder, or digestive problems; and dizziness or light-headedness caused by changes in blood pressure. Other symptoms include:

- Nausea, vomiting, or abdominal bloating after meals
- Urinary symptoms, such as incontinence, difficulty beginning to urinate, or feeling that the bladder does not empty completely
- Impotence (erectile dysfunction) in men
- Dizziness or fainting, constipation or diarrhea, blurred vision, heat intolerance or decreased ability to sweat.

Causes and Risk Factors

Nerve damage may be caused by different diseases, injuries, infections, metabolic problems, exposure to toxins, exposure to certain drugs, or vitamin deficiency states.

Most cases of neuropathy are found in people who have the metabolic disorder diabetes; the problem here is then called *diabetic neuropathy*.

Other conditions can also lead to:

- Chronic liver or kidney disease
- HIV infection and AIDS

- Toxic substances and drug causes
- Long-term excessive alcohol intake
- Nutritional deficiencies
- Cancer (lymphoma or multiple myeloma)
- Lyme disease, a tick-borne bacterial infection
- Charcot-Marie-Tooth disease, a genetic cause of nerve damage, particularly in the lower limbs
- Guillain-Barré syndrome, a rare condition that damages peripheral nerves
- Diphtheria, a common bacterial infection in developing countries such as Haiti and Vietnam, but rare in other parts of the world (Medical News Today 2016).
- Amyloidosis
- Uremia-a high concentration of waste products in the blood due to kidney failure

Idiopathic neuropathy is neuropathy with no known cause.

Diagnostic Procedures

The exams and tests performed will depend on the patient's symptoms and medical history. A physical examination may be conducted to determine the cause and severity of neuropathy and may include testing the reflexes and function of sensory and motor nerves.

Blood tests and imaging studies such as x-rays, CT scans, and MRI scans may be performed to identify where and how nerves may be damaged.

Other tests of nerve function include:

- *Electromyography* measures the function of the nerves using a very thin needle inserted through the skin into the muscle to measure the electrical activity of the muscle.
- A *nerve conduction velocity test* measures the speed at which signals travel through the nerves; it is often used along with electromyography.
- In some cases, a *nerve biopsy* may be recommended where the surgical removal of a small piece of tissue is examined under a microscope.

Treatments

The treatment of neuropathy is aimed at reducing the cause of the problem and managing the symptoms and depends on the cause of the problem, the type of condition, and the length of time the condition has prevailed. Medical treatments of the underlying disease can reduce or eliminate the symptoms of neuropathy. In other cases, especially those involving compression or nerve entrapment by a tumor or other condition, surgery may be beneficial.

Prognosis

The outlook for nerve damage depends upon its cause. If the underlying medical condition or cause can be effectively treated with medicine or surgery and severe damage has not occurred, the prognosis can be excellent or very good. Nerves that have been affected by neuropathy can take time to recover, even when the underlying cause is appropriately treated. In other conditions, such as genetic conditions, there may be no effective treatment. Severe nerve damage from any cause is typically not reversible.

In sensory peripheral neuropathy, the loss of sensory input from the foot may cause blisters and sores on the feet to develop rapidly, and these may go unnoticed. Because there is a reduced sensation of pain, these sores may become infected, and the infection may spread to deeper tissues, including bone. In severe cases, amputation may be necessary.

Prevention

Neuropathy is preventable if the underlying condition or cause is preventable. For example, in those with diabetes, long-term control of blood glucose levels can help prevent or reduce any prevailing neuropathy and other diabetic complications. Neuropathy that arises due to poor nutrition or alcohol abuse may be preventable, as may those caused by toxins or excess medication usage. Genetic or inherited causes of neuropathy are not preventable.

Prognosis

The outcome of having a neuropathy depends on the cause and the early diagnosis of the condition. If it is caused by a genetic factor, the prognosis may be less favorable than if it is caused by a health issue that can be reduced or eliminated.

Future

Clinical trials are under way to help find new and more effective treatments for neuropathy. For example, treatments that involve electrical nerve stimulation or magnetic nerve stimulation are being studied.

Ray Marks

See also: Diabetes, Type 1; Diabetes, Type 2; Kidney Diseases; Kidney Failure; Peripheral Nerve Disorders

Further Reading

Foundation for Peripheral Neuropathy. (2016). Neuropathy. Retrieved from https://www.foundationforpn.org/.

Latov, N. (2007). *Peripheral Neuropathy: When the Numbness, Weakness, and Pain Won't Stop.* American Academy of Neurology (AAN) quality of life guides. Saint Paul, MN: AAN Press.

Medical News Today. (2016, March 18). Neuropathy: Causes, symptoms and treatments. Retrieved http://www.medicalnewstoday.com/articles/147963.php.

NON-HODGKIN LYMPHOMA

Non-Hodgkin lymphoma originates in the lymphatic system and refers to any group of cancers involving white blood cells. According to the National Cancer Institute (2016), there will be 71,850 new cases of non-Hodgkin lymphoma and about 19,790 deaths. It is more common than the general type of lymphoma, or Hodgkin disease. The main problem is that there are too many white blood cells in this disease, and they crowd into the lymph nodes and cause swelling of these nodes. The condition is more common in people over 60 years of age, but it can occur in younger people. It is the sixth most common cancer in the United States.

Subgroups or Types

There are different types of non-Hodgkin lymphoma: aggressive or fast-growing or indolent or low-grade slow-growing. According to the National Cancer Institute (2007), these can occur either with respect or T or B white blood cells. B-cells fight infection by producing antibodies that neutralize foreign invaders. Examples of B-cell non-Hodgkin lymphomas include Burkitt lymphoma, chronic lymphocytic leukemia/small lymphocytic lymphoma (CLL/SLL), and diffuse large B-cell lymphomas. Examples of T-cells involved in killing foreign invaders directly in T-cell non-Hodgkin lymphomas include mycosis fungicides, anaplastic large cell lymphoma, and precursor T-lymphoblastic lymphoma. Lymphomas that occur after bone marrow or stem cell transplantation are usually B-cell non-Hodgkin lymphomas.

Symptoms

The symptoms include abdominal pain, abdominal swelling, trouble breathing or coughing, chest pain, fever, fatigue, weight loss, and night sweats. The lymph glands may be swollen, but not necessarily painful; the skin may be itchy; and there may be bone and joint pain, recurring infections, a lack of energy, and red patches on the skin as well.

There are four non-Hodgkin lymphoma stages of severity based on how far the disease has spread:

Stage I (early disease): occurs in a single lymph node or one area external to the lymph node.

Stage II (locally advanced disease): occurs in two or more lymph node regions on one side of the diaphragm.

Stage III (advanced disease): involves lymph nodes both above and below the diaphragm.

Stage IV (widespread disease): occurs in several parts of one or more organs or tissues (in addition to the lymph nodes). Or, it is in the liver, blood, or bone marrow. (Lymphoma Research Foundation 2015)

Key Causes and Risk Factors

Medications that suppress the immune system may increase the risk of the condition according to the Mayo Clinic (2013). Other factors that may cause this condition are bacterial and viral infections, exposure to chemicals, and being of an older age. Others include having a family history of the condition or a recent organ transplant.

Diagnostic Procedures

The diagnostic procedures commonly include blood test, a medical history and physical examination, imaging tests, bone marrow samples being withdrawn with a needle for microscopic examination, excisional biopsies, or tissue removal from the lymph nodes that are examined microscopically.

Treatment

Treatment will depend on what type of lymphoma is present and what stage of development the cancer is categorized as, as well as the patient's age and general health status. Typical treatments include chemotherapy, radiation therapy, stem cell transplants, medications to boost the immune system, and medications that deliver radiation to the affected cells.

Prognosis

The outcome depends on the stage of the cancer. Some patients may relapse, and some may become resistant to the treatments.

Prevention and Future

There is no way to prevent non-Hodgkin's lymphoma, but researchers suggest that there may be a link between obesity and developing non-Hodgkin's lymphoma. Researchers are constantly developing new and improved approaches to curing the disease. Today, the percentage of people who are cured is about 70 percent or higher (Powell 2012).

Ray Marks

See also: Brain Cancer; Cancer Survivorship; Childhood Cancer; Hodgkin Disease; Leukemia; Lymphatic Disorders; Lymphoma

Further Reading

DeVita, V. T., Jr., & DeVita-Raeburn, E. (2015). *The Death of Cancer: After 50 Years on the Front Lines of Medicine, a Pioneering Oncologist Reveals Why the War on Cancer Is Winnable & How We Can Get There.* New York: Sarah Crichton Books/Farrar Straus and Giroux.

Lymphoma Research Foundation. (2004). *Understanding Non-Hodgkin's Lymphoma: A Guide for Patients.* Los Angeles, CA.

Lymphoma Research Foundation. (2015). Non-Hodgkin lymphoma. Retrieved from http://www.lymphoma.org/site/pp.asp?c=bkLTKaOQLmK8E&b=6300139.

Mayo Clinic. (2013). Non-Hodgkin lymphoma. Retrieved from http://www.mayoclinic.com/health/non-hodgkins-lymphoma/DS00350.

National Cancer Institute. (2007). What you need to know about non-Hodgkin lymphoma. Retrieved from http://www.cancer.gov/publications/patient-education/wyntk-non -hodgkin-lymphoma.

National Cancer Institute. (2016). SEER stat fact sheets: Non-Hodgkin lymphoma. Retrieved from http://seer.cancer.gov/statfacts/html/nhl.html.

Powell, J. L. (2012). Non-Hodgkin lymphoma. KidsHealth. Retrieved from http://kidshealth .org/teen/diseases_conditions/cancer/non_hodgkins.html.

0

OBESITY

Obesity is a complex and serious disorder that involves an excessive amount of body fat, which increases the risk of heart disease, high blood pressure, stroke, diabetes, gallstones, some types of cancer, osteoarthritis, sleep apnea and breathing problems, depression, anxiety, and pain and difficulty with physical movement. It is also associated with an increased risk of disability and premature death. It is caused by consuming more calories than are expended through exercise and normal daily activities, which the body stores the calories as fat. For adults 35 and older, obesity is categorized as having a BMI, or body mass index, of 30 or higher; BMI is calculated based on a healthy body weight for a specific height. Obesity affects millions of people in the United States, including children: Nearly 35 percent of adults (notably between 40 and 59 years old) and 17 percent of children and adolescents are obese, which is considered an epidemic. Difficult to treat, obesity can benefit from weight-loss programs and other interventions; losing 5 to 10 percent of total weight can prevent or delay associated health problems.

Symptoms

In addition to overt or obvious signs of weight gain and any weight-related health problems, obesity is diagnosed in adults with a BMI, or body mass index, that is 30 or higher. BMI describes body weight relative to height, and it is calculated by dividing weight in kilograms by height in meters squared. BMI for children and adolescents compares height and weight against growth charts that account for age and sex; called BMI-for-age percentile, it compares a BMI with others of the same age and sex.

Causes and Risk Factors

Obesity is caused when more calories are consumed from foods and beverages, including alcohol, than are expended through exercise and normal daily activities; the body then stores the excess calories as fat. A high-calorie diet that lacks adequate fruits and vegetables, fast food, high-calorie beverages, and oversized portions contribute to the risk of obesity.

Genetics and family history play a role in some people becoming obese; chances are greater if one or both of parents are overweight or obese. Genes may also determine the amount of fat a person stores and where on the body it is carried. One genetic cause of obesity is the deficiency of the hormone leptin, which is produced in fat cells and signals the brain to eat less when stores of body fat are too high. Obesity occurs when this hormone malfunctions and can't signal the brain. Other hormone disorders such as underactive thyroid, Cushing's syndrome, and polycystic ovarian syndrome may also cause obesity.

Behavior can influence body weight: Those who are physically inactive and eat high-calorie foods increase the chance of becoming obese, and children who adopt unhealthy habits of their parents also increase the risk of obesity. Other causes of obesity may include medications that slow the rate of calorie burning, increase appetite, or cause water retention; emotional eating; smoking; aging; lack of sleep; and pregnancy.

Diagnosis

In adults, obesity is diagnosed with a BMI, or body mass index, that is 30 or higher. BMI describes body weight relative to height, and it is calculated by dividing weight in kilograms by height in meters squared. BMI for children and adolescents compares height and weight against growth charts that account for age and sex; called BMI-for-age percentile, it compares a BMI with others of the same age and sex. A physician will also take a medical history; perform a physical exam; and may conduct tests for high blood pressure, diabetes, cholesterol levels, and thyroid and liver function. Measuring waist circumference helps screen for health risks associated with obesity in adults. People who carry too much fat around the middle are more likely to experience coronary heart disease and Type 2 diabetes. For women, the risk increases with a waist size of 35 inches or greater and for men, 40 inches or more.

Treatments

The goal of obesity treatment is reaching and maintaining a healthier weight; a modest weight loss of 5 to 10 percent along with long-term maintenance of that weight loss results in significant health benefits. Other treatments include reducing calories and practicing healthier eating habits, increasing physical activity or exercise, and behavior modification to help make permanent lifestyle changes. Medication may be prescribed for those who have obesity-related health problems that increase their risk of developing heart disease. Weight-loss surgery may be an option for those with extreme obesity (BMI of 40 or higher) and for whom other strategies have not been successful.

Prevention

The steps to preventing weight gain are the same as those to losing weight: choosing a lifestyle that includes a healthful diet that includes low-calorie, nutrient-dense foods and balances the number of calories consumed with the number of calories expended; daily physical activity and exercise; regularly monitoring weight; getting adequate sleep; and a lifelong commitment to adopting healthy habits.

Prognosis and Outcomes

Reaching and staying at a healthy weight is a long term, but with appropriate treatment, motivation, and support, those with obesity can lose weight and lower their long-term risk of many other serious and chronic diseases. In the United States, more than 100,000 deaths are directly related to obesity each year; most in people with a BMI over 30. Those who have a BMI that is over 40 face a significantly reduced life expectancy.

Ray Marks

See also: Cardiovascular Disease; Cholesterol; Diabetes, Type 1; Diabetes, Type 2; Diet and Nutrition; Food Guides from the USDA; Heart Diseases; Obesity, Morbid; Prediabetes; Stroke

Further Reading

Centers for Disease Control and Prevention (CDC). (2013). Overweight and obesity. Retrieved from http://www.cdc.gov/obesity/.

Centers for Disease Control and Prevention (CDC). (2015). Prevention strategies & guidelines. Retrieved from http://www.cdc.gov/obesity/resources/strategies-guidelines.html.

Goldman, L. (2015). *Too Much of a Good Thing: How Four Key Survival Traits Are Now Killing Us.* New York, NY: Little, Brown and Company.

Lustig, R. H. (2013). *Fat Chance: Beating the Odds against Sugar, Processed Food, Obesity, and Disease.* New York, NY: Hudson Street Press.

Mayo Clinic. (2015, June 10). Obesity. Retrieved from http://www.mayoclinic.org/diseases-conditions/obesity/basics/definition/con-20014834.

National Heart, Lung, and Blood Institute. (2012, July 13). What are overweight and obesity? Retrieved from http://www.nhlbi.nih.gov/health/health-topics/topics/obe.

National Institute of Diabetes and Digestive and Kidney Diseases. (2012, December). Understanding adult overweight and obesity. Retrieved from http://www.niddk.nih.gov/health-information/health-topics/weight-control/understanding/Pages/understanding-adult-overweight-and-obesity.aspx.

Power, M. L., & Schulki, J. (2009). *The Evolution of Obesity.* Baltimore: Johns Hopkins University Press.

Taubes, G. (2011). *Why We Get Fat and What to Do about It.* New York, NY: Alfred A. Knopf.

World Health Organization (WHO). (2013). Obesity. Retrieved from http://www.who.int/topics/obesity/en/.

OBESITY, MORBID

Obesity is classified based on one's body mass index (BMI), which is the mathematical relationship between one's weight and height. Obesity refers to having excess body fat and has been associated with a variety of medical concerns, including diabetes and coronary heart disease. The names used to denote the highest BMIs include morbid obesity, class III obesity, and extreme obesity. The BMI for obesity begins at 30; morbid obesity refers to those with a BMI of 40 or more or those who have a BMI of at least 35 and who are also diagnosed with what are considered to be obesity-related health conditions, such as high blood pressure and diabetes.

According to the National Institute of Diabetes and Digestive and Kidney Diseases, based on data gathered in a survey conducted in 2009–2010, just over 6 percent of adults 20 years or older have a BMI of 40 or higher. There are twice as many women as men in this group. Overweight and obesity are also measured in children based on BMI; however, classification of overweight or obesity is based on percentile. A child with a BMI at the 85th percentile or higher is overweight, while a child with a BMI at the 95th percentile or higher is considered to be obese. Further classification of obesity is not made in children.

Obesity has been scientifically linked to a variety of diseases, including diseases of the cardiovascular system, diabetes, sleep apnea, some types of cancer, asthma, and osteoarthritis. The most serious health concerns are more strongly connected with morbid obesity and can lead to an earlier death. Thus, although some research has indicated that those who are moderately obese are at greater risk for these diseases in comparison to those who are overweight, those who are morbidly obese have been found to live shorter lives by an average of 8 to 10 years. Due to the concern for the overall health and longevity of those identified as morbidly obese, the recommendation is usually that they need to lose weight. For some, this may mean weight loss surgery.

Critics of the focus placed on weight point to the fact that a causal link between obesity and these diseases has not been found; rather, obesity is correlated to (co-occurs with) these conditions but may not be the root cause. While this may be the case, there is clear evidence that those who are classified as morbidly obese have a much greater chance of suffering from these conditions than those at a lower BMI.

Christine L. B. Selby

See also: Cardiovascular Disease; Diabetes, Type 2; Obesity; Sleep Disturbances and Sleep Disorders

Further Reading

Baesser, G. A., & Blair, S. N. (2002). *Big Fat Lies: The Truth about Your Weight and Your Health.* Carlsbad, CA: Gürze Books.

Brethauer, S., Kashyap, S., & Schauer, P. (2013, March). Obesity. Cleveland Clinic: Disease Management. Retrieved from http://www.clevelandclinicmeded.com/medicalpubs /diseasemanagement/endocrinology/obesity/.

Haslam, D. W., & James, P. T. (October 2005). Obesity. *Lancet, 366*(9492), 1197–1209.

Lustig, R. H. (2012). *Fat Chance: Beating the Odds Against Sugar, Processed Food, Obesity, and Disease.* New York: Hudson Street Press.

Naheed, A. (2012). *The Obesity Reality: A Comprehensive Approach to a Growing Problem.* Baltimore, MD: Rowman & Littlefield.

National Institute of Diabetes and Digestive and Kidney Diseases. (2012). Overweight and obesity statistics. Retrieved from http://www.niddk.nih.gov/health-information/health -statistics/Pages/overweight-obesity-statistics.aspx.

O'Connell, J. (2011). *Sugar Nation: The Hidden Truth Behind America's Deadliest Habit and the Simple Way to Beat It.* New York: Hachette.

Sugerman, H. J., & Nguyen, N. (2005). *Management of Morbid Obesity.* Boca Raton, FL: CRC Press.

University of Pittsburgh Medical Center. (2016). Morbid obesity-related health concerns. Retrieved from http://www.upmc.com/Services/bariatrics/candidate/Pages/obesity-con cerns.aspx.

OBSESSIVE COMPULSIVE DISORDER

Obsessive compulsive disorder (OCD) is a chronic disorder of the brain and behavior that causes severe anxiety. Formerly classified as an anxiety disorder, it is now considered a unique disorder characterized by obsessions, or unwanted and intrusive thoughts, that often compel people toward compulsions, or repeated ritualistic behaviors and routines performed in an attempt to ease anxiety. OCD usually starts during childhood or the teen years, and most people receive a diagnosis by age 19. About 2.2 million adults of all races and socioeconomic backgrounds in the United States are affected, both men and women equally; about one-third of adults experience symptoms during childhood.

Symptoms

The symptoms of this disorder are the obsessions and compulsions, which may vary or come and go. Most people are aware that their obsessions and compulsions are irrational, but they cannot stop them. Some spend hours performing complicated rituals such as hand-washing, counting, or checking to ward off persistent, unwelcome thoughts, feelings, or images.

Common obsessions, or unwanted intrusive thoughts, include constant worry about dirt, germs, or contamination; excessive concern with order, arrangement, or symmetry; fear that negative or blasphemous thoughts or impulses will cause personal harm or harm to a loved one; excessive concern about accidentally or purposefully injuring another person; and distasteful religious and sexual thoughts or images.

Common compulsions, or ritualistic behaviors to ease anxiety, include repeated hand-washing, bathing, or cleaning household items, often for hours at a time; checking and rechecking several to hundreds of times a day that, for example, doors are locked, the stove is turned off, the hairdryer is unplugged; the inability to stop repeating a name, phrase, or simple activity (such as going through a doorway over and over again); touching and arranging. These behaviors also include mental rituals such as endlessly reviewing conversations or counting, repetitively calling up "good" thoughts to neutralize "bad" thoughts, or excessive praying and saying special words or phrases to neutralize obsessions.

Causes and Risk Factors

A combination of biological and environmental factors are thought to contribute to the cause of OCD. Having a family member with OCD increases the risk, but it is not known why some people have the disorder while others do not. Some research shows that OCD comes from problems in the brain pathways that link areas involved with judgment and planning with the area that involves body movements. Other causes may include an infection caused by the streptococcus bacteria or environmental factors, which can trigger or worsen OCD in those at high risk, including abuse, illness, excessive stress caused by changes in relationships, school, work, or living conditions.

Diagnosis

A clinician or other therapist trained in treating OCD makes a diagnosis based on a person having obsessions or compulsive behaviors or both, as well as the amount of time the obsessions and compulsions take and how much they interfere with daily functioning.

Treatments

OCD can be effectively treated with psychotherapy (talk therapy), medication, or both. Cognitive-behavioral therapy, or CBT, teaches people how to change their thinking, behaving, and reacting to situations to lessen anxiety without having obsessive thoughts or acting compulsively. For OCD specifically, a type of CBT called exposure and response prevention (ERP) is very effective as a person who is gradually exposed to a feared situation or object becomes less sensitive to it over time.

Anti-anxiety medications and antidepressants may be prescribed along with therapy. For OCD that does not respond to other treatments, the relatively new technique of deep brain stimulation (DBS) has been shown to relieve symptoms in some people.

Prognosis and Outcomes

Untreated, OCD can interfere with all aspects of life, including daily routines, school and work, jobs, family, and social activities. But most people who receive treatment see significant improvement and enjoy an improved quality of life. In most cases, OCD can be treated successfully with cognitive-behavioral therapy, medication, or both, providing lasting relief from symptoms and a return to normal or near-normal functioning.

Future

Many research studies are under way to uncover the causes of OCD, such as using brain imaging to look for biomarkers, as well as to identify new ways to treat the disorder using medications, therapies, and novel treatments.

Ray Marks

See also: Anxiety Disorders; Neurological Diseases

Further Reading

Anxiety and Depression Association of America. (2016). Obsessive-compulsive disorder (OCD). Retrieved from http://www.adaa.org/understanding-anxiety/obsessive-comp ulsive-disorder-ocd.

International OCD Foundation. (2015). What is OCD? Retrieved from https://iocdf.org /about-ocd/.

Mayo Clinic. (2013, August 9). Obsessive-compulsive disorder (OCD). Retrieved from http://www.mayoclinic.org/diseases-conditions/ocd/basics/definition/con-20027827.

McGrath, P. (2008). *The OCD Answer Book.* Naperville, IL: Sourcebooks.

National Institutes of Mental Health. (2015). Obsessive-compulsive disorder, OCD. Retrieved from http://www.nimh.nih.gov/health/topics/obsessive-compulsive-disorder -ocd/index.shtml.

OCCUPATIONAL HEALTH

Occupational health is a professional field concerned with the health and safety of people in the workplace. It is a broad and diverse field incorporating several different types of occupations, ranging from scientists, technicians, and physicians to government inspectors and regulators. The primary goal in occupational health is to eliminate or reduce workplace conditions that cause health or safety problems (including cancer) and chronic diseases (such as respiratory illnesses, circulatory diseases, musculoskeletal disorders, hearing loss, and stress-related disorders) in addition to infectious diseases, accidents, and deaths.

Every year, thousands of people in the United States are killed while at work as a result of preventable accidents or illnesses. According to the Occupational Safety and Health Administration (OSHA), an agency of the U.S. Department of Labor, 4,585 workers were killed on the job in 2013 in the United States. That is the equivalent of 12 deaths every day—a seemingly large amount, but actually the second lowest total since such statistics began to be recorded. By comparison, an average of 38 workers died every day in 1970.

OSHA reported that injuries involving construction activities accounted for about 20 percent of all fatal work injuries in private industry in 2013. Of the more than 800 construction deaths, about 37 percent were caused by falls, 10 percent by being struck by objects, 9 percent by electrocutions, and 3 percent by being caught in or between objects.

Types of Hazards

Potential health-related problems vary depending on the type of workplace. Although statistics suggest that construction sites are the most dangerous worksites because of the risk of serious injuries, all places of work—including factories, offices, laboratories, clinics, farms, and even houses—have certain possible hazards.

Physical hazards, such as those at construction sites, include loud noises as well as injuries from equipment and falls. These types of hazards are also common in factories and on farms. Other physical hazards are ergonomic in nature, ranging from repetitive strain injuries caused by frequent computer keyboard use to back problems caused by frequent lifting of heavy objects.

Examples of biological hazards include infectious diseases that can be spread from patients to health care workers in clinics and hospitals, as well as illnesses spread by contaminated equipment in laboratories. Chemical hazards include such toxic substances as certain chemicals used in research labs; industrial compounds used in factories; and indoor pollutants emanating from ventilation systems, copying equipment, wall and floor coverings, and other materials in offices.

Electrical hazards, which might be present anywhere, include frayed electrical cords that carry the risk of fire and accidents causing electrocution. Other fire and explosion risks are present in the compressed tanks of oxygen and other gases used in many laboratories, factories, and health care centers.

Psychosocial hazards include a variety of psychological factors, such as stress from too many responsibilities, tiredness during late shifts, and fear of violence from coworkers in hostile work environments. These hazards are among the most important, though also among the more difficult, ones to address because they tend to lead to progressively worsening health, along with high absentee rates, reduced productivity, "burnout," and early retirement.

In 2014, OSHA ranked the top 10 most frequently cited workplace hazards and problems as the following:

1. Inadequate fall protection in construction
2. Inadequate communication of hazard risks in general industry
3. Poorly made scaffolding in construction
4. Inadequate respiratory protection against particles or gases
5. Hazards related to industrial trucks
6. Lack of control of hazardous energy sources, such as electrical, mechanical, hydraulic, pneumatic, chemical, and thermal sources
7. Ladder hazards in construction
8. Problems with electrical wiring, components, or equipment in general industry
9. Hazards with machines and inadequate machine guarding
10. Problems with electrical systems design in general industry

According to rankings by the World Health Organization (WHO), occupational hazards cause 37 percent of all cases of back pain worldwide, 16 percent of hearing loss cases, 13 percent of chronic obstructive pulmonary disease, 11 percent of asthma, 9 percent of lung cancer, 8 percent of injuries, 8 percent of depression, and 2 percent of leukemia.

OSHA Responsibilities

OSHA has the primary responsibility of ensuring that working conditions in the United States are safe and healthful. The federal agency meets these responsibilities through the development and enforcement of regulations over employers covering everything from the design of hand railings and stairways to the prevention of fire and explosions to the use of protective eyewear and other clothing. OSHA also establishes the maximum exposure levels that are legally allowed for all sorts of workplace hazards, including noise from machinery, toxins in industrial chemical compounds, and various forms of indoor air pollution.

To enforce its regulations, OSHA has a team of about 2,200 inspectors or compliance officers—amounting to roughly one officer for every 59,000 workers. These inspectors are charged with checking the more than 8 million workplaces around the country for violations of OSHA regulations and standards. Employers must correct all violations found by the inspectors or risk being charged large fines or being temporarily or permanently shut down.

In addition to the federal OSHA agency, states have their own departments of occupational health to partner with OSHA in the enforcement of health and safety standards. Between 1970 and 2015, the efforts of OSHA and its state partners reduced both worker fatality rates and injury/illness rates by about 66 percent.

WHO Global Plan of Action

WHO has implemented a Global Plan of Action on Workers' Health to improve the diagnosis, reporting, and management of work-related health problems in countries around the world. The plan is meant to address the fact that workers in many poor nations have little or no access to occupational health services. Only about one-third of nations have programs to address occupational diseases, and more than half the workforce in many countries is employed informally with no forms of social protection against health problems caused by work.

Specific WHO activities in its Plan of Action include making estimates of the prevalence of work-related health problems according to cause, such as accidents, carcinogenic substances, ergonomic issues, and noise. The plan is also designed to advise companies about ways to improve occupational conditions and to help physicians and other health care workers successfully detect, diagnose, and treat occupational health problems.

A. J. Smuskiewicz

See also: Asthma; COPD (Chronic Obstructive Pulmonary Disease); Lung Cancer; Occupational Cancer; Secondhand Smoke

Further Reading

Occupational Safety & Health Administration. (2015). Commonly used statistics. Retrieved from https://www.osha.gov/oshstats/commonstats.html.

Occupational Safety & Health Administration. (2016). Retrieved from http://www.osha.gov.

U.S. Environmental Protection Agency. (2016). An introduction to indoor air quality. Retrieved from http://www.epa.gov/indoor-air-quality-iaq/introduction-indoor-air-quality.

World Health Organization. (2015). Health topics: Occupational health. Retrieved from http://www.who.int/topics/occupational_health/en/.

World Health Organization. (2014, April). Protecting workers' health. Retrieved from http://www.who.int/mediacentre/factsheets/fs389/en/.

ORAL CANCER

As with any cancer, oral cancer is associated with the abnormal growth of cells in the mouth or throat area. That is, oral cancer is associated with an uncontrollable growth of cells from the inside of the mouth, but it can occur anywhere in the areas of the lips, cheeks, tongue, floor of the mouth—the most common area—sinuses, hard and soft palette or tonsil areas, and the throat. Current estimates are that about 37,000 new cases of oral cancer are diagnosed every year. If this type of cancer is not diagnosed early, it may prove fatal. It is also called *mouth cancer* or *oral cavity cancer*.

Symptoms

Among the many symptoms of oral cancer are jaw pain, tongue pain, loose teeth, difficult or painful chewing or swallowing, sore throat, unexplained mouth bleeding, white or reddish patches on the inside of the mouth, unexplained numbness or pain in the facial or mouth area, ear pain, dramatic weight loss, or some form of lump or thickening in the mouth or throat area.

Key Causes and Risk Factors

While anyone can develop oral cancer, most commonly males over age 40—especially African American males with a smoking history—or those with an excessive alcohol-, snuff-, or chewing tobacco-related usage history are susceptible to this condition. Another risk factor is exposure to the HPV sexually transmitted virus. There is also the possibility that the mouth area will be more susceptible to cancer if the brain or related areas of the face and mouth are already cancerous. Having a family history of oral cancer may also increase the risk, as may excessive exposure of the lips to sunlight.

Diagnostic Procedures

The diagnostic approaches include a physical examination and a medical history. Some form of tissue biopsy procedure may follow to search for cancerous cells in the laboratory. A test known as endoscopy, where the doctor examines the throat with a lighted scope, may be conducted as well. Other tests include imaging tests such as computerized tomography, positron emission tomography, and magnetic resonance imaging.

Treatment

The treatment for oral cancer will depend on the site of the problem and the stage of the disease and may involve surgery, radiation therapy, chemotherapy, or targeted drug therapy.

Prognosis

There is a high survival rate of about 80 percent if the cancer problem is detected early on.

Prevention

Avoiding excess tobacco usage, as well as excess alcohol usage is recommended. Learning about safe sexual practices may also be helpful as may reduce exposure of the mouth area to excess sunlight.

Seeing a dentist regularly and knowing the signs of oral cancer are also indicated.

Future

In the future, a simple saliva test might be used for early detection of oral cancer, given that certain protein biomarkers are found to be present in the saliva of most people with oral cancer.

Ray Marks

See also: Cancer; HPV (Human Papillomavirus); Sexually Transmitted Diseases; Tobacco Addiction

Further Reading

Crosby, R. A., DiClemente, R. J., Salazar, L. F., Nash, R., Younge, S., & Head, S. (2012, January). Vaccine intention among college men: What's oral sex got to do with it? *Journal of American College Health, 60*(1), 8–12.

Mayo Clinic. (2015). Mouth cancer. Retrieved from http://www.mayoclinic.org/diseases-conditions/mouth-cancer/home/ovc-20157214.

MedlinePlus. (2014). Oral cancer. Retrieved from http://www.nlm.nih.gov/medlineplus/oralcancer.html.

National Cancer Institute. (2013). Oral cancer. http://www.cancer.gov/cancertopics/types/oral.

Oral Cancer Foundation. (2016). Retrieved from http://oralcancerfoundation.org/.

Research Portfolio Online Reporting Tools (RePORT). (2013, March 29). Oral cancer. Retrieved from https://report.nih.gov/nihfactsheets/ViewFactSheet.aspx?csid=106.

ORAL HEALTH

Overview

Oral health refers to the mouth, teeth, and gums, and it is linked closely to the body's general health. The mouth is filled with bacteria, although most of them are not harmful and can be controlled with daily tooth brushing and flossing, as well as a healthy body's natural defenses. If not, the bacteria can cause tooth decay and gum disease, including severe gum disease called periodontitis.

A common chronic childhood illness is tooth cavities, which can negatively affect school, social relationships, and success as an adult. Toothaches are very common among adults, and the pain can affect eating, swallowing, and talking. Many adults have some evidence of gum disease, or gingivitis, and some experience severe disease, called periodontitis, which in an advanced state is responsible for bleeding gums, painful chewing, and eventual tooth loss; smoking is its most significant risk factor.

Those with diabetes, HIV/AIDS, and weakened immune systems have an increased risk for tooth and gum infections. The following illnesses may contribute to oral health problems, or they may be part of the cause: gastroesophageal reflux disease (GERD), osteoporosis, Alzheimer's disease, Parkinson's disease, eating disorders, and Sjögren's syndrome, a disease that causes dry mouth. Patients undergoing chemotherapy often experience mouth ulcers, dry mouth, and an impaired sense of taste. Some people taking steroids also are at higher risk of oral health problems; decongestants, antihistamines, painkillers, and diuretics—medications that reduce the flow of saliva—may also contribute to bacterial growth and possible disease.

Chronic facial pain (called TMJ for temporomandibular joint) refers to disorders of the temporomandibular joint and muscles that cause pain and dysfunction. These are characterized by jaw tenderness or popping, as well as headaches and neck aches, which is caused by teeth grinding (bruxism) or jaw clenching; these can also increase the risk for gum disease, tooth erosion, and cracked teeth.

Because the mouth affects the body's overall health, poor oral health may lead to heart disease, including endocarditis, a serious infection; respiratory diseases, including pneumonia; and pregnancy complications, including delivery of premature babies. A history of periodontal disease has also been associated with an increased risk of pancreatic cancer.

History

Since fluoride was added to public water systems in the United States in the 1960s, the oral health of most Americans has improved. Scientific studies show that it prevents tooth decay by up to 40 percent. Dental sealants protect the chewing surfaces of molars from decay. Sealant programs in schools, focused on treating children in low-income families, have been successful in preventing tooth decay in up to 60 percent of tooth decay in the treated teeth.

Treatments

In addition to identifying cavities and other oral health problems, a dentist conducting a routine check-up can see signs of disorders associated with poor hygiene and nutrition, jaw problems, and other overall health issues. For example, worn tooth enamel may indicate stress due to bruxism, or tooth-grinding; receding or swollen gums may suggest diabetes; long-lasting mouth sores that aren't healing may signal oral cancer; and moderate or severe gum disease may show an increased risk for heart and vascular diseases. People with these symptoms should be referred to the appropriate specialist for further treatment.

Prevention

Maintaining good oral health can contribute to keeping the rest of body in overall good health. Regular dental check-ups, including prophylaxis (or professional teeth cleaning), help detect serious oral and other health problems. Daily, thorough tooth brushing with a fluoride toothpaste and flossing help prevent mild gum disease by reducing plaque. Other precautions are drinking fluoridated water; avoiding tobacco in all forms; limiting alcohol; and eating a healthful diet, especially avoiding sugar- and starch-filled foods. Dry mouth caused by medications may respond to different medications; if not, drinking water and other activities to stimulate saliva production can help symptoms. Controlling blood sugar in diabetes helps prevent the development of gum disease. For those beginning treatment for cancer, an oral health check-up and appropriate remedies may forestall further complications.

Ray Marks

See also: Alzheimer's Disease; Bruxism; Diabetes; Eating Disorders; Gastroesophageal Reflux Disease (GERD); Heart Diseases; Oral Cancer; Sjögren's Syndrome

Further Reading

Centers for Disease Control and Prevention. (2013, July 10). Adult oral health. Retrieved from http://www.cdc.gov/oralhealth/publications/factsheets/adult_oral_health/adults.htm.
Everyday Health. (2015). Dental health and overall health. Retrieved from http://www.everydayhealth.com/dental-health/101.aspx.
HealthyPeople.gov (2014). Oral health. Retrieved from http://www.healthypeople.gov/2020/topics-objectives/topic/oral-health.
Mayo Clinic. (2013, May 11). Oral health: A window to your overall health. Retrieved from http://www.mayoclinic.org/healthy-lifestyle/adult-health/in-depth/dental/art-20047475.
National Institute of Dental and Craniofacial Research. (2014, February 26). Oral health diseases and conditions. Retrieved from http://www.nidcr.nih.gov/oralhealth/OralHealth Information/DiseasesandConditions/.

ORAL PHARYNGEAL DISORDERS

Oral pharyngeal disorders are disorders of the mouth and the back of the throat and upper part of the esophagus. They include sore throat, strep throat and gastric reflux disorders, tonsillitis, pharyngitis, swallowing disorders, and oral cancers. Nasopharyngeal cancer is common in Asian populations.

Signs and Symptoms

Signs and symptoms of a problem in this area of the body may include fever, redness in the mouth, bleeding, inflammation, mouth ulcers, difficulty swallowing, mouth sores, pharyngitis, pain, and lumps in the oral cavity. Postnasal drainage, cough and sore throat, painful swallowing, nasal obstruction, and lymph node swelling in the neck region may be additional symptoms.

Causes and Risk Factors

Viral or bacterial infections are common causes of throat-related disorders. Neurological and systemic conditions such as scleroderma, diabetes, and rheumatoid arthritis are also common causes. Cancers may be caused by excess tobacco use.

Diagnostic Procedures

A diagnosis may involve a clinical evaluation, radiographic tests, blood tests, as well as biopsy examinations. In cases where there is a neuromuscular disease, the physician might assess oral, pharyngeal, and esophageal motor function.

Treatment and Prognosis

Treatment depends on the cause and may include antibiotics and analgesics. The underlying condition may need to receive treatment as well. Other remedies may include rest, antihistamines, gargling, attention to oral hygiene, and, in some cases, surgery. Swallowing problems or throat problems related to neurological problems may require a respiratory therapist, nursing assistance, and physical therapy. Prognosis may depend on the cause, as well as on early treatment.

Ray Marks

See also: Gastroesophageal Reflux Disease (GERD); Oral Cancer; Oral Health; Swallowing Disorders; Throat Cancer; Throat Disorders

Further Reading

American Academy of Pediatrics. (2015). When a sore throat is a more serious infection. Retrieved from https://www.healthychildren.org/English/health-issues/conditions/ear-nose-throat/pages/When-a-Sore-Thoat-is-a-More-Serious-Infection.aspx.

MedlinePlus. (2015). Throat disorders. Retrieved from https://www.nlm.nih.gov/medlineplus/throatdisorders.html.

Wise, J. L., & Murray, J. A. (2006). Oral, pharyngeal and esophageal motility disorders in systemic diseases. *G.I. Motility Online*. doi:10.1038/gimo40.

OSTEOARTHRITIS

Osteoarthritis is a common degenerative joint disease associated with aging. Involving the breakdown of key joint structures such as the articular cartilage lining of the joint and the underlying bone, the condition is very painful and disabling. Among the most commonly affected joints are the hands, hips, knees, and spinal joints. People of all ages can have osteoarthritis, although the most common finding is that the condition occurs more in older adults than in younger adults. Women are generally diagnosed more often than men with the condition. It is different from rheumatoid arthritis, which is an autoimmune disease in which the immune system attacks healthy cells, often the membrane around the joints, called the *synovium*. In some cases, rheumatoid arthritis can lead to problems with the lung and heart, unlike osteoarthritis.

Symptoms

Key symptoms of osteoarthritis are pain; stiffness; tenderness; and loss of flexibility, mobility, balance, and dexterity.

Key Causes and Risk Factors

The causes of osteoarthritis remain unknown, although age is thought to be an important risk factor. Other factors thought to lead to osteoarthritis are trauma, joint malalignment, obesity, heredity, muscle weakness, and inflammatory conditions of the joint. Other possible risk factors are estrogen deficiency and deficits in vitamins C, E, and D. Certain occupations that involve repetitive stress and other diseases such as diabetes may predispose an individual to osteoarthritis.

Diagnostic Procedures

Osteoarthritis is usually diagnosed with x-rays following a clinical and medical examination. Other tests may involve blood tests to rule out other diseases, joint aspiration and serum joint fluid tests, and ultrasound or MRI scans.

Treatment

Treatments may involve nonoperative strategies, operative strategies, or both. Heat, cold, and exercise are examples of nonoperative treatments. Joint replacement surgery is an example of the most common surgical procedure. Medication, weight control, joint injections, alternative medicines, supplements, joint protection, assistive devices, physical therapy, shoe inserts, braces, rest, massage, lubrication or hyaluronic injections, and acupuncture are other forms of treatment or interventions designed to promote function and decrease pain that are commonly applied.

Prognosis

Osteoarthritis is a progressive disease, but it is not usually life-threatening, It can be managed successfully using a combination of nonsurgical and surgical approaches.

Prevention

There is no known preventive intervention against osteoarthritis, although maintaining a healthy weight and avoiding trauma might be helpful.

Future

Scientists are examining if stem cells can be used to promote joint repair of the damaged joint. They are also searching for biomarkers of osteoarthritis.

Ray Marks

See also: Arthritis; Inflammation; Musculoskeletal Disorders; Paget's Disease of the Bone; Rheumatoid Arthritis

Further Reading

Arthritis Foundation. (2013). Osteoarthritis. Retrieved from http://www.arthritis.org /conditions-treatments/disease-center/osteoarthritis/.

Centers for Disease Control and Prevention. (2015). Osteoarthritis. Retrieved from www .cdc.gov/arthritis/basics/osteoarthritis.htm.

Chang-Miller, A. (2013). *Mayo Clinic on Arthritis*. Rochester, MN: Mayo Clinic.

Healthy Women. (2013). Osteoarthritis. Retrieved from http://www.healthywomen.org /condition/osteoarthritis.

Levine, H. (2015, November). Your joints: A user's manual. *Health, 29*(9), 99–104.

Lorig, K., & Fries, J. F. *The Arthritis Helpbook: A Tested Self-Management Program for Coping with Arthritis and Fibromyalgia*, 6th ed. New York: Da Capo Press.

Mayo Clinic. (2013). Osteoarthritis. Retrieved from http://www.mayoclinic.com/health /osteoarthritis/DS00019.

National Institute of Arthritis and Musculoskeletal and Skin Diseases (NIAMS). (2015). Osteoarthritis. Retrieved from http://www.niams.nih.gov/Health_Info/Osteoarthritis/.

Osteoarthritis: Symptoms and treatment. (2006, March). *Harvard Men's Health Watch, 10*(8), 3–6.

OSTEOMYELITIS

Osteomyelitis, which is a disorder of bone infections, can be caused by a fracture that pierces the skin or other open bone injury or wound; an infection from the lung, bladder, or elsewhere in the body that is spread by the blood or from nearby skin or muscles; and minor trauma and secondary infection.

It is an uncommon condition, occurring in about 2 of every 10,000 people, but it can affect male and female infants, children, and adults of all races. In children, bone infections occur predominantly in the adjacent ends of long bones. In adults, these infections tend to occur in the spine or pelvis.

If a bone infection is left untreated, it can diminish the blood supply to the bone, which can eventually die. This can lead to permanent deformity, possible fracture, and other chronic problems, especially if the bone marrow swells and presses against the bone's blood vessels. The severity can range from mild to severe.

Symptoms

Bone infections may not present obvious symptoms, or they may be similar to other conditions. The symptoms most commonly include pain, redness, or tenderness, as well as swelling and warmth in the infected area; a change in the gait, or walking pattern, when the legs are affected; fever, lethargy, nausea, and a general feeling of illness or discomfort; and oozing or drainage of pus through the skin.

Causes

People with diabetes, weakened immune systems, poor circulation, sickle cell disease, and HIV (human immunodeficiency virus) are at risk for bone infections. Also at risk are older adults, intravenous drug users, those undergoing kidney dialysis or orthopedic repair surgery, and people who have had recent bone injuries.

Diagnosis

Bone infections are first diagnosed with a physical examination and medical history. No single blood test definitively diagnoses a bone infection, but a test revealing an elevated level of white blood cells suggests that the body is fighting an infection, and the C-reactive protein test can also indicate bone infection. Samples of pus, joint fluid, bone, or bone tissue help identify the cause of an infection, as does a blood culture study. A bone biopsy, considered one of the most reliable diagnostic methods, reveals the type of organism that has infected the bone. X-rays show bone damage, computed tomography (CT) scans show detailed cross-sectional views of the bones, and magnetic resonance imaging (MRI) creates highly detailed images of bones and the surrounding tissues.

Prevention

Keeping skin wounds and bone injuries clean and sterile so they won't get infected is the best prevention technique, as well as remaining aware of redness, tenderness, swelling, pain, discharge, and other signs of infection. Immediate medical care can prevent chronic problems requiring ongoing treatment.

Treatments

The goal of treatment is to eliminate an infection and prevent its recurrence. Treatment depends on the extent and severity of the condition. Antibiotic medications that kill or reduce the bacteria are a common treatment. Common surgeries include draining the infected wound, removing infected or dead bone portions, and restoration of blood flow with tissue grafting. In extreme cases, amputation may be necessary for those who develop chronic infections that do not clear up with medical intervention. For those with stubborn chronic infections, hyperbaric oxygen therapy often gets more oxygen to the bone to promote healing.

Prognosis and Outcomes

It is possible to make a full recovery without prolonged complications, but the prognosis depends on overall health, age, and type of infection. If a bone infection can be controlled or eliminated early on, the outlook is positive. If an infection spreads to other parts of the body, it can reduce limb or joint function.

Ray Marks

See also: AIDS; Bone Diseases; Diabetes, Type 1; Sickle-Cell Disease

Further Reading

Cleveland Clinic. (2014, September 3). Osteomyelitis. Retrieved from http://my.cleveland clinic.org/disorders/Osteomyelitis/hic_Osteomyelitis.aspx.

Johns Hopkins Medicine Health Library. (2014/2015). Osteomyelitis (bone infection). Retrieved from http://www.hopkinsmedicine.org/healthlibrary/conditions/bone_disorders /osteomyelitis_bone_infection_134,150/.

Mayo Clinic. (2012, November 20). Osteomyelitis. Retrieved from http://www.mayoclinic .org/diseases-conditions/osteomyelitis/basics/definition/CON-20025518.

PDR Health. Physicians' Desk Reference. (2015). Bone infection. Retrieved from http://www .pdrhealth.com/diseases/bone-infection.

OSTEONECROSIS

Osteonecrosis is the term used to describe a health condition in which blood flow to the joints—especially the large joints such as the shoulder, hip, knee, elbow, and ankle—is reduced. The lack of blood supply weakens the bone, which may cause the joint to ultimately collapse. If it is not treated appropriately, the joint can develop severe arthritis. It is also termed *aseptic necrosis, avascular necrosis, ischemic necrosis,* or *ischemic bone necrosis.*

Symptoms

The condition may be asymptomatic early on, with pain developing in the later stages. The joint may move less well than normal and in a limited range. Leg or upper limb dysfunction may occur depending on the affected site.

Key Causes and Risk Factors

Osteonecrosis can be produced as a result of trauma, such as a fracture or a dislocation; prolonged usage of steroids; radiation therapy; decompression illness after deep-sea diving; and health conditions such as sickle cell anemia, HIV, lupus, and diabetes. But, sometimes, no cause seems present. In children and adolescents, the condition can occur as a result of Legg-Calve-Perthes disease.

Diagnosis and Treatment

A detailed history, physical examination, x-ray examination, bone scan, bone biopsy, and MRI or CT scan may be conducted. Treatment may include medication; treating the underlying health condition; surgery such as core decompression, or drilling small holes in the affected bone to stimulate healing; total joint replacement; transplanting a small piece of healthy bone from another area along with its blood supply onto the affected bone area; the use of crutches; and limiting the use of the affected joint.

Prognosis and Prevention

The outcome may depend on age, health status, stage of the condition, and degree of osteonecrosis. Preventing severe trauma, excessive alcohol and steroid usage may be helpful.

Future

In the future, drugs may be developed that help prevent osteonecrosis. Bone grafts and the use of stem cells and blood platelet applications, plus electrical stimulation to replace dead bone or stimulate bone growth, are being studied.

Ray Marks

See also: Arthritis; Lupus; Sickle-Cell Disease

Further Reading

American Academy of Orthopedic Surgeons. (2011). Osteonecrosis of the hip. Retrieved from http://orthoinfo.aaos.org/topic.cfm?topic=a00216.

American College of Rheumatology. (2015). Osteonecrosis. Retrieved from http://www.rheumatology.org/Practice/Clinical/Patients/Diseases_And_Conditions/Osteonecrosis/.

Cleveland Clinic. (2016). Osteonecrosis. Retrieved from http://my.clevelandclinic.org/orthopaedics-rheumatology/diseases-conditions/osteonecrosis.aspx.

National Osteonecrosis Foundation. (2013). Osteonecrosis. Retrieved from http://nonf.org/osteonecrosis.html.

New York Times. (2013). Osteonecrosis. Retrieved from http://www.nytimes.com/health/guides/disease/aseptic-necrosis.

OSTEOPOROSIS

A highly common bone disease, *osteoporosis* means "porous bone" or bone that has lost density or mass, making its tissue abnormal and more likely to break. Bone tissue is always breaking down and being replaced, but when new bone tissue does not adequately replace the old, osteoporosis takes place. As people age, the creation of bone mass slows, and it is lost faster than it can be replaced.

In the United States, more than 40 million people have either osteoporosis or low bone mass, meaning they are at high risk for the disease. It is most common in people age 50 and older, but it can affect anyone; Caucasian and Asian women past menopause are at higher risk. It is estimated that 50 percent of women and 25 percent of men older than age 50 will experience a bone fracture due to osteoporosis. Because weakening bones have no outward signs, a break may be the first indication of the disease. Most fractures occur in the hip, spine, and wrist, but a break in any part of the body could signal weak bones in an older person; loss of height and a curved spine are other indications. Treatments for osteoporosis include medications as well as changes in lifestyle that can reduce risk factors for losing bone mass.

Symptoms

Initial symptoms of osteoporosis may not be evident, but breaking a bone is often the first obvious symptom. Those of weakening bones may include a dull pain or muscle fatigue in the low back or neck; stooped posture; losing an inch or more in height over time; and bones that fracture unexpectedly or more easily than normal. As the disease progresses, sharp sudden pains may occur; they may worsen with activity or be accompanied by surrounding tenderness. These pains may lessen in about a week, or they may last for months.

Causes and Risk Factors

No specific cause of osteoporosis is known, and bone loss usually takes place over a very long period of time. The primary cause is aging and the subsequent loss of estrogen in women and androgen in men. Other contributing causes are changes in other hormone function; some medications prescribed for depression, cancer, endometriosis, seizures, and transplant rejection, as well as steroids for arthritis and asthma; low calcium and vitamin D; hypothyroidism and Cushing's disease; and bone cancer.

Common risk factors include being a Caucasian or Asian woman; having a small or very thin frame; low body weight; poor diet; family history of osteoporosis; history of a previous fracture; having osteopenia (low bone density); smoking; and engaging in no physical activity, especially weight-bearing exercise.

Diagnosis

In addition to a medical history and physical examination, a bone density test is the most widely recognized one for diagnosing osteoporosis before a person breaks a bone; it measures bone strength, which can help predict the risk for a fracture. A DEXA (dual-energy x-ray absorptiometry) scan, which is the most common such test, measures density at the hip and spine, and it also monitors changes in bone density over time. Lab tests such as blood calcium, thyroid function, and testosterone levels may also be used to diagnose an underlying condition that may be a cause of bone loss. CT scans, MRIs, and other imaging tools may detect bone changes caused by diseases, inflammation, and other broken bones.

Treatments

Osteoporosis has no cure, so treatments aim to slow or stop the loss of bone minerals, increase bone density, prevent future breaks, and control pain. Medications may be prescribed for women and men who are at increased risk of fracture; antiresorptive drugs decrease the activity of bone-dissolving cells to slow bone loss, while anabolic medications increase the rate of bone formation. Hormone-related therapy is also a common treatment, along with maintaining a diet high in vitamin D and calcium (or taking supplements) and engaging in weight-bearing exercises. Strategies to prevent falling and protect joints as well as physical therapy are often helpful.

Prevention

Weight-bearing exercise, which makes muscles pull on bones, can build bone density, including hiking, jogging, tennis, brisk walking, dancing, and lifting weights. A diet rich in calcium and vitamin D keeps bones strong, while smoking increases the rate of bone loss, and more than two alcoholic drinks daily for men and one for women may contribute to the decrease of bone formation. Falls can be prevented by wearing low-heeled shoes with nonslip soles and keeping rooms brightly lit and free of clutter or slippery rugs on the floor.

Prognosis

Osteoporosis is a slowly progressive disorder, but early detection and treatment improve the prognosis for living with it. It can be managed effectively by regular weight-bearing and muscle-strengthening exercises, good nutrition, maintaining a healthy weight, and not smoking or consuming excessive alcohol. Bone density tests are recommended, and medications, taken when necessary, significantly reduce the risk of bone breaks in those who have osteoporosis.

Future

Researchers are studying which genes and bone formation mechanisms will lead to targeted therapies and prevention strategies that will be based on each person's individual characteristics.

Ray Marks

See also: Bone Cancer; Bone Disease

Further Reading

HealthLine. (2014, October 6). What do you want to know about osteoporosis? Retrieved from http://www.healthline.com/health/osteoporosis.

Hodgson, S. (2003). Mayo Clinic on osteoporosis: Keeping bones healthy and strong and reducing the risk of fracture. Rochester, MN: Mayo Clinic.

Mayo Clinic. (2014). Osteoporosis. Retrieved from http://www.mayoclinic.org/diseases -conditions/osteoporosis/basics/definition/con-20019924.

National Osteoporosis Foundation. (2014). Learn about osteoporosis. Retrieved from http:// nof.org/learn.

NIH Senior Health. (2013, March). Osteoporosis. Retrieved from http://nihseniorhealth.gov /osteoporosis/whatisosteoporosis/01.html.

OVARIAN CANCER

Ovarian cancer is the abnormal, uncontrolled multiplication of cells within one or both of a woman's ovaries. Most commonly, ovarian cancer originates in the epithelial tissue that covers the ovaries. In some cases, the cancer develops in other ovarian tissues.

Prevalence and Mortality

Ovarian cancer is most prevalent in women who have experienced menopause, especially women who are older than age 60. The disease is more prevalent among women in developed, Western nations than in the less developed nations of Asia and Africa. In 2014, there were about 22,000 newly diagnosed cases of ovarian cancer in the United States. Some 14,000 American women died from ovarian cancer that year.

The earlier a diagnosis for ovarian cancer is made and the earlier treatment is begun, the more successful the outcome is likely to be. Unfortunately, this cancer is typically diagnosed after it has spread beyond the ovaries, resulting in high mortality rates. On average, 45 percent of women are alive five years after diagnosis. If the cancer remains localized in the ovaries at the time of diagnosis, the five-year survival rate rises to about 92 percent. If the cancer has already metastasized to distant tissues of the body at the time of diagnosis, the five-year survival rate falls to about 22 percent.

Risk Factors

A woman's risk for ovarian cancer is increased by the inheritance of mutations in either of two genes, known as BRCA1 and BRCA2. Approximately 1 in 200 women have at least one of these mutated genes, which also increase the risk of breast cancer (much more common than ovarian cancer). Blood tests can detect the presence of BRCA1 and BRCA2. A woman with either of these genes may choose to have her ovaries and/or breasts surgically removed to prevent the possible development of cancer.

Only 10 percent of ovarian cancer cases are associated with the BRCA1 and BRCA2 genes. Other cases have causes that are not fully understood. However, factors that are believed to increase the risk of ovarian cancer include a diet high in fat, never being pregnant, going through menopause relatively late in life (after age 50), and having had a relatively early onset of menstruation (before age 12). Some studies suggest that women who use hormone replacement therapy to relieve the symptoms of menopause are at an elevated risk for ovarian cancer.

Research indicates that certain factors may lower a woman's risk of ovarian cancer. These factors include having given birth, having breastfed their infant, and having undergone a tubal ligation or a hysterectomy. The use of oral contraceptives may also lower ovarian cancer risk, but such use may increase breast cancer risk.

Symptoms and Diagnosis

Women with ovarian cancer may notice chronic pain or cramps in the abdominal or pelvic areas, as well as frequent nausea, bloating, abnormal vaginal bleeding, and an abnormally frequent need to urinate. Such symptoms can also be associated with less serious conditions. If the symptoms are noticed almost every day for two or three weeks, the woman should see a doctor. The doctor is likely to perform a pelvic examination, looking for signs of abnormal lumps on the ovaries. Lumps may also be detected with an ultrasound examination.

A suspicion of ovarian cancer is usually followed up with a blood test and biopsy. The blood will be analyzed for elevated levels of a protein called cancer antigen 125 (CA-125). High levels of CA-125 could suggest any of various pathological conditions, including ovarian cancer, endometriosis, and uterine fibroids. To determine the precise condition, an ovarian tissue sample must be collected for biopsy. Additional tests, such as computed tomography (CT), can be used to determine the stage of cancer development.

Treatment

If the presence of cancer is confirmed, surgery is usually performed to remove one or both ovaries. In many cases, the uterus and Fallopian tubes are also removed to try to ensure that all the cancer is gone. These procedures will make it impossible for the woman to become pregnant, and they will cause a younger woman to immediately enter menopause.

In the most advanced cases of ovarian cancer, additional tissues may be removed, including part of the intestines, the lining of the abdominal wall, and the spleen. Chemotherapy and radiation therapy may also be used in a patient's treatment.

Follow-up therapy often includes routine blood tests to monitor levels of CA-125 and other substances that could indicate a recurrence of cancer.

As with breast cancer treatment, treatment for ovarian cancer sometimes results in emotional problems regarding a woman's perception of her body and her sexuality. Psychological counseling may be incorporated into follow-up therapy.

A. J. Smuskiewicz

See also: Breast Cancer; HPV (Human Papillomavirus); Pelvic Inflammatory Disease; Women's Health

Further Reading
Benedict, B. B. (2013). *The Ultimate Guide to Ovarian Cancer: Everything You Need to Know About Diagnosis, Treatment, and Research*. Atlanta, GA: Sherryben Publishing House.
Centers for Disease Control and Prevention. (2016). Basic information about ovarian cancer. Retrieved from http://www.cdc.gov/cancer/ovarian/basic_info/.
Friedman, S., Sutphen, R., & Steligo, K. (2012). *Confronting Hereditary Breast and Ovarian Cancer: Identify Your Risk, Understand Your Options, Change Your Destiny*. Baltimore, MD: Johns Hopkins University Press.
McKay, J., & Schacher, T. (2009). *The Chemotherapy Survival Guide: Everything You Need to Know to Get through Treatment*. Oakland, CA: New Harbinger Publications.
Montz, F. J., Bristow, R. E., & Anastasia, P. J. (2005). *A Guide to Survivorship for Women with Ovarian Cancer: A Johns Hopkins Press Health Book*. Baltimore, MD: Johns Hopkins University Press.
National Cancer Institute. (2015). SEER stat fact sheets: Ovary cancer. Retrieved from http://seer.cancer.gov/statfacts/html/ovary.html.

National Ovarian Cancer Coalition. (2016). What is ovarian cancer? Retrieved from http://www.ovarian.org/what_is_ovarian_cancer.php.

Office in Women's Health. (2016). Ovarian cancer fact sheet. Retrieved from http://www.womenshealth.gov/publications/our-publications/fact-sheet/ovarian-cancer.html.

Salani, R., & Bristow, R. (2009). *Johns Hopkins Patients' Guide to Ovarian Cancer*. Burlington, MA: Jones & Bartlett Learning.

OVERWEIGHT AND OBESITY IN CHILDREN

Childhood obesity and overweight is a serious health challenge affecting more than 43 million preschool children worldwide (6.7 percent), with studies showing it could have adverse effects on later health. The percentage of children aged 6 to 11 years in the United States who were obese increased from 7 percent in 1980 to nearly 20 percent in 2008. Similarly, the percentage of adolescents aged 12 to 19 years who were obese increased from 5 to 18 percent over the same period. In 2008, more than one-third of children and adolescents were overweight or obese.

Overweight is defined as having excess body weight for a particular height from fat, muscle, bone, water, or a combination of these factors. *Obesity* is defined as having excess body fat. Overweight and obesity are the result of "caloric imbalance"—too few calories expended for the amount of calories consumed—and are affected by various genetic, behavioral, and environmental factors.

Childhood obesity occurs when a child is well above the normal weight for his or her age and height. Obesity is a serious medical condition that affects children and adolescents. According to various studies, some of the problems within the populations include low socioeconomic status, poverty, high unemployment rate, and unhealthy lifestyle leading to adverse health outcomes.

Causes

Some of the causes leading to the concern of the built environment include limited amount of safe space available for physical activities, lack of healthy food sources in the area, the abundance of fast-food chain restaurants, poverty level, and low socioeconomic status. Although there are some genetic and hormonal causes of childhood obesity, most of the time it is caused by children eating too much and exercising too little.

Risk factors

Many factors increase a child's risk of becoming overweight:

- *Diet.* Regularly eating high-calorie foods, such as fast foods, baked goods, and vending machine snacks, can easily cause a child to gain weight. Loading up on soft drinks containing sugar, candy, and desserts also can cause weight gain.
- *Lack of exercise.* Children who don't exercise much are more likely to gain weight because they don't burn calories through physical activity.

- *Family history.* If a child comes from a family of overweight people, he or she may be more likely to put on excess weight,
- *Psychological factors.* Some children overeat to cope with problems or to deal with emotions, such as stress.
- *Family factors.* If family buys their groceries from convenience foods, such as cookies, chips, and other high-calorie items, this can contribute to child's weight gain.
- *Socioeconomic factors.* Frozen meals, crackers, and cookies often contain a lot of salt and fats. These foods are often less expensive or an easier option than fresher, healthier foods.

Diagnosis

As part of regular well-child care, the doctor calculates a child's body mass index (BMI) and determines where it falls on the national BMI-for-age growth chart. The BMI helps indicate if a child is overweight for his or her age and height.

Using the growth chart, a doctor determines the child's percentile, meaning how the child compares with other children of the same sex and age. Cutoff points on these growth charts, established by the Centers for Disease Control and Prevention (CDC), help identify overweight and obese children:

- BMI-for-age between 85th and 94th percentiles—overweight
- BMI-for-age 95th percentile or above—obesity

In addition to BMI and charting weight on the growth charts, the doctor also evaluates:

- The family's history of obesity and weight-related health problems, such as diabetes
- The child's eating habits
- The child's activity level
- Other health conditions that child may have

Health Effects of Childhood Obesity

Childhood obesity has both immediate and long-term effects on health and well-being.

Immediate health effects:

- Obese youth are more likely to have risk factors for cardiovascular disease, such as high cholesterol or high blood pressure.
- Obese adolescents are more likely to have prediabetes, which lead to develop diabetes in adulthood.
- Children and adolescents who are obese are at greater risk for bone and joint problems, sleep apnea, and social and psychological problems such as stigmatization and poor self-esteem.

Long-term health effects:

- Children and adolescents who are obese are likely to be obese as adults and are, therefore, more at risk for adult health problems such as heart disease, Type 2 diabetes, stroke, several types of cancer, and osteoarthritis. One study showed that children who became obese as early as age two were more likely to be obese as adults.

- Overweight and obesity are associated with increased risk for many types of cancer, including cancer of the breast, colon, endometrium, esophagus, kidney, pancreas, gall bladder, thyroid, ovary, cervix, and prostate, as well as multiple myeloma and Hodgkin's lymphoma.

Prevention

- Healthy lifestyle habits, including healthy eating and physical activity, can lower the risk of becoming obese and developing related diseases.
- The dietary and physical activity behaviors of children and adolescents are influenced by many sectors of society, including families, communities, schools, child care settings, medical care providers, faith-based institutions, government agencies, the media, and the food and beverage industries and entertainment industries.
- Schools play a particularly critical role by establishing a safe and supportive environment with policies and practices that support healthy behaviors. Schools also provide opportunities for students to learn about and practice healthy eating and physical activity behaviors.

In summary, overweight and obesity in childhood (including adolescence) is associated with serious physiological, psychological, and social consequences. Many of these consequences manifest during childhood; others appear later in life. Of great concern is that children who are overweight or obese are also more likely to be overweight or obese as adults. And, perhaps even more disturbing, today's youth may have a shorter life expectancy than their parents because of the high prevalence of obesity.

Ray Marks

See also: Diet and Nutrition; Family Health; Obesity; Obesity, Morbid; Physical Activity; Poverty; Prediabetes

Further Reading

Centers for Disease Control and Prevention. (2011). National diabetes fact sheet: National estimates and general information on diabetes and prediabetes in the United States, Atlanta, GA: U.S. Department of Health and Human Services.

Food Research and Action Center. (2012). Consequences of childhood overweight and obesity. Retrieved from http://frac.org/initiatives/hunger-and-obesity/what-are-the-consequences-of-childhood-overweight-and-obesity/.

Dolnick, S. (2010, March 12). The obesity-hunger paradox. *The New York Times*, MB4.

Grier, S., & Kumanyika, S. (2008). The context for choice: Health implications of targeted food and beverage marketing to African Americans. *American Journal of Public Health*, 98(9), 1616–1629.

Guo, S. S., & Chumlea, W. C. (1999). Tracking of body mass index in children in relation to overweight in adulthood. *American Journal of Clinical Nutrition*, 70, S145–S148.

Heinrich, K., Lee, R., Regan, G., & Reese-Smith, J. (2008). How does the built environment relate to body mass index and obesity prevalence among public housing residents? *American Journal of Health Promotion*, 22(3), 187–194.

Isaacs, S., & Schroeder, S. (2004). Class: The ignored determinant of the nation's health. *The New England Journal of Medicine*, 351(11), 1137–1142.

Kushi, L. H., Byers, T., & Doyle, C., et al. (2006). American Cancer Society guidelines on nutrition and physical activity for cancer prevention: reducing the risk of cancer with healthy food choices and physical activity. *CA: A Cancer Journal for Clinicians, 56,* 254–281.

Lynch, J., Smith, G., Kaplan, G., & House, J. (2000). Income inequality and mortality: Importance to health of individual, psychosocial environment, or material conditions. *British Medical Journal, 320,* 1200–1204.

Maantay, J. (2001). Public health matters: Zoning, equity, and public health. *American Journal of Public Health, 91*(7), 1033–1041.

Matte, T., Ellis, J. A., Bedell, J., & Selenic, D. (2007). *Obesity in the South Bronx: A Look across Generations.* New York, NY: The New York City Department of Health and Mental Hygiene, Bronx District Public Health Office. Retrieved from http://www.nyc.gov/html /doh/downloads/pdf/dpho/dpho-bronx-obesity.pdf.

Moore, L., & Roux, A. (2006). Associations of neighborhood characteristics with the location and type of food stores. *American Journal of Public Health, 96*(2), 325–331.

P

PAGET'S DISEASE OF THE BONE

Paget's disease is an uncommon chronic disease that affects bone and is associated with a disruption in the normal cycle of new bone buildup and old bone removal in isolated areas of the body. Basically, the condition is associated with rapid remodeling of bone, instead of slower modeling due to age, and this rebuilt bone is softer, or more brittle and weaker, than regular bone or results in enlarged bones or bones that bend easily or fit together haphazardly. The bones commonly affected are the skull, spine, clavicle or collarbone, the upper arm bone or humerus, pelvis, and thigh and shin bones. Complications of Paget's disease of the bone include osteoarthritis, fractures, bone cancer, pinching of adjacent nerves, hearing and vision loss, and heart failure with widespread disease due to the stress placed on the heart to shunt blood to the bones that are overactive. The disease may also lead to bone cancer in the area affected by the disease if pain is severe and unremitting. Normally affecting adults over the age of 40 at a rate of 1 percent of the population in the United States, there is a rare form of Paget's disease known as juvenile Paget's disease. It is also known as *osteoitis deformans*.

Symptoms

The condition may present with no symptoms or symptoms of pain in one or more bones. There may be a feeling of tingling or numbness associated with the condition, as well as deformities of the affected bones; broken bones; osteoarthritis of the affected joints; loss of facial muscle strength, vision, or hearing; and headaches. In some cases, the condition results in an overelevated level of calcium in the blood, and this can cause weakness, fatigue, appetite loss, or abdominal problems and pain.

Key Causes and Risk Factors

Advancing age, being male, being of British or northern European descent, and having a family history are risk factors for Paget's bone disease, but the precise cause remains unknown. Genetic disturbances, and some form of viral infection affecting certain bone cells may also increase the risk of this condition.

Diagnosis

Diagnostic procedures for Paget's bone disease include a physical exam, a medical history, and x-rays. Other tests may include bone scans, bone biopsies, and a test to measure the extent of alkaline phosphatase in the blood, which is normally elevated.

Treatment

Medications known as bisphosphonates are used to treat Paget's disease of the bone. In rare cases, surgery—such as joint replacements, joint realignment, and decompression of a joint to reduce and pressure on the nerves due to abnormal bone growth—may be indicated. A good healthy diet, as well as regular exercise, is also recommended.

Prognosis

Medical interventions, plus prevention of fractures, and arthritis disability has improved the outlook for most people with this condition. In 1 percent of cases, the disease may result in bone cancer or Paget's sarcoma, which is associated with a very poor outcome.

Prevention

People with Paget's disease of the bone should be educated about how to prevent falls because their bones may be very brittle.

Future

Researchers are examining genetic causes of Paget's bone disease and may be able at some point to predict who will be at risk for the condition, as well as how to better treat the condition. The goal is to reverse the destructive bone process, rather than slow it down, or treat the condition symptomatically.

Ray Marks

See also: Bone Cancer; Bone Diseases; Osteoarthritis

Further Reading

American College of Rheumatology. (2015). Paget's disease of the bone. Retrieved from http://www.rheumatology.org/Practice/Clinical/Patients/Diseases_And_Conditions /Paget_s_Disease_of_Bone/.

Mayo Clinic. (2013). Paget's disease of the bone. Retrieved from http://www.mayoclinic.com /health/pagets-disease-of-bone/DS00485/METHOD=print.

MedlinePlus. (2013). Paget's disease of the bone. Retrieved from http://www.nlm.nih.gov /medlineplus/ency/article/000414.htm.

National Institute of Arthritis and Musculoskeletal and Skin Diseases. (2015). What is Paget's disease of the bone? NIH Osteoporosis and Related Bone Diseases, National Resource Center. Retrieved from http://www.niams.nih.gov/Health_Info/Bone/Pagets /patient_info.asp.

PAGET'S DISEASE OF THE BREAST

Overview

Paget's breast disease is a form of cancer that affects the dark area of the skin around the nipple of the breast, called the areola. Starting in the nipple and extending to the areola area, women and men who acquire this rare disease may also experience the presence of one or more tumors within the same breast.

Paget's disease of the breast was named after a 19th-century British doctor, Sir James Paget, who noted the relationship between the changes in the nipple and breast cancer, specifically the skin cell changes that led to the formation of large round cells called Paget cells that occurred singly or in groups around the skin of the nipple and areola. Although Sir James Paget had believed the cells he discovered were not cancerous, later research showed the cells were cancer cells, and their presence indicated the presence of underlying breast cancer.

The disease can occur in young people as well as people in their 90s, but the most common age is around 57. More women than men are affected by the disease, and most women who develop Paget's breast disease have a form of cancer called ductal breast cancer, which can occur in situ, meaning it started in the breast,; less commonly, they may have breast cancer that has spread to the breast from another site. If untreated, it may prove fatal.

Symptoms

Possible signs and symptoms of Paget's breast disease include the presence of a flaky or scaly skin area or rash on one nipple; oozing, thickened, or hardened skin on either the nipple, areola, or both; itching and redness or burning of the skin in the area of the breast and nipple; as well as pain and increased skin sensitivity, one or more lumps in the breast, bloody or yellow colored discharge from the nipple, and an inverted or flattened nipple.

The skin changes may wax and wane in the early disease stages, so often a diagnosis is put off because it seems the skin is healing.

Key Causes and Risk Factors

The factors causing Paget's disease of the breast are unclear. The most well-accepted explanation is that the disease results from the presence of an underlying ductal form of breast cancer, and these cancer cells in the breast then travel through the milk ducts to the nipple and the surrounding skin area. Another explanation states that the disease can develop independently, which could explain why some people with the disease do not have a tumor inside the breast. In some cases, it may be possible for Paget's breast disease to develop independently of tumors inside the same breast.

Risk factors affecting the likelihood of developing Paget's breast disease are similar to those associated with breast cancer such as older age; having a cancer history, especially breast cancer or breast conditions; and having a family history of breast or ovarian cancer or both.

Genetic factors, such as having defective genes, especially the BRCA1 or BRCA2 gene, can place a person at increased risk of developing breast cancer as well as ovarian and other cancers. Other risk factors are the presence of dense breast tissue, radiation exposure, being overweight, being on hormone replacement therapy, and being white rather than black or Hispanic.

Diagnosis

Tests to evaluate the presence of Paget's disease of the breast may include a clinical breast and physical exam, mammography or x-ray exam of the breast tissue, and a magnetic resonance imaging (MRI) test of the breast to detect cancer not visible on a mammogram. Other tests include a biopsy of the breast tissue, microscopic examination of cells from the skin surface of the nipple and areola, and/or lab tests of any fluid discharge.

Treatment

Surgical options include having a simple mastectomy or breast removal, without removing the lymph nodes in the armpit in case the breast cancer has not spread to the lymph nodes.

A lumpectomy involves removing only the portion of the breast containing the tumor, with follow-up radiation therapy, and possible nipple reconstruction after treatment.

Anticancer drugs or chemotherapy, along with radiation therapy or hormone therapy, may be used in conjunction with surgery to prevent a breast cancer reoccurrence.

Prognosis

The outlook for people with Paget's breast disease depends on several factors, including whether or not a tumor is present in the affected breast.

Prevention

Risk factors that are within the control of the individual include getting enough exercise, limiting alcohol intake, eating healthy meals, and maintaining a healthy weight.

Some high-risk women may decide to undergo a preventive mastectomy or removal of one or both breasts in the hope of preventing or reducing their breast cancer risk.

Ray Marks

See also: Breast Cancer; Male Breast Cancer; Ovarian Cancer

Further Reading

Breast Cancer.org. (2015). Paget's disease of the nipple. http://www.breastcancer.org /symptoms/types/pagets.

Mayo Clinic. (2013). Paget's disease of the breast. Retrieved from http://www.mayoclinic .org/diseases-conditions/pagets-disease-of-the-breast/basics/definition/con-20025786.

Medical News Today. (2016, February 18). Paget's disease of the breast: Causes, symptoms and diagnosis. Retrieved from http://www.medicalnewstoday.com/articles/192362.php.

National Cancer Institute. (2012). Paget disease of the breast. Retrieved from http://www .cancer.gov/typs/breast/paget-breast-fact-sheet.

PAIN, CHRONIC

Pain is physical suffering or distress due to injury or illness and is expressed as a distressing sensation in a particular part of the body. Sometimes, we use the term to identify mental or emotional suffering.

As kids growing up, we skinned our knees, got stung by a bee, hit our thumb with the hammer, had a belly ache, or bumped our "funny bone." Sometimes, we knew what caused the pain—the fall, the sunburn, that extra piece of pie, or bumping into the coffee table. Other times, we did not know the cause and our parents took us to the doctor. In either case, we were fortunate: Our body informed us that something was not as it should be. According to Ehrenberg (2012), "pain is usually protective, prompting us to pull our hands off a hot stove . . . but not all pain is alike, and not all pain [is] helpful" (23). Generally speaking, pain can be divided into *protective* and *unhelpful*. Pain can also be chronic, lasting for weeks and up to years or even forever.

Protective pain is recognized as a response to intense stimulus (nociceptive) and an immune system response (inflammatory). *Nociceptive* pain (from the Latin *nocere*, to hurt or injure) is protective and alerts you to actual or impending injury. Once activated, these nerve endings respond instantaneously. *Inflammatory* pain occurs as a response to the injury. Our immune system warns us not to move or to rest the twisted ankle or broken arm. One form of unhelpful pain is *dysfunctional* pain, which is generally the result of genetic abnormalities. *Neuropathic* pain is pain due to injury to the nerve endings.

Pain that results from metabolic disorders, autoimmune disease, or viruses is not helpful—it is assaulting the nerve endings. These over stimulated, "trigger-happy" nerve endings continually fire pain warnings. Other causes of unhelpful pain include cancer, HIV, antiviral medications, diabetes, shingles (a secondary infection of herpes zoster), and compressed or crushed nerve endings. The following list—while not exhaustive—highlights some the more common causes of pain, which is usually chronic:

- Acute injury (broken bone, laceration, sprain)
- Cancer
- Carpal tunnel
- Chronic back pain (slipped discs, fractures, soft-tissue injury)
- Depression

- Diabetes nerve pain
- Dental disease
- Fibromyalgia
- Lupus
- Migraines
- Osteoporosis
- Psychogenic pain
- Rheumatoid arthritis

Tests. Pain is complex and the diagnosis of the cause of pain, whether acute or chronic, takes patience and the skill of an empathetic diagnostician. Several tests are useful in determining the cause of pain. These include:

CT or CAT scan: Computed tomography (CT) or computed axial tomography (CAT) scans use x-rays and computers to produce an image of a cross-section of the body. Sometimes, an intravenous (injected into a vein) contrast material is required for a CAT scan.

MRI: Magnetic resonance imaging (MRI) produces clear pictures of the body without the use of x-rays. This test uses a large magnet, radio waves, and a computer to produce images. Certain MRI exams require an injection of a contrast material called gadolinium, which helps identify certain anatomic structures on the scan images.

EMG: This procedure allows doctors to evaluate the activity of the muscles. During the procedure, very fine needles are inserted in muscles to measure the muscles' response to signals from the brain or spinal cord.

Quality of life scale: Physicians often use this psychometric scale to better understand how a patient is affected by his or her pain. For more information, see https://www.theacpa.org/uploads/documents/Life_Scale_3.pdf.

Pain Management and Treatment. There are multiple options to treat and/or manage pain, including traditional or Western medicine and complementary and alternative medicine (CAM). Western medicine typically employs physical therapy, bioelectric therapy, nerve blocks, and medication. In extreme (intractable) cases, surgery is an option. Complementary and alternative medicine includes acupuncture, acupressure, chiropractic care, massage, herbs, therapeutic touch, Reiki, yoga, and the mind-body therapies of progressive relaxation, meditation, guided imagery, biofeedback, and hypnosis.

Analgesics (Pain Killers). Both short- and long-term pain can be managed with over-the-counter (OTC) and prescribed medications. Analgesic medications are either nonnarcotic or narcotic. OTC medications are *per se* nonnarcotic, which means they do not require a physician's prescription.

Three basic types include acetaminophen, also known as Tylenol and Aspirin Free Excedrin, is widely acknowledged as an effective pain killer; nonsteroidal anti-inflammatory drugs (NSAIDs) include aspirin, Motrin and Aleve; and topical corticosteroids (e.g., Cortaid, Cortisone). Acetaminophen and NSAIDs reduce fever and relieve pain. However, only NSAIDs can reduce inflammation (swelling and irritation). These two classifications of drugs work differently: NSAIDs relieve pain by reducing the production of prostaglandins—hormone-like substances that cause pain; acetaminophen works on the parts of the brain that receive the "pain messages." Opioids are narcotic pain medications (prescription only) used for acute pain, such as short-term pain after surgery. Some examples include Percocet, Vicodin, methadone, morphine, fentanyl, oxycodone, and codeine. While these medications are effective pain relievers, they must be used with the greatest of caution: They are habit-forming—in other words, addictive. In some cases, they can lead to addictions to such illegal drugs as heroin and can lead to death from overdoses.

Living with and Managing Chronic Pain. Living with chronic pain can be challenging. With these tips, the good days can outnumber the bad days. Some basics include:

- Reduce and manage stress levels through deep breathing, meditation, and guided imagery.
- Learn how to distract yourself.
- Be physically active—which sounds counterintuitive—but is actually is a natural way to raise endorphin levels.
- Join a support groups.
- Learn biofeedback.
- Keep a pain journal and discover what triggers or reduces your pain level.
- Don't drink.
- Don't smoke.
- Eat healthily.
- Work with your doctor.

Linda R. Barley

See also: Cancer; Carpal Tunnel; Chronic Disease Management; Depression; Diabetes, Type 1; Fibromyalgia; Lupus; Osteoporosis; Rheumatoid Arthritis

Further Reading

American Chronic Pain Association. (2016). Quality of life scale. Retrieved from http://www.theacpa.org/uploads/documents/life_scale_3.pdf.

Ehrenberg, R. (2012, June 30). Hurt blocker: The next big pain drug may soothe sensory firestorm with outside effects. *Science News*, 20–25.

National Center for Complementary and Integrative Health (NCCIH). (2015). Health. Retrieved from http://nccam.nih.gov/.

Schneider, J. P. (2006–2007). Opioids, pain management and addiction. *Pain Practitioner*, *16*, 17–24.

Sutherland, S. (2014, December). "Pain That Won't Quit." *Scientific American*, *311*(6), 60–67.

Woolf, C. J., & Salter, M. W. (2000). Neuronal plasticity: Increasing the gain in pain. *Science News*, *288*, 1765–1768.

PANCREATIC CANCER

The pancreas is a gland between the stomach and the spine. Its exocrine cells produce enzymes to help the body digest food, and its neuroendocrine cells produce the hormones insulin and glucagon, which help control blood sugar levels. Pancreatic cancer usually develops in the exocrine cells, which do not secrete hormones or cause any symptoms; this makes it difficult to diagnose and treat successfully. Cancer in the pancreatic neuroendocrine cells offers a better prognosis than exocrine cancers. The causes for either type of pancreatic cancer are unknown, but they appear to be based in gene mutations, either inherited or acquired.

Symptoms often do not show up until the disease is advanced, and they typically include upper abdominal pain, loss of appetite and weight, blood clots, and jaundice. Most people who develop pancreatic cancer are men over age 45; African Americans face a higher risk. Other risk factors include smoking, having diabetes or chronic pancreatitis, being overweight, and a personal or family history of certain genetic disorders.

Treatments for pancreatic cancer include surgery, radiation therapy, and chemotherapy and targeted therapy drugs. But for most people who have exocrine pancreatic cancer, treatments do not cure the disease. Estimates are that in 2015 nearly 49,000 people will receive a diagnosis of pancreatic cancer (American Cancer Society 2015), usually after the age of 45. Because exocrine pancreatic cancer spreads quickly and is difficult to find, it the fourth deadliest cancer diagnosis, and about 40,560 people were expected to die of it in 2015.

Symptoms

Symptoms of pancreatic cancer may not appear until the disease is in an advanced stage. When they do appear, they typically include pain in the upper abdomen that radiates toward the spine, jaundice (yellowing of the skin and whites of the eyes), loss of appetite, unexplained weight loss, clay-colored stools, dark urine, and fatigue.

Causes and Risk Factors

The causes for exocrine and neuroendocrine pancreatic cancers are unknown, but they appear to be based in gene mutations, either inherited or acquired. Most people who develop pancreatic cancer are older than 45; men and African Americans also face an increased risk. A significant risk factor for pancreatic cancer is tobacco use: About 20 to 30 percent of exocrine cancer may be caused by smoking cigarettes; smoking cigars and pipes and using smokeless tobacco are also significant risk factors. Other risk factors include obesity, chronic diabetes or pancreatitis (inflammation of the pancreas), cirrhosis of the liver, ulcer-causing bacteria causing stomach infections, and heavy exposure to certain chemicals, as well as a family history of pancreatic cancer or genetic disorders that include a mutation in the BRCA2 gene, Lynch syndrome, familial atypical mole malignant melanoma, Peutz-Jeghers syndrome, and Von Hippel-Lindau syndrome.

Diagnosis

Pancreatic cancer is often difficult to diagnose, and no screening tests exist that can detect the disease in those without symptoms. Often, it is not found until it has spread elsewhere in the body. A doctor performing a physical exam will look for masses or fluid accumulation in the abdomen, as well as an enlarged gallbladder, liver, or lymph nodes. Further diagnostic tools may include a CT scan; MRI; abdominal or endoscopic ultrasound; and a cholangiopancreatogram, an imaging test that looks for blockages in the pancreatic and bile ducts. For neuroendocrine pancreatic cancer, a somatostatin receptor scintigraphy, often called octreoscan, is very helpful. Blood tests that examine liver function and search for tumor markers can be useful for confirming a diagnosis of both types of pancreatic cancer. If diagnostic tests suggest pancreatic cancer, a biopsy is often to only way to confirm the disease.

Treatments

A variety of standard treatments are used for pancreatic cancers: surgery to remove all or part of the tumor; ablative treatments that destroy tumors with extreme heat or cold; radiation therapy to destroy cancer cells with high-energy x-rays; chemotherapy, or medications to destroy cancer cells by stopping their ability to grow and divide; chemoradiation, a combination of chemotherapy and radiation to increase the effects of both; and targeted therapy, which uses substances that attack cancer cells without harming normal cells.

Prevention

Because the causes of pancreatic cancer are not known, it is difficult to prevent. But quitting smoking and reducing other avoidable risk factors helps limit the chance of developing the disease.

Prognosis and Outcomes

Pancreatic cancer often has a poor prognosis, even when diagnosed early. Rarely detected in its early stages, it usually spreads rapidly. For most people with exocrine pancreatic cancer, standard treatments do not cure the disease; some types of neuroendocrine pancreatic tumors respond to treatment and offer a better prognosis. The one-year survival rate of people with pancreatic cancer is about 28 percent, and the five-year survival rate is 7 percent. Pancreatic cancer accounts for about 3 percent of all cancers in the United States and for about 7 percent of all cancer deaths.

Future

Researchers are testing new types of treatments, including surgeries, in clinical trials. Scientists are also studying how the changes in DNA cause pancreatic cells to become cancerous and increase the risk of developing pancreatic cancer. They have discovered that the cancer develops over many years, and they are working to develop tests for detecting noninherited gene changes in pancreatic cancer precancerous conditions. Although more research is needed, two recent scientific studies report that scientists have identified a blood protein and developed a urine test that may detect pancreatic cancer at early stages.

Ray Marks

See also: Abdominal Diseases; Cancer; Inflammation; Pancreatic Diseases; Tobacco Addiction

Further Reading

American Cancer Society. (2015, January 9). Pancreatic cancer. Retrieved from http://www .cancer.org/cancer/pancreaticcancer/.
Cancer.net (2014, November). Pancreatic cancer overview. Retrieved from http://www.cancer .net/cancer-types/pancreatic-cancer/overview.
Mayo Clinic. (2014, November 22). Pancreatic cancer. Retrieved from http://www.mayoclinic .org/diseases-conditions/pancreatic-cancer/basics/definition/con-20028153.
National Cancer Institute. (2015, July 2). Pancreatic cancer: For patients. Retrieved from http://www.cancer.gov/types/pancreatic.

PANCREATITIS

Overview

Pancreatitis refers to an inflammation of the pancreas. The pancreas releases powerful enzymes that help with digestion, and pancreatic damage happens when the digestive enzymes are activated before they are released into the small intestine and begin attacking the pancreas.

The two forms of pancreatitis, *acute* and *chronic*, refer to the short-term inflammation of the pancreas versus the long-term inflammation of the pancreas (which occurs after an initial acute attack), respectively.

Pancreatitis commonly occurs in adults ages 30 to 40 and is rare in children, but it can occur secondary to hereditary disease or pancreatic trauma; often, in these rare instances, the cause is unknown.

Signs and Symptoms

In acute pancreatitis, the patient looks ill and feels ill, and the symptoms can range from a mild discomfort to a severe, life-threatening illness. As well, in an acute state of pancreatitis, the abdomen may be swollen and tender and there may be pain referred to the back, fever, nausea, an increased heart rate, and vomiting.

In chronic pancreatitis, patients often experience constant upper abdominal pain that radiates to the back. They may lose weight, and the pain may become disabling.

Causes and Risk Factors

Causes of acute pancreatitis are gallstones or excess usage of alcohol. Medications, infections, injuries, metabolic disorders, and surgery may be other causes.

One cause of chronic pancreatitis is drinking. Others are gallstones, certain autoimmune conditions, hereditary pancreatic disorders, cystic fibrosis, high triglycerides, high levels of blood fat, and certain medications.

In both acute and chronic cases, the cause may be unknown.

Risk factors are having gallstones and heavy regular drinking.

Diagnosis

The diagnosis of acute pancreatitis may involve blood enzyme test for amylase and lipase. If there are high levels of these two enzymes, this may confirm the presence of acute pancreatitis. Other tests include pancreatic function tests, ultrasound or CT scans, biopsies of the pancreas, x-rays of the pancreas and bile ducts, and a glucose tolerance test. Other tests are blood, endoscope ultrasound through a tube into the throat to look at the stomach, magnetic resonance imaging tests, and urine tests and stool tests.

Treatment

People with acute pancreatitis are treated with IV fluids and pain medications in the hospital. An acute attack of pancreatitis usually lasts a few days. An acute attack of pancreatitis caused by gallstones may require surgery to remove the gallbladder or surgery of the bile duct.

For people with chronic pancreatitis, the doctors will commonly try to relieve the patient's pain and improve their nutrition. They be given pancreatic enzymes or insulin, and a low-fat diet may be recommended.

Surgery may be used to relieve abdominal pain and restore drainage of pancreatic enzymes or hormones. Patients should stop smoking and drinking alcohol and take the medications recommended in order to have fewer and milder attacks.

Prognosis or Outcome

Most cases of acute pancreatitis recover completely. In severe cases, acute pancreatitis can cause bleeding into the pancreas, serious tissue damage, infection, and cyst formation. Severe pancreatitis can also harm the heart, lungs, and kidneys.

Prevention

People who consume a great amount of alcohol should try to quit.

Future

Research at the National Institutes of Health is being undertaken to further understand the causes of pancreatitis and to develop treatments.

Ray Marks

See also: Autoimmune Diseases; Cystic Fibrosis; Digestive Diseases; Gall Bladder Disease; Pancreatic Cancer

Further Reading
Mayo Clinic. (2014). Pancreatitis. Retrieved from http://www.mayoclinic.org/diseases -conditions/pancreatitis/basics/definition/con-20028421.
MedlinePlus. (2014). Pancreatitis. Retrieved from https://www.nlm.nih.gov/medlineplus /pancreatitis.html.
National Institute of Diabetes and Digestive and Kidney Diseases. (2012). Pancreatitis. Retrieved from http://www.niddk.nih.gov/health-information/health-topics/liver-disease /pancreatitis/Pages/facts.aspx.
National Pancreas Foundation. (n.d.). Chronic pancreatitis. Retrieved from https://www .pancreasfoundation.org/patient-information/chronic-pancreatitis/.

PARASITIC DISEASES

The term *parasitic disease* refers to a variety of health conditions that occur as a result of being infected by parasites, including worms, insects, and single-celled organisms called protozoa that reside inside the body. These types of diseases are especially common in developing countries in the regions of Africa, Asia, India, and Central and South America and affect children as well as adults. Many children and adults can die as a result, although being infected may not cause any problems in many cases. Among the most common forms of parasitic disease that can cause serious problems are malaria, river blindness, sleeping sickness, and schistosomiasis.

Some parasites also occur in wealthier nations such as the United States. These include pinworms; whipworms; protozoa such as *Giardia lamblia*, which causes intestinal problems; ticks that cause fever and chills; *Trichomonas vaginalis*, which infects the genital tracts of men and women; and *Cryptosporidium parvum*, which has caused diarrheal illness in some U.S. cities.

Each parasite thus causes a different disease, and parasites are classified into four types. Approximately 30 percent live in the digestive system of the body; the remaining 70 percent live in other parts such as the brain, eyes, and sinus cavities.

While some parasites live in the body and do not cause harm, in some places, especially undeveloped countries, parasitic diseases can make many people weak, ill, or unable to work. This, in turn, can partially explain the slow economic development in many of these regions and why they remain impoverished. They can also cause health problems such as asthma, stomach ulcers, and allergies.

Signs and Symptoms

The symptoms that arise if one is infected by a parasitic organism vary widely, but many parasitic infections cause fever, fatigue, weakness, headaches, joint pain, and/ or intestinal problems such as diarrhea or obstruction of the intestines. In cases where the brain is affected, there may be confusion, reduced coordination, sleep disturbances, and mental deterioration.

Causes and Risk Factors

In most cases, people become infected by bathing in, swimming in, or drinking water containing parasites. The can also be infected as a result of eating uncooked or inadequately cooked food; not washing their hands when exposed to infectious materials, or coming into contact with untreated sewage.

Both insects and animals can spread some parasitic diseases; for instance, malaria is spread by a mosquito, and the African tsetse fly spreads sleeping sickness. As well, domestic animals such as cows and pigs can spread tapeworms.

Diagnosis

Parasitic diseases are difficult to diagnose without special blood tests because many parasites do not show up on the routine blood tests. In addition, people with parasites are often susceptible to bacterial infections, so the physician may think this is what is making them ill. Parasites can sometimes be detected if samples of the stool are examined microscopically.

Treatment

Although medication can be used to kill most parasites, some are not destroyed by medications.

Prognosis or Outcome

Although progress has been made in the last 10 years to develop vaccines against parasites, this is very difficult because the organisms are very complex. The only areas of significant progress in the past five years have occurred in the development of vaccines against malaria and leishmaniasis. According to one report, the problem of Chagas disease has responded to an improved ability to control the spread of the transmission more directly.

Prevention

Prevention is key to controlling the onset and prevalence of parasitic diseases, and public health strategies to build sewage and water treatment systems and prevent the breeding of the infective agent are very important. Basic education such as teaching people to wash their hands thoroughly after using the bathroom and before handling food is strongly indicated as well.

Future

Research to understand the organisms and to develop a vaccine against this is proceeding slowly.

Ray Marks

See also: Centers for Disease Control and Prevention (CDC); Malaria; Public Health; Waterborne Diseases; World Health Organization

Further Reading

Centers for Disease Control and Prevention. (2014). About parasites. Retrieved from http://www.cdc.gov/parasites/about.html.
MacKenzie, D. (2013, December 14). America's hidden epidemic. *New Scientist, 220*(2947), 8–9.
MedlinePlus. (2014). Parasitic diseases. Retrieved from http://www.nlm.nih.gov/medlineplus/parasiticdiseases.html.

PARKINSON'S DISEASE

Overview

Parkinson's disease is progressive disease of the motor system or neurodegenerative disease that principally results in a loss of brain cells that produce the important brain chemical that transmits nerve messages, called *dopamine*. This loss of dopamine produces many problems, including the ability to control movements of the legs and arms, as well as to use the muscles of the face normally. In the early disease stages, the problems may be less noticeable and isolated to a hand or leg area. As the condition progresses, and the symptoms worsen, the movement problems and the inability to speak coherently may become more obvious and disabling.

The first descriptions of Parkinson's disease have been traced back as far as 5000 BCE when an ancient Indian civilization identified the disorder and gave it the name Kampavata. Later, the term *Parkinson's disease* was used after a British doctor, James Parkinson, described the disorder as a "shaking palsy" in 1817.

Although Parkinson's disease is not curable, medications exist that can reduce the symptoms, as may surgery in selected cases.

The rate of disease progression of Parkinson's and the extent of the emerging disability may vary from individual to individual, however. Some may be able to live a long productive life, while others may become disabled quite rapidly.

According to the Parkinson's Disease Foundation, about 1 million people in the United States are affected by Parkinson's disease, and most are at least 60 years old.

Symptoms

Parkinson's disease is characterized by a slow progressive loss of muscle control that often causes the limbs and head to tremble at rest. There may also be stiffness of the body parts, movement slowness, and balance problems. As the symptoms worsen, difficulties in walking, talking, and completing simple tasks may be seen.

The four key symptoms of Parkinson's disease are thus the presence of a tremor in the hands, arms, legs, jaw, and face area at rest; rigidity, or stiffness of the muscles of the limbs and trunk; pain and slowness of movement, postural instability, or poor balance; and lack of coordination. Other related problems may include swallowing difficulties, difficulties chewing and speaking, bladder and bowel problems, and skin and sleep disturbances. There may also be a loss of the ability to carry out automatic movements such as blinking, smiling, or arm swinging when walking, as well as speech changes and writing changes.

Additional problems include cognitive problems such as dementia and thinking difficulties, which usually occur in the later disease stages, depression and emotional changes, and a decrease in sexual desire or performance

Causes and Risk Factors

The cause of Parkinson's disease is unknown, but several factors appear to play a role, including genetic factors, triggers in the environment, and the presence of Lewy bodies (protein deposits) in the brain.

Specific risk factors include age, having a family history of the disease, being male, and having had exposure to toxins such as pesticides.

Diagnosis

There are currently no blood or laboratory tests that can diagnose Parkinson's disease. A diagnosis is usually based on a medical history and a comprehensive neurological examination that may involve the use of brain scans or laboratory tests in order to rule out other diseases. The earlier a diagnosis is made, the better the prognosis.

Treatment

Although there is no cure for Parkinson's disease, medications that can reduce many of the symptoms mentioned earlier are usually given or recommended. Most of these medications try to increase or substitute for a specific signaling chemical or neurotransmitter in the brain known as dopamine.

In some cases, surgery may be tried if the disease is not helped by drugs. For example, a form of therapy called deep brain stimulation, which uses electrodes implanted into the brain and connected to a small electrical pulse generator, can be programmed to try to reduce the need for drugs and to improve movement and reduce symptoms of tremor.

Lifestyle changes, including aerobic exercises and physical therapy to improve balance, may also be helpful.

Prognosis

The outcome of Parkinson's disease depends on the severity of the condition and how long it has existed. However, its symptoms generally worsen over time.

Prevention

There is no known preventive strategy against Parkinson's disease, but some research suggests eating more high-fiber foods, fish, and omega-3 rich oils may be somewhat protective.

Future

Current research programs using animal models aim to examine the causes of Parkinson's disease and how it progresses, including the possible role of environmental toxins and genetic factors that may trigger the disorder. Other scientists are trying to develop new drugs to prevent, slow, or reverse Parkinson's disease.

Ray Marks

See also: Environment; Neurodegenerative Diseases; Neurological Diseases

Further Reading

Mayo Clinic. (2015). Parkinson's disease. Retrieved from http://www.mayoclinic.com/health/parkinsons-disease/DS00295.

The Michael J. Fox Foundation for Parkinson's Research. (2016). Retrieved from https://www.michaeljfox.org/.

National Institute of Neurological Diseases and Stroke. (2016). Parkinson's disease. National Institutes of Health. Retrieved from http://www.ninds.nih.gov/disorders/parkinsons_disease/parkinsons_disease.htm.

Palfreman, J. (2015, September/October). Cracking the Parkinson's puzzle. *Scientific American Mind, 26*(5), 54–61.

Parkinson's Disease Foundation. (2016). What is Parkinson's disease? Retrieved from http://www.pdf.org/en/about_pdParkinson's.

Sharma, N., & Richman, E. (2005). *Parkinson's Disease and the Family: A New Guide.* Cambridge, MA: Harvard University Press.

Weiner, W. J., Shulman, L. M., & Lang, A. E. (2013). *Parkinson's Disease: A Complete Guide for Patients and Families,* 3rd ed. Baltimore, MD: Johns Hopkins University Press.

PELVIC INFLAMMATORY DISEASE

Pelvic inflammatory disease (PID) is a serious medical complication that develops from bacteria that travel from the vagina or cervix to the uterus, Fallopian tubes, and ovaries. It is typically caused by sexually transmitted diseases (STDs), but other there are other causes for it as well, including using an IUD (intrauterine device). Because PID involves the uterus, Fallopian tubes, and ovaries, it has the potential of being permanently life-changing and scarring. PID is not an uncommon disease. In fact, it is estimated that approximately 750,000 women are diagnosed with PID each year in the United States, with an estimated total number of 1.5 million affected women. Up to 10 to 15 percent of these women may become infertile as a result of PID.

Being between 16 and 25 years of age is a generalized risk factor for PID. The other risk factors include the presence of an STD, a previous episode of PID, sexual intercourse at an early age, high number of sexual partners or a partner with multiple sex partners, and alcohol or drug use. In addition, several other risk factors have been identified for urban adolescents, such as having older sex partners (who may be more sexually experienced and thus more likely to have and spread STDs) and previous involvement in child protective services or attempted suicide (which may indicate a history of abuse or rape).

Oftentimes, PID is not diagnosed because the symptoms are too subtle. If a woman waits too long to get treated for symptoms related to gonorrhea, chlamydia, or the organisms that cause bacterial vaginosis (BV), then she will be at increased risk of developing PID. The symptoms that most women complain about are lower abdominal pain, pelvic or vaginal pain, fevers greater than 100.4°F, chills, foul-smelling or discolored vaginal discharge, and nausea or vomiting. PID may also present with painful intercourse (dyspareunia), back pain, abnormal uterine or vaginal bleeding, painful urination (dysuria), or itching and burning in the vagina.

PID can inflame and scar the uterus (endometritis), cervix (cervicitis), ovaries (tubo-ovarian abscess), and Fallopian tubes (salpingitis). These events can place the patient at increased risk for having ectopic pregnancies and can also make the woman infertile. With PID, the inflammation can cause abdominal inflammation (peritonitis) and scar tissue formation in the abdomen called adhesions. These adhesions can lead to continuous abdominal and pelvic pain and can also cause strictures (narrowing) of the gastrointestinal, reproductive, and urinary systems. When the stricture involves the gut, this can cause bowel obstructions and constipation and increase the risk of abdominal surgeries. The adhesions also can cause urinary obstruction, leading to enlargement of the kidney and more severe UTIs, possibly causing kidney infection. The only way to reduce or improve adhesions is to remove them surgically. If a woman is pregnant and develops PID, the stakes are even higher, including the risk of dying, premature delivery of the baby, or death of the unborn infant. In such cases, the woman is hospitalized, treated, and monitored closely throughout the rest of her pregnancy.

On occasion, the infection can be so bad, or go untreated for so long, that the woman can develop severe medical conditions that put her at risk for further problems. A very late complication of PID is sepsis, which is an infection that invades the bloodstream and goes to all of the other organs, such as the heart, lungs, and kidneys. Another medical condition could develop, called Fitz-Hugh–Curtis syndrome, in which the PID infection continues to progress through the abdomen and invades the liver, placing the patient at risk of liver failure and death.

The diagnosis of PID is confirmed with collection of laboratory data from the woman's blood and cultures from her vagina or cervix. Radiological studies such as ultrasound or CT scans are not 100 percent accurate in diagnosing PID. In order to diagnose PID, a speculum exam must be performed that includes a cervical culture and wet prep, looking for vaginal discharge, sores in the vagina, odors, and a cervix that is fragile (bleeds easily). The speculum exam is followed by palpating (feeling) each ovary, the uterus, and the cervix.

PID is treated with antibiotics. Treatment for PID depends on the findings from the cervical culture and wet prep. The standard therapy is an intramuscular injection of ceftriaxone (Rocephin) or cefotetan, plus two weeks of oral doxycycline. Another antibiotic that may be used is azithromycin (Z-Pak), and there are also other medication combinations.

The best "treatment" for PID, however, is to prevent the transmission of STDs because PID is simply an extension of a typical vaginal or cervical STD that advances upward in the reproductive tract. Annual STD screening for any woman with new sexual partners since prior testing is another method of prevention, though PID can certainly progress from a "silent" STD in less than 12 months. Sexually active men and women should always use STD-protective barrier devices, like condoms, in addition to other forms of birth control, because the barrier methods are the only birth control that also protect against STDs. Early treatment at first sign of an STD is critical to avoid complications such as PID. If an STD is identified, then the individual should be treated and notify her or his sexual partners for STD testing and treatment in order to prevent further transmission.

Howard MacLennan

See also: Abdominal Diseases; Ovarian Cancer; Sexually Transmitted Diseases; Vaginal Diseases; Women's Health

Further Reading

Centers for Disease Control and Prevention. (2016). Pelvic inflammatory disease (PID) fact sheet. Retrieved from http://www.cdc.gov/std/pid/stdfact-pid.htm.

Fletcher, Kenneth, et al. (2003). Identification of symptoms that indicate a pelvic examination is necessary to exclude PID in adolescent women. *Journal of Pediatric Adolescent Gynecology, 16*(1), 25–30.

Grimes, J. A., Smith, L. A., & Fagerberg, K., eds. (2013). *Sexually Transmitted Disease: An Encyclopedia of Diseases, Prevention, Treatment, and Issues.* Santa Barbara, CA: Greenwood.

Mayo Clinic. (2016). Pelvic inflammatory disease. Retrieved from http://www.mayoclinic .org/diseases-conditions/pelvic-inflammatory-disease/basics/definition/con -20022341.

Office on Women's Health. (2016). Pelvic inflammatory disease. Retrieved from http://www .womenshealth.gov/publications/our-publications/fact-sheet/pelvic-inflammatory -disease.html.

Peipert, J., et al. (2001). Clinical predictors of endometritis in women with symptoms and signs of pelvic inflammatory disease. *American Journal of Obstetrics and Gynecology, 184*, 856–863.

PEPTIC ULCERS

Peptic ulcers are holes or open sores in the lining of the stomach or the duodenum, the upper part of the small intestine that connects to the stomach. Ulcers in the stomach are called *gastric ulcers*; those in the duodenum known as called *duodenal ulcers*, which are more common. Symptoms of both are burning pain and other gastrointestinal symptoms, and they are distinguished only by when they occur: A gastric ulcer causes pain while food is still in the stomach or shortly afterward, while pain from a duodenal ulcer takes place on an empty stomach, many hours after eating, and it may even improve after eating. Both types are commonly caused by infection with the *Helicobacter pylori* (*H. pylori*) bacterium or the frequent use of nonsteroidal anti-inflammatory drugs (NSAIDs). Treatment of ulcers is achieved with medications, lifestyle changes, and sometimes surgery.

Peptic ulcers are very common, affecting about 10 percent of the population in the United States every year. Both men and women can get peptic ulcers at any age, but rarely as children or teens. The rate of duodenal ulcers has declined for younger men, but it has increased for older women—trends thought to reflect the prevalence of *H. pylori* bacterium that can cause peptic ulcers as well as the use of painkillers in older populations.

Symptoms

Having a peptic ulcer may not produce any symptoms, but a gnawing or burning pain in the middle or upper stomach is the most common. Gastric ulcer pain occurs while food is still in the stomach or shortly afterward; duodenal ulcer pain happens on an empty stomach. Other symptoms may include bloating, heartburn, nausea, and vomiting. The symptoms of a bleeding ulcer, which is severe, can include dark or black stool, vomiting blood (that may look like coffee grounds), changes in appetite, and unintended weight loss. Symptoms may disappear and recur every few days or weeks. Bleeding from an ulcer can occur slowly, going unnoticed until it causes anemia, indicated by fatigue, shortness of breath with exercise, and pale skin color, and it can be life-threatening.

Causes and Risk Factors

Most peptic ulcers are caused by an infection with the *Helicobacter pylori,* or *H. pylori,* bacterium, which lives in the stomachs of infected people. Another common cause is long-term use of nonsteroidal anti-inflammatory medicines. Called NSAIDs, this group of medications treats pain and includes aspirin, ibuprofen, and naproxen. Stress and spicy foods, once thought to cause ulcers, can make symptoms worse.

Other risk factors that increase the likelihood of getting peptic ulcers include diseases that produce excess stomach acid; smoking or chewing tobacco; regular excessive alcohol consumption; family history of ulcers; age 50 or older; radiation treatment to the stomach; and liver, kidney, or lung disease.

Diagnosis

In addition to a physical examination and a medical and family history, diagnostic tools for peptic ulcers include blood, stool, and breath tests that check for the presence of the *H. pylori* bacterium. CT scans can show if a peptic ulcer has made a hole in the lining of the stomach or small intestine. A doctor may use an endoscopy or x-ray to locate an ulcer because symptoms for gastric and duodenal ulcers are similar. A barium x-ray, or barium swallow, provides images to help evaluate the esophagus, stomach, and duodenum. An endoscopy allows entry into these organs with an endoscope, a thin, flexible, lighted tube; a sample of tissue for a biopsy can be removed with this instrument.

Treatments

Peptic ulcers worsen without treatment, which may include medicines that reduce levels of stomach acids as well as antibiotics to fight *H. pylori* infection. Elimination of substances such as NSAIDs, tobacco, and alcohol that cause an ulcer is also key. Bleeding ulcers may be treated with endoscopy, in a procedure using an endoscope, a thin, flexible viewing instrument. Inserted through the mouth to the stomach, an endoscope can be used to stop bleeding or inject steroid medications into the tissue. Surgery may be required to repair perforations in the stomach lining or control bleeding that does not respond to an endoscopy. Once considered effective home remedies, antacids and milk cannot heal peptic ulcers.

Prevention

Diet and nutrition do not have a significant role in either causing or preventing peptic ulcers. But it may be possible to prevent them from occurring or recurring by avoiding alcohol, smoking tobacco, NSAIDs, and other substances that break down mucous membranes of the stomach lining and increase stomach acid levels. Avoiding contaminated water and foods and adhering to strict personal hygiene habits can help prevent *H. pylori* infection.

Prognosis and Outcomes

With appropriate treatment, most peptic ulcers heal, especially if medication to fight *H. pylori* bacterium is taken as prescribed. Untreated ulcers can cause severe complications, including bleeding, perforation of the intestinal wall, and obstruction due to inflammation.

Ray Marks

See also: Abdominal Diseases; Bleeding Disorders; Digestive Diseases

Further Reading

Healthline. (2013, September 9). Gastric ulcers. Retrieved from http://www.healthline.com/health/gastric-and-duodenal-ulcers#Overview1.

Mayo Clinic. (2013, July 26). Peptic ulcer. Retrieved from http://www.mayoclinic.org/diseases-conditions/peptic-ulcer/basics/definition/con-20028643.

National Institute of Diabetes and Digestive and Kidney Diseases. (2014, November 13). Peptic ulcer disease. Retrieved from http://digestive.niddk.nih.gov/ddiseases/pubs/pepticulcers_ez/.

PERICARDIAL DISORDERS/PERICARDITIS

Overview

Pericardial diseases are those that affect the pericardium or the sac that surrounds the heart. The term *pericardial disease*, or *pericarditis*, refers to the presence of inflammation of any of the layers of the pericardium. Pericarditis can be acute (occurring suddenly) or chronic (long standing). Chronic pericarditis refers to long-standing inflammation that begins gradually and results in fluid accumulation in the pericardial space around the heart or in the actual thickening of the pericardium.

Signs and Symptoms

Signs and symptom of pericarditis include chest pain, low-grade fever, and an increased heart rate. Constrictive pericarditis is a related condition to pericarditis, but it is also accompanied by:

- Shortness of breath
- Fatigue
- Heart failure symptoms such as leg (swelling, unexplained weight gain)
- Atrial fibrillation or an irregular heartbeat

Causes and Risk Factors

The cause of pericarditis is often hard to determine. In most cases, doctors are either unable to determine the cause or may suspect a viral infection is the cause.

Pericarditis can also develop shortly after a major heart attack, due to the irritation of the underlying damaged heart muscle. In addition, a delayed form of pericarditis may occur weeks after a heart attack or heart surgery because of antibody formation. This delayed form of pericarditis is known as Dressler's syndrome in which the body carries out an incorrect inflammatory response and sees its own tissues as foreign—in this case, the heart and pericardium.

Other causes of pericarditis include:

- Systemic inflammatory disorders such as lupus and rheumatoid arthritis
- Injury to the heart or chest as a result of a motor vehicle crash or another accident
- Other health disorders such as kidney failure, AIDS, tuberculosis, and cancer
- Certain medications
- Radiation exposure

Diagnostic Procedures

Diagnosis may require a medical history, a medical exam, an electrocardiogram (EKG or ECG), and a physical exam.

Other diagnostic tests used for constrictive pericarditis include:

- A chest x-ray and/or echocardiogram to view an image of the heart and its structures, and any fluid accumulation around the heart. Computerized tomography (CT) and CT scanning may also be done to rule out other causes of acute chest pain.
- Magnetic resonance imaging (MRI) might also be performed along with blood tests.

Treatment

Treatment of pericarditis is based on the cause and may include medications to reduce the inflammation and swelling associated with pericarditis. When a bacterial infection is the underlying cause of pericarditis, antibiotics and drainage may be used. Surgical procedures include pericardiocentesis, which uses a needle to remove fluid from the heart cavity, or removal of the pericardium, called a pericardiectomy.

Prognosis or Outcome

Most patients recover from pericarditis in two to four weeks.

Mild cases may improve on their own. Early diagnosis and treatment may help to reduce the risk of long-term complications.

Complications of pericarditis include constrictive pericarditis that that can lead to severe swelling of the legs and abdomen and shortness of breath. Cardiac tamponade is another complication that can occur as a result of unresolved pericarditis and can cause a sudden drop in blood pressure.

Prevention

A person with this condition should get prompt treatment and follow up the treatment as indicated to prevent complications.

Ray Marks

See also: AIDS; Cancer; Heart Diseases; Kidney Failure; Tuberculosis

Further Reading

American Heart Association. (2016). Symptoms and diagnosis of pericarditis. Retrieved from http://www.heart.org/HEARTORG/Conditions/More/Symptoms-and-Diagnosis-of-Pericarditis_UCM_444932_Article.jsp.

Cedars-Sinai. (2016). Chronic pericarditis. Retrieved from https://www.cedars-sinai.edu/Patients/Health-Conditions/Chronic-Pericarditis.aspx.

Kagan, H. L. (2014, June). Teenage heartache [case study]. *Discover, 35*(5), 26–28.

Mayo Clinic. (2011). Pericarditis. Retrieved from http://www.mayoclinic.com/health/pericarditis/DS00505/METHOD=print.

Merck Manual. (2015). Chronic pericarditis. Home Health Book. Retrieved from http://www.merckmanuals.com/home/heart-and-blood-vessel-disorders/pericardial-disease/chronic-pericarditis.

National Heart, Lung, and Blood Institute. (2012). What is pericarditis? Retrieved from https://www.nhlbi.nih.gov/health/health-topics/topics/peri.

PERIPHERAL ARTERIAL DISEASE

The term *peripheral arterial disease* refers to a health condition in which blood flow to the tissues and limbs is reduced due to the narrowing of the arteries in those areas. As result, the person with this condition experiences pain when he or she walks, and the term used to describe this pain is *intermittent claudication*. The disease affects about 8 to 10 million Americans and can occur suddenly, without any previous symptoms. Men are affected slightly more frequently than women. It is also called *atherosclerotic peripheral arterial disease, peripheral arterial disease,* or *peripheral vascular disease.*

Signs and Symptoms

Pain or cramping in the arms, feet, calves, thighs, buttock, or hip areas when walking for a long period of time is the most typical feature of the condition, which may be severe and very disabling, although some people may have no symptoms or very mild symptoms. There may also be numbness in the limbs, tiredness or weakness and/or wasting of the limb muscles, skin changes, and changes in the pulses of the limbs, which might be weakened. Nail and hair growth might be affected detrimentally as well, and wounds may heal slowly. Most of the time, the pain experienced may diminish when the person stops the activity, but in severe cases, the pain and discomfort may be present even when the person is not moving or walking.

Causes and Risk Factors

One cause of peripheral arterial disease may be related to the buildup of fatty substances or plaque in the arteries due to a disease called *atherosclerosis*. Limb injury, inflammation of the blood vessels, and exposure of the blood vessels to radiation may be additional causes.

Poor diet, being overweight, having a family history of the condition, having diabetes or high blood pressure, being over age 70, smoking, having high cholesterol, and a lack of exercise may all be risk factors for this condition.

Diagnosis

A medical history and physical exam may be conducted, plus a physical examination, including pulse testing and listening to the heart with a stethoscope. A specific test called angiography that involves injected dye into the blood vessels and scanning these with x-rays or MRI machines may be helpful. Blood tests to assess glucose levels, homocysteine, and cholesterol; treadmill tests; Duplex ultrasound tests or scans; and a test called the ankle-brachial index test can be used to compare the blood pressure in the leg to the arm.

Treatment

Managing the symptoms is important and may involve the use of medications called statins to control cholesterol levels, high blood pressure medication, diabetes medications, pain relievers, and medications to prevent blood clots. Lifestyle changes, such as giving up smoking, supervised exercise, careful foot care, and surgery may be helpful, including angioplasty surgery, bypass surgery to reroute the blood flow, amputation, and surgery to remove blood clots.

Prognosis or Outcome

Having peripheral arterial disease raises the risk for limb infection and, if this does not heal, for gangrene, which can require amputation. It also raises the risk of acquiring coronary heart disease, stroke, and reducing the blood flow to the kidneys. The disease is treatable, however, and can be managed by lifestyle adaptations and medications. In severe disease, a person may develop sores on the feet and toes, or a condition called *critical ischemia*, which is dangerous and refers to the lack of oxygen being transported to the limbs.

Prevention

Heart-healthy lifestyle changes such as eating healthy foods and maintaining a normal blood sugar level can help to prevent the condition or to reduce complications.

Future

New treatments for the condition are being sought, including the role of exercise in helping to reduce or prevent the disease.

Ray Marks

See also: Atherosclerosis; Cholesterol; Heart Diseases; Hypertension; Vascular Disorders

Further Reading

American College of Cardiology. CardioSmart. (2015). Peripheral artery disease. Retrieved from https://www.cardiosmart.org/Heart-Conditions/Peripheral-Arterial-Disease-of-the-Legs.

American Heart Foundation. (2016). Peripheral artery disease. Retrieved from http://www.heart.org/HEARTORG/Conditions/More/PeripheralArteryDisease/Peripheral-Artery-Disease-PAD_UCM_002082_SubHomePage.jsp.

Mayo Clinic. (2015). Peripheral artery disease (PAD). Retrieved from http://www.mayoclinic.com/health/peripheral-arterial-disease/DS00537.

MedlinePlus. (2015). Peripheral artery disease. Retrieved from http://www.nlm.nih.gov/medlineplus/peripheralarterialdisease.html.

National Heart, Lung and Blood Institute. (2015). What is peripheral artery disease? National Institutes of Health. Retrieved from http://www.nhlbi.nih.gov/health/health-topics/topics/pad/.

Peripheral artery disease. (2012, April). *Harvard Women's Health Watch, 19*(8), 4–6.

Society for Vascular Surgery. Vascular Web. (2010). Peripheral artery disease. Retrieved from http://www.vascularweb.org/vascularhealth/Pages/peripheral-artery-disease-(-pad-)-.aspx.

PERIPHERAL NERVE DISORDERS

Peripheral nerve disorders refer to many health conditions that affect the peripheral nervous system, or nerves that lie outside of the brain and spinal cord, and transmit messages from the brain and spinal cord to muscles and information about temperature and body or limb position to the brain and spinal cord. The problems that arise from damage or pressure on one or more nerves or nerve trunks lead to one or more of the symptoms associated with these conditions, which will vary according to the nerves involved and the severity of the problem, among other factors. Examples of the more than 100 different peripheral nerve conditions are various neuropathies, which commonly affect the arms and feet or facial areas; sciatica caused by an irritation of the sciatic nerve; brachial plexus injuries; thoracic outlet syndrome; poliomyelitis; and post-herpetic neuralgia to name a few. The problems that exist may be located on one or both sides of the body and may increase in extensiveness and severity over time, even though some forms of peripheral nerve disorders may recover over time.

Signs and Symptoms

Some typical problems that are indicative of nerve damage are temporary or permanent numbness, tingling, and sensations of discomfort, including an increased sensitivity to touch. Other problems may be related to severe burning pain, which can be unrelenting; paralysis; organ dysfunction; and muscle cramps, or the wasting and cramping of muscle. Functions including digestive functions, breathing, and keeping a safe blood pressure level may be affected by nerve damage to any of these areas. If muscles to the limbs are affected, walking, coordination, balance, and grasping may be affected as well. Changes in hair, nails, and skin can occur, as well as bone degeneration and loss of reflexes.

Causes and Risk Factors

A peripheral nerve disorder may be determined by genetic factors or hereditary factors. It can also be acquired due to injury, exposure to toxins or chemicals, alcoholism, nutritional deficiencies, tumors, exposure to radiation, diabetes, blood diseases, hormonal imbalances, chronic inflammation, infections, repetitive stress, and medications used to treat HIV/AIDS and autoimmune disorders.

Diagnosis

A medical history and a neurological examination may be used to diagnose the presence of a peripheral nerve disorder. Nerve conduction tests; electrical testing of muscle function; reflex testing; muscle strength testing; balance testing; nerve, muscle, and skin biopsies; spinal taps; and sensory nerve tests may be conducted as well. Computed tomography or magnetic resonance imaging may help to detect muscle and nerve problems. Other tests include blood tests, urine analysis tests, autonomic nervous system tests, thyroid function tests, and posture and coordination tests.

Treatment

Treatments will depend on the cause of the condition and could include efforts to protect the affected areas from trauma, along with adopting healthy lifestyle habits and specific forms of exercise. Controlling the symptoms of health conditions, such as diabetes and inflammatory diseases, and using pain medications to control pain may be helpful as well. In severe cases, anesthetic injections or surgery to alleviate severe pain and other forms of nerve-related disability may be tried. In some cases, protective mechanical devices or orthopedic aids and footwear may be helpful.

Prognosis or Outcome

Some peripheral neurological disorders are self-limiting; others are progressive. Some ongoing neuropathies can result in emotional problems and low life quality.

Prevention

Preventing further nerve injury is indicated in most cases of peripheral nerve damage. Avoiding excess alcohol and obtaining medical help for underlying health conditions is also very important. Early diagnosis can help prevent unwarranted complications.

Future

Current studies are under way to examine the genetic basis of nerve disorders and the development of new therapies to reduce the symptoms of nerve or neuropathic pain that often accompany nerve damage. Understanding how nerves are generally protected so they can function normally is also being studied more intently.

Ray Marks

See also: Alcoholism; Diabetes, Type 1; Diabetes, Type 2; Neurological Diseases; Neuropathy

Further Reading

Kuritzky, L. (2010, May). Managing diabetic peripheral neuropathic pain in primary care. *Journal of Family Practice. Diabetes Supplement, 59*(5), S15–S22.

Mayo Clinic. (2016). Neurology research: Peripheral nerve disorders. Retrieved from http://www.mayo.edu/research/departments-divisions/department-neurology/programs/peripheral-nerve-disorders.

National Institute of Neurological Disorders and Stroke. (2016). Peripheral neuropathy fact sheet. Retrieved from http://www.ninds.nih.gov/disorders/peripheralneuropathy/detail_peripheralneuropathy.htm.

PERITONEAL DISORDERS

Peritoneal disorders include anything that creates excessive fluid in the peritoneal cavity, which is located inside the abdominal cavity. Here, the *peritoneum*, a layer of tissue, lines the abdominal wall and covers most of the organs in the abdomen: the intestines, the stomach, the liver, and the ovaries in women. Lubricating the surface of this tissue is the peritoneal fluid. Disorders of this area are not common; those experienced most often include peritonitis, complications resulting from peritoneal dialysis, peritoneal cancer, and peritoneal mesothelioma, a rare but aggressive cancer.

Excess fluid that accumulates in the peritoneal cavity usually signals a peritoneal disease, causing swelling in the abdomen that can put pressure on the lungs and make breathing difficult. Infections in the fluid can spread rapidly through the bloodstream and become life-threatening. Many peritoneal diseases cause liver or kidney failure; those at most risk have liver disease or are being treated for kidney failure with peritoneal dialysis, which provides a small percentage of normal kidney function. Peritonitis is an inflammation of the peritoneum that is caused by infection from an injury, other medical condition, or a peritoneal dialysis catheter. Peritoneal mesothelioma is caused only by exposure to asbestos, a microscopic natural fiber used in construction and manufacturing. Peritoneal cancer is rare, starting in the peritoneum and affecting the surface of the organs inside the peritoneal cavity.

Symptoms

The symptoms common to peritoneal disorders, regardless of the type, are abdominal tenderness, discomfort, pain, bloating, and swelling. Peritonitis symptoms may also include fever, nausea and vomiting, fatigue, excessive thirst, poor appetite, diarrhea, constipation, passing little or no gas and only small amounts of urine, racing heart, and shortness of breath.

Peritoneal cancer symptoms are similar and may also include an unexplained weight gain or loss, rectal bleeding, or abnormal vaginal bleeding. In addition, those with peritoneal mesothelioma may experience bowel obstruction, anemia, and swelling in the legs or feet. People on peritoneal dialysis may see fluid that is cloudy or with white flecks or clumps, as well as redness or pain around the catheter.

Causes and Risk Factors

Peritonitis is caused by an infection of the fluid in the peritoneal cavity and by liver or kidney failure; those on peritoneal dialysis for kidney failure face an increased risk. The buildup of fluids may be caused by a wound or injury to the abdomen, as well as a ruptured appendix, ulcer, or perforated colon; diverticulitis, pancreatitis, cirrhosis of the liver, and Crohn's or other bowel diseases; infections in the gallbladder, intestines, or blood; pelvic inflammatory disease in women; and infections associated with dialysis catheters or feeding tubes. Those with these disorders or conditions are at higher risk of developing peritonitis.

Only those exposed to asbestos face a risk for peritoneal mesothelioma. Women, especially those who are older, are more likely to develop peritoneal cancer, particularly those at risk for ovarian cancer or who have two breast cancer genetic mutations, but it is not known what causes it.

Diagnosis

A medical history and complete physical examination, which includes pressing on a swollen abdomen, helps diagnose a peritoneal disorder. Analysis of peritoneal fluid helps diagnose the cause of fluid accumulation. For peritonitis, blood tests can also identify the infection-causing bacteria, and a CT scan or x-ray may show holes or other damage to the peritoneum. A diagnosis for those on peritoneal dialysis may be based on the appearance of the dialysis fluid.

In addition to fluid analysis, CT scans, and specific blood tests, diagnostic tools for peritoneal cancer may include ultrasounds, barium enema tests, and biopsies. Fluid analysis also diagnoses peritoneal mesothelioma when it identifies the presence of malignant cells.

Treatment

Treatment for peritoneal disorders must start promptly to avoid complications. But before treatment can begin, the underlying cause of a peritoneal disorder must be identified. Medication for pain and infection-fighting antibiotics are usually the first options for peritonitis. Surgery may be required to remove infected tissues. Those on kidney dialysis who also have peritonitis may need to stop dialysis temporarily. The accumulation of fluid may also be treated with bed rest, a low-salt diet, and diuretic drugs, which may be prescribed to help the kidneys drain excess fluid into the urine.

Chemotherapy is the most common treatment for peritoneal mesothelioma, and surgery may be an option for those diagnosed early, often accompanied by radiation therapy. Treatments for peritoneal cancer include surgery, chemotherapy, and palliative care in advanced stages.

Prevention

Once symptoms appear, getting prompt medical attention for peritonitis helps prevent the spread of infection and dangerous complications. Improved technology and training have reduced the risk of peritonitis from dialysis. Practicing hygienic techniques, including using antibiotic cream, lowers the risk.

Peritoneal mesothelioma, caused by exposure to asbestos, is only prevented by reducing any exposure to asbestos fibers. Because the cause of peritoneal cancer is not known, it is not possible to prevent its development.

Prognosis

Prognosis depends largely on the cause of the disease, its progression, and a person's overall health. Relatively recent development of improved antibiotics, aggressive intensive care, and earlier diagnosis and treatment have contributed to a significant reduction in deaths related to peritoneal disorders. Depending on its cause, peritonitis can be cured with medications and surgery, if needed. Even with the risk of infection, peritoneal dialysis is thought to improve quality of life because the procedure is done at home instead of in a dialysis center. No cure exists for peritoneal mesothelioma, and prognosis is poor, although early diagnosis and surgical intervention may add years.

Jean Kaplan Teichroew

See also: Abdominal Diseases; Kidney Diseases, Kidney Failure; Liver Diseases

Further Reading

Healthline. (2012, July 18). Peritonitis. Retrieved from http://www.healthline.com/health/peritonitis#Overview1.

Mayo Clinic. (2015, March 31). Peritonitis. Retrieved from http://www.mayoclinic.org/diseases-conditions/peritonitis/basics/definition/con-20032165.

PHENYLKETONURIA

Phenylketonuria, or PKU, is a rare genetic disorder in which the body is missing an enzyme that is necessary to break down the amino acid phenylalanine, which is in foods containing protein. This leads to a harmful buildup in the blood and tissues that results in damage to the brain and central nervous system and leads to intellectual, developmental, and behavioral delays, as well as physical abnormalities.

In the United States, it is estimated that PKU occurs in 1 of 10,000 to 15,000 newborns, most commonly in those with European or Native American ancestry. Babies must undergo a screening test when they are born in a U.S. hospital. PKU is treatable by strictly following a diet that avoids high-protein foods and aspartame, an artificial sweetener.

Symptoms

A buildup of phenylalanine takes a few months, so newborns do not show symptoms, which can range from mild to severe. But without treatment, symptoms may include intellectual disability, developmental and social delays, psychiatric illnesses, behavioral and emotional problems, and seizures and other neurological disabilities. Physical problems may include slow or stunted growth; eczema and other skin disorders; microcephaly, or an abnormally small head; a musty odor in the urine, breath, or skin as a result of the buildup of phenylalanine; and fair skin and blue eyes because the body can't transform phenylalanine into melanin, the pigment that colors hair and skin.

Causes and Risk Factors

PKU is caused by mutations in the gene that helps make the enzyme phenylalanine hydroxylase (PAH), which is necessary to convert the amino acid phenylalanine into other substances required for a healthy body. A mutated, or defective, PAH gene means the body cannot break down phenylalanine.

PKU is an inherited disorder, passed down through families. Even if both parents carry the defective gene, their child has a 25 percent chance that he or she will pass on the normal PAH gene and child will not have the disorder. There is also a 25 percent chance that both carrier parents will pass on the mutated gene, and their child will have PKU. But a child has a 50 percent chance of inheriting a normal gene from one parent and a defective gene from the other, which makes the child a carrier, too.

Diagnosis

Babies born in hospitals in all 50 states must undergo a screening test for PKU, which involves taking a few drops of blood from the heel. The blood sample is tested for too much phenylalanine.

Treatments

Treatment for PKU is a lifelong diet of low-protein foods, including special formulas for babies. The diet for older children and adults includes fruits and vegetables, as well as low-protein breads, pastas, and cereals. High-protein foods that must be avoided include dairy products, nuts, beans and legumes, most meats and fish, and beer. To provide necessary nutrients not available in their diet, all those with PKU must consume a special supplementary formula.

Prevention

As an inherited disorder, it is not possible to prevent PKU. But people with PKU can take measures to minimize its effects. In addition to following a strict diet, the artificial sweetener aspartame must be avoided; it is found in some foods, drinks, medications, and vitamins. After digestion, aspartame releases phenylalanine, raising its level in the blood. An enzyme test can determine if parents are carriers for the PKU gene, and chorionic villus sampling (CVS) during pregnancy can screen the unborn baby. Women who have PKU must follow a strict, low-phenylalanine diet before conception and throughout the pregnancy; a buildup of phenylalanine will harm a developing baby even if the fetus has not inherited the defective gene.

Prognosis or Outcome

With very careful, lifelong adherence to their diet, those with PKU can lead normal lives, and mothers who have the disorder can give birth to healthy children. Those who continue the diet into adulthood have been shown to have better physical and mental health.

Future

The U.S. Food and Drug Administration (FDA) has approved the drug sapropterin dihydrochloride, which helps some people reduce the level of phenylalanine in their blood. Alone, it does not reduce the phenylalanine enough, so it must be taken with the PKU diet. Research continues on its long-term safety and effectiveness.

Scientists and researchers are exploring new treatments for PKU, including large neutral amino acid supplementation, which may help prevent phenylalanine from entering the brain, and enzyme replacement therapy, which uses a substance similar to the enzyme that usually breaks down phenylalanine. They are also examining ways to use gene therapy, or injecting new genes to break down phenylalanine, that would decrease its level in the blood.

Ray Marks

See also: Genetics and Genomics; Metabolic Disorders; Tay-Sachs Disease; Thyroid Disorders

Further Reading

Eunice Kennedy Shriver National Institute of Child Health and Human Development. (2013, October 23). Phenylketonuria (PKU): Overview. Retrieved from http://www.nichd.nih .gov/health/topics/pku/Pages/default.aspx.

Mayo Clinic. (2014, November 26). Phenylketonuria (PKU). Retrieved from http://www .mayoclinic.org/diseases-conditions/phenylketonuria/basics/definition/con -20026275.

PHYSICAL ACTIVITY

Physical activity, important for the health and well-being of all, is defined as any body movement that uses the muscles and requires the use of more calories than when the muscles are not moving. Some examples of common everyday physical activities are walking, jogging, biking, dancing, swimming, tennis, and gardening. Physical activity can also be carried out as part of one's recreational activities, work activities, and house chore activities and does not have to be formally structured. Exercise is, however, a form of physical activity.

Physical activity is very important because research shows physical inactivity, or too little physical activity, is a leading risk factor for chronic diseases and for premature death and disability. In addition to being the key cause of many common diseases such as breast and colon cancers, diabetes, and ischemic heart disease burden, people who do very little physical activity may find it hard to regulate their weight.

On the other hand, both adults and children who regularly participate in physical activity can potentially:

- Reduce the risk of incurring high blood pressure and can reduce their risk of a heart attack, stroke, diabetes, breast and colon cancer, depression, and anxiety, as well as the risk of falls and fracturing a hip
- Improve bone, muscle, and joint health, as well as the ability to function physically
- Increase energy supply and reduce fatigue, as well as excess weight and body fat
- Increase chances of living longer
- Lower health care costs and number of doctor visits
- Promote psychological well-being and quality of life
- Promote self-esteem and academic performance in young people
- Improve teamwork, self-discipline, sportsmanship, leadership, and socialization skills

Physical activity is thus very important for preventing chronic diseases, as well as for those with chronic diseases such as asthma, Alzheimer's disease, heart disease, arthritis, diabetes, and osteoporosis. The best way to start being active is slowly. For those individuals who have health conditions, or might have to pursue careful physical activity regimens, a formal check-up by a doctor before starting is recommended. Physical activity can be pursued in the school, community, household, or the worksite. About 30 minutes of moderate physical activity five days a week is recommended, but young people should try to be active for one hour at least each day of the week. Different types of physical activity are encouraged because the benefits are additive. Choosing pleasant activities that can be carried out regularly are the best.

Ray Marks

See also: Diet and Nutrition; Family Health; Food Guides from the USDA; Genetics and Genomics; Health; Healthy Lifestyles and Risky Behaviors; Healthy People 2020; Men's Health; Prediabetes; Substance Abuse; Wellness; Women's Health

Further Reading

Centers for Disease Control and Prevention (CDC). (2015). Physical activity statistics. Retrieved from http://www.cdc.gov/physicalactivity/data/index.html.

Centers for Disease Control and Prevention (CDC). (2015). Physical activity and health. Retrieved from http://www.cdc.gov/physicalactivity/everyone/health/index.html.

Healthy People 2020. (2016). Physical activity. Retrieved from http://www.healthypeople.gov/2020/topicsobjectives2020/overview.aspx?topicid=33.

Kruk, J. (2007). Physical activity in the prevention of the most frequent chronic diseases: An analysis of the recent evidence. *Asian Pacific Journal of Cancer Prevention, 8,* 325–338.

Mayo Clinic. (2015). Exercise and chronic disease. Retrieved from http://www.mayoclinic.com/health/exercise-and-chronic-disease/MY02165.

National Heart, Lung, and Blood Institute. (2015). What is physical activity? Retrieved from http://www.nhlbi.nih.gov/health/health-topics/topics/phys/.

World Health Organization. (2016). Physical activity. Retrieved from http://www.who.int /dietphysicalactivity/pa/en/index.html.

PHYSICAL THERAPY

Physical rehabilitation and *physical therapy* are both names for a course of treatment that can help people restore or improve muscle and joint movements that have been impaired. Injuries, surgeries, and various diseases and conditions can leave muscles weakened and joints stiff. During physical rehabilitation, patients follow planned exercise programs designed to strengthen their muscles and increase their range of motion. The treatment is overseen by trained medical specialists called physical therapists.

The medical definition of *rehabilitate* is "to restore or bring to a condition of health or useful and constructive activity." The success of physical rehabilitation is hugely dependent on patient participation and cooperation. Moving injured or debilitated (weakened) muscles and joints can be painful and may require a great deal of effort. Patients must be willing to tolerate some discomfort to perform physical therapy. Those who are highly motivated to regain their mobility skills have the best outcomes. As a result, physical therapists often take on a cheerleading role to encourage and coax patients to work through the process. In the United States, physical therapists must have a master's or doctorate degree from an accredited university and be licensed in the state in which they practice. They are specialists in the biomechanical processes involved in movement.

Physical rehabilitation is typically recommended after serious injuries or surgeries involving the musculoskeletal (muscular and skeletal) system. Immediately after an injury or surgery, there is a time of rest to allow healing to begin. However, too much rest leads to deconditioning—loss of muscle tone, strength, and endurance. Unused muscles will begin to atrophy, meaning that they shrink in size and become weaker. There is also a chance that inflexible scar tissue will form at the site of an injury, rather than healthy tissue, and reduce mobility in the future. For all of these reasons, movement is considered a key part of the recovery process.

Physical therapy can benefit people who suffer damage to the nervous system, which includes the brain, spinal cord, and nerves. For example, a stroke occurs when brain cells are harmed by loss of oxygen or sudden bleeding in the brain. Patients recovering from strokes or other neurological problems can have severe movement challenges. They may have lost their kinesthetic sensitivity (or proprioception), which is awareness of the positions of the body parts and how to coordinate their movements, especially with regard to force and direction. Exercise programs tailored to improve balance and coordination can help overcome these disabilities.

Some people need physical therapy because of the damaging effects of chronic diseases. These are persistent and long-lasting diseases that cannot be cured but can be managed. Some chronic diseases, such as arthritis (joint inflammation), obesity, and diabetes, can reduce a person's range of motion over time. Supervised exercise may be incorporated into the health management regimen for these patients to enhance their mobility and reduce or slow deterioration in their movement skills.

Physicians recognize the value of physical therapy as a treatment method. The process typically begins with a physician referring a patient to a specialist trained in physical rehabilitation. With the physician's input, the physical therapist devises a treatment plan for the patient that includes both short-term and long-term goals. These goals are highly individualized and depend on the type of disability involved and the level of mobility that is physically achievable and desired by the patient. For example, injured athletes typically seek to regain the high level of functioning that is key to success in their sport. Other patients may strive to restore their everyday abilities to walk, climb stairs, or enjoy their recreational pastimes, such as jogging or playing tennis.

Physical therapy sessions may be recommended one or more times per week and last for many weeks. The total duration is based, in part, on the prognosis (predicted outcome) and selected course of treatment, but it may be limited by the patient's health insurance coverage. Physical rehabilitation sessions take place in different settings. Some hospitals and nursing homes operate onsite physical therapy centers. There are also stand-alone facilities that patients can visit. In some cases, physical therapists travel to patient's homes to conduct the sessions. This is most common for patients who lack access or transportation to a rehabilitation facility.

Exercise is the most prominent type of physical therapy. Patients may be directed through movements and stretches while standing, being seated, or lying down. One of the keys to building muscle strength is to increase the level of resistance that muscles must overcome in order to move joints. For some recovering patients, simply moving a limb against the force of gravity is difficult. Gradually, the resistance can be increased by adding stretchy exercise bands or using pulleys and weights or other apparatus to build muscle strength to the desired level. Pool exercises are another option. The buoyancy provided by the water helps relieve the pain and impact of movement on joints.

Some patients undergo physical therapy to become ambulatory—to be able to walk—or to improve their ambulatory skills. Their course of treatment often includes workouts on a set of parallel bars that provide support to the upper body while a patient concentrates on maneuvering the hips, legs, and feet. These sessions benefit muscle strength, coordination, and balance. Physical therapy facilities often include other aids, such as practice stairs, on which patients can exercise and train for mobility challenges that they encounter in everyday life. Various types of exercise equipment, such as stationary bicycles or treadmills, may also be used.

Physical therapists may provide manual assistance during exercise, for example, by supporting a limb as a patient moves or stretches it. Assistance is especially needed when a patient is reluctant to move for fear of injury. Physical therapists know the range of motion that is safely achievable and desirable for the best outcomes. They can manually assist in these movements and in those patients find painful but are willing to do with gentle help. Even patients unable to move their limbs on their own benefit from exercise therapy. Physical therapists can manually manipulate muscle groups, for example, by bending the arms or legs back and forth. This is called passive therapy because the patient does not actively participate in the exercise.

Physical rehabilitation sessions can also include massages and heat or cold treatments. The purpose is to increase blood circulation to muscles and other tissues and reduce pain, stiffness, inflammation, swelling, and muscle spasms. Whirlpool bath soaks combine massage and heat application. Another physical therapy modality (method) is the therapeutic use of electrical stimulation for pain relief and other purposes. Very mild electrical currents cause muscles to contract, basically forcing them to exercise. This helps prevent atrophy and can build muscle strength and subsequently improve joint range of motion.

Some high-tech tools for diagnosing and treating musculoskeletal disabilities have emerged in the field of physical rehabilitation. Electronic sensors placed on a patient's body and on the floor can collect data about muscle and joint movements and measure the forces exerted on the floor as the person walks. Reflective body markers can also be used with specialized cameras that record detailed information about how a person moves during various activities. Computer and robotics technology is also being incorporated into aids that physical therapists use to help patients regain or improve muscle manipulation and coordination. For example, a small, sensor-equipped device with a video screen can be strapped to a patient's hand to allow him or her to play interactive "video games" specially designed to work hand and finger muscles.

Kim Masters-Evans

See also: Carpal Tunnel Syndrome; Charcot-Marie-Tooth Disorder; Inflammation; Stroke

Further Reading

American Physical Therapy Association. (2016). The role of a physical therapist. Retrieved from http://www.apta.org/PTCareers/RoleofaPT/.

Cleveland Clinic: Diseases & Conditions. (2016). What can physical therapy do for your back & neck pain? Retrieved from https://my.clevelandclinic.org/health/diseases_conditions/hic_your_back_and_neck/hic_What_Can_Physical_Therapy_Do_For_Your_Back_and_Neck_Pain.

Kujala, U. M. (January 2006). Benefits of exercise therapy for chronic diseases. *British Journal of Sports Medicine, 40*(1), 3–4.

Pacifica Orthopedics. (2015). The importance of rehabilitation after orthopedic surgery. Retrieved from http://www.pacificaorthopedics.org/wp10/orthopedics/the-importance-of-rehabilitation-after-orthopedic-surgery/.

Vickery, S., & Moffat, M. (1999). *The American Physical Therapy Association Book of Body Maintenance and Repair: Hundreds of Stretches and Exercises for Every Part of the Human Body*. New York: Holt Paperbacks.

PITUITARY DISORDERS

The pituitary gland is a small gland located in the region of the brain near the base of the skull. It is an endocrine gland that regulates all other endocrine glands in the body. There are many problems that arise when the pituitary gland functions abnormally, including acromegaly (where bone growth is abnormally affected), Type 1 diabetes, Cushing's syndrome, reproductive problems, and pituitary tumors—the most common problem. Some disorders are caused by too little hormone secretion, while others are caused by excessive hormone secretion. Symptoms may also occur if there is pressure placed in the pituitary gland by surrounding structures of the brain or trauma. Anyone, at any age, can be affected.

Signs and Symptoms

The signs and symptoms may depend on the cause of the problem and the target endocrine gland affected.

Causes and Diagnosis

There are three possible causes of pituitary symptoms. First, a tumor could cause the pituitary gland to secrete an excess amount of a particular hormone. Second, a tumor near the gland could press on the gland and cause it to secrete an excess amount of pituitary hormones. Finally, in addition to trauma, a tumor near the gland can press on nerves responsible for vision or eye movement.

Diagnosis includes various lab tests to measure the presence of certain hormones as well as brain imaging through CT and MRI procedures.

Treatment and Prognosis

Although most pituitary tumors are not malignant, surgery may be carried out to remove these if they are producing adverse, long-term health effects. In other cases, medications or radiation therapy may be sufficient to minimize the symptoms. For hormonal disorders, medications are prescribed.

Prognosis for those with these disorders depends on the type of disorder. Most pituitary tumors are non-life-threatening in themselves.

Ray Marks

See also: Diabetes, Type 1

Further Reading

Hormone Health Network. (2013). Pituitary disorders. Retrieved from http://www.hormone .org/diseases-and-conditions/pituitary.

Mayo Clinic. (2015). Pituitary tumors. Retrieved from http://www.mayoclinic.org/diseases -conditions/pituitary-tumors/home/ovc-20157627.

The pituitary patient resource guide, revised 4th ed. (2007). Thousand Oaks, CA: Pituitary Network Association.

University of California San Francisco Medical Center. (2010). Interview with Dr. Lewis Blevins: Pituitary disorders. Retrieved from http://www.ucsfhealth.org/education /interview_blevins_pituitary_disorders/.

PLATELET DISORDERS

Platelets form an important constituent of blood. Disorders of platelets are relatively rare, and when they do occur, they may be mild and include various medical disorders that either affect the development of platelets or the production of platelets. These disorders, which can occur at any age, may result in excess bleeding because the blood fails to coagulate. Examples of these conditions are thrombocytopenia, where the number of platelets in the blood is lower than it should be normally; adhesion blood platelet disorders, where platelets are unable to clump together; and Scott syndrome, where blood clotting is disturbed.

Signs and Symptoms

Common symptoms of platelet dysfunction include bleeding gums, bleeding in the joints, nose bleeds, bruising, and defective wound healing.

Causes and Risk Factors

Some causes include failure of the bone marrow to make enough platelets or if the body destroys or uses platelets at an excessive rate (despite normal rates of production), if the spleen retains too many platelets, or a combination of these factors. Direct causes may include certain autoimmune disorders, bone marrow cancers, infections, and drugs such as aspirin. Other causes are deficiencies of certain B vitamins, chronic alcoholism, various genetic defects, chemotherapy, and radiation therapy.

Diagnosis

Diagnostic procedures include a physical examination and laboratory analysis of the blood and bone marrow samples. Imaging studies, bone marrow examinations, platelet aggregation tests, and tests of bleeding time are also used in this regard.

Treatment and Outcome

Treatment may involve steroid therapy, splenectomy, and selected medications and depends on the platelet count and extent of any bleeding. Patients may have to avoid use of drugs that affect platelet production. In serious cases, transfusions of platelets may be required.

Severe bleeding can prove fatal.

Prevention

There are no known forms of preventing these disorders.

Ray Marks

See also: Alcoholism; Bleeding Disorders

Further Reading

WebMD. (2014). Bleeding or Clotting Disorders That Cause Bruising. Retrieved from http://
    www.webmd.com/skin-problems-and-treatments/bleeding-or-clotting-disorders-that
    -cause-bruising.
Margolis, S. (2011). Platelet function disorders. *John Hopkins Symptoms and Remedies: The
    Complete Home Medical Reference.* HealthCommunities.com. Retrieved from http://www
    .healthcommunities.com/blood-disorders/platelet-function-disorders.shtml.
MedlinePlus. (2016, August 30). Platelet disorders. Retrieved from http://www.nlm.nih.gov
    /medlineplus/plateletdisorders.html.

PLEURAL DISORDERS

The pleura is a membrane that consists of two large, thin layers of tissue covering the lungs and inside of the chest cavity.

Between the layers of tissue is a very thin space called the *pleural space*. Normally, this space is filled with a small amount of fluid. Many diseases affect the pleura in children and adults such as pneumonia, cancer, and heart disease.

Pleurisy occurs if the two layers of the pleura become irritated and inflamed. Instead of gliding smoothly past each other, they rub together every time a breath is taken, causing sharp pain.

Many conditions can cause pleurisy, including viral infections.

Other pleural disorders include:

Pneumothorax occurs as a result of air or gas building up in the pleural space due to a lung disease or injury.

Pleural effusion is when excess fluid builds up in the pleural space making it hard to breathe. This extra fluid can get infected and turn into an abscess or empyema. It may be caused by heart disease, pneumonia, liver disease, and cancer.

Hemothorax occurs when blood builds up in the pleural space; it can put pressure on the lung and cause it to collapse.

Symptoms and Causes

General symptoms of pleural disorders include a cough, shortness of breath, and fever. Diseases, injuries, and exposure to asbestos can increase the risk for pleural disorders.

Diagnosis

A physical exam, a pleural fluid test, chest x-rays, and various scanning devices and laboratory tests may be used for diagnosis.

Treatment

Treating the medical condition may be helpful. Medications and drainage of the lung in the presence of pleural effusion may be helpful.

Prognosis

Pleurisy and other pleural disorders can be serious, depending on their causes. If the condition that caused the pleurisy or other pleural disorder isn't too serious and is diagnosed and treated early, a full recovery can be expected.

Prevention

Because there are many causes, it is uncertain how to prevent pleural disorders. Preventing injury, tuberculosis, and asbestos exposure may be helpful, however.

Ray Marks

See also: Cancer; Heart Diseases; Liver Diseases; Lung Diseases; Pneumonia

Further Reading

American Thoracic Society. (2014). Pleural disease. Retrieved from http://thoracic.org /education/breathing-in-america/resources/chapter-14-pleural-disease.pdf.

MedlinePlus. (2014). Pleural disorders. Retrieved from http://www.nlm.nih.gov/medlineplus /pleuraldisorders.html.

National Heart Blood and Lung Institute. (2011). What are pleurisy and pleural disorders? Retrieved from http://www.nhlbi.nih.gov/health/health-topics/topics/pleurisy/.

PNEUMONIA

The term *pneumonia* refers to the presence of a lung infection that inflames the air sacs of one or both lungs. It can occur among older adults, as well as in children and babies, either alone or in combination with a chronic illness. It can be mild to life-threatening in severity and can prevent the required level of oxygen from circulating in the body. Pneumonia can be chronic and recurring in both adults and children.

Symptoms

Symptoms of pneumonia include coughing, fever, and having a hard time breathing. Sweating, as well as chills, may be present, as may chest pain, headaches, muscle pain, fatigue, nausea, and vomiting.

Causes and Risk Factors

Pneumonia is commonly caused by viruses, bacteria, or fungi. Chronic diseases, a weaker immune system, being of older age, being a smoker, and being exposed to viruses in either the hospital or community are common risk factors.

Diagnosis

Radiographs, physical examinations, and blood tests, along with the history of the patient, may be used to arrive at a diagnosis. Other tests include the use of a pleural fluid culture or a sputum test to sample the fluid from the lungs to pinpoint the infection type and a test method called pulse oximetry to measure blood oxygen levels. Bronchoscopy via the throat can be used to try to view the lung through a long thin tube with camera at the end to envision the cause of the problem.

Treatments

Treatment may occur at home or in a hospital and will depend on the cause of the problem and its severity. Antiviral drugs and antibiotics may be used. Fever reducers and cough medicine may be helpful.

Prognosis

Pneumonia is usually treatable and can resolve in two to three weeks. This depends on the underlying health status of the patient, however, and whether prompt treatment was received. Pneumonia can be a serious and life-threatening, though, in the elderly as well as in children and those with serious medical problems, such as chronic obstructive airways disease, diabetes, heart disease, and certain cancers.

High-risk groups such as the elderly may also acquire:

- Bacteremia or bacteria in the bloodstream; these bacteria can spread the infection to other organs, possibly resulting in organ failure
- A lung abscess
- A pleural effusion or a collection of fluid around the lungs
- Breathing difficulties

Prevention

Getting vaccinated against pneumococcal pneumonia for those at high risk of getting pneumonia is useful. According to the Centers for Disease Control and Prevention (CDC), pneumococcal conjugate vaccine (PCV13) is recommended for all children younger than five years old, all adults 65 years or older, and people six years or older with certain risk factors. Pneumococcal polysaccharide vaccine (PPSV23) is recommended for all adults 65 years or older. People 2 through 64 years old who are at high risk of pneumococcal disease should also receive PPSV23. (CDC 2015). Not smoking, eating well, and washing one's hands frequently is helpful as well.

Ray Marks

See also: Legionnaires' Disease; Lung Cancer; Lung Diseases; Pleural Disorders; Pollution; Respiratory Diseases; Secondhand Smoke; Tobacco Addiction; Whooping Cough

Further Reading

American Lung Association. (2016). Pneumonia. Retrieved from http://www.lung.org/lung
-disease/pneumonia/.

Be alert to pneumonia this winter. (2015, January) *Harvard Women's Health Watch*, 22(5), 6.

Centers for Disease Control and Prevention. (2015). Pneumococcal vaccination. Retrieved
from http://www.cdc.gov/vaccines/vpd-vac/pneumo/default.htm?s_cid=cs_797.

Mayo Clinic. (2015). Pneumonia. Retrieved from http://www.mayoclinic.org/diseases
-conditions/pneumonia/basics/definition/CON-20020032.

PNEUMOTHORAX

A *pneumothorax*, or a collapsed lung, refers to a collection of air in the chest that causes the lung to collapse. This problem arises when air leaks into the space between the lungs and chest wall and the air pushes on the outside of the lung and makes the whole lung or, more commonly, only a portion of the lung collapse.

Types

A pneumothorax that occurs spontaneously is called a primary pneumothorax, and this occurs in the absence of any trauma to the chest or any existing lung disease. A secondary pneumothorax is the situation that occurs as a consequence of an underlying condition.

Symptoms

Common symptoms of a pneumothorax are the presence of sudden chest pain and shortness of breath.

Causes and Risk Factors

Common causes of a pneumothorax are chest injuries that are blunt or penetrating, certain medical procedures involving the lungs, as well as damage from an underlying chronic disease. They may also occur for no obvious reason. They can arise as a result of ruptured air blisters on the surface of the lung because, if these burst, air may leak into the space surrounding the lungs. Sometimes, the inappropriate use of a mechanical ventilator can produce a pneumothorax. Common risk factors are being a male, being a smoker, being between 20 and 40 years of age with air blisters, as well as being very tall and thin.

- Genetics and lung diseases, especially chronic obstructive pulmonary disease make a collapsed lung more likely.
- People who need mechanical ventilation to assist their breathing are at higher risk of pneumothorax.
- A history of pneumothorax places one at increased risk of another, usually within one to two years of the first episode.

Diagnosis

A diagnosis usually involves a chest x-ray or computerized tomography (CT) scan or a combination of CT scans with x-ray images from different angles.

Treatments

If only a small portion of the lung collapses, the doctor may simply monitor the condition with a series of chest x-rays. The recovery process normally takes a week or two, and supplemental oxygen may be used to speed up the absorption process. If a large area of the lung has collapsed, a flexible needle or tube or syringe may be inserted into the chest wall to help get rid of the excess air from the chest cavity. If all this fails, surgery may be attempted.

Prognosis

Many people who experience one pneumothorax experience another, usually within one to two years of the first. Air may sometimes continue to leak if the opening in the lung will not close. However, a small, uncomplicated pneumothorax may heal quickly on its own.

Ray Marks

See also: COPD (Chronic Obstructive Pulmonary Disease); Lung Diseases; Men's Health; Tobacco Addiction

Further Reading

Mayo Clinic. (2014). Pneumothorax. Retrieved from http://www.mayoclinic.org/diseases-conditions/pneumothorax/basics/definition/con-20030025.
MedlinePlus. (2014). Collapsed lung (pneumothorax). Retrieved from https://www.nlm.nih.gov/medlineplus/ency/article/000087.htm.

POLIO AND POST-POLIO SYNDROME

Polio, often called *poliomyelitis*, is a highly contagious illness spread by the poliovirus, and it primarily affects children under five years old. The virus can attack the body's nervous system and cause diminished use of limbs, paralysis, difficulty breathing, and occasionally death. The virus is transmitted from person to person, where it multiplies in the throat and intestines. Polio appears as asymptomatic (no symptoms) or as symptomatic in three forms: abortive, a mild form; nonparalytic polio, associated with neurological symptoms; and the severe form known as paralytic polio.

Most people (about 70 percent) are infected with the asymptomatic form of virus and do not exhibit symptoms. But for the one in four who contract symptomatic polio, the symptoms can include fever, sore throat, fatigue, headache, diarrhea, vomiting, stiff neck, and pain in the limbs. About 1 in 200 infections may result in irreversible paralysis, usually the legs. There is no cure for polio, and treatment focuses on managing symptoms. Polio has been eliminated in the United States; about 99 percent of children who receive the vaccine are protected. Those who have not been vaccinated are at greatest risk of contracting the disease.

Those who recover from polio are at risk of developing post-polio syndrome, or PPS, decades later. They may slowly experience progressive weakening in the muscles that were originally affected, as well as joint pain followed by long periods of stability. PPS is not contagious: Survivors of polio are the only ones at risk of developing it.

History

Today's widely used polio vaccine became available in 1955. During the last polio epidemic in the United States in 1952, nearly 60,000 cases were reported, including more than 3,000 deaths. Thanks to the vaccine, polio was eliminated in the United States by 1979 and in the Western hemisphere by 1991. Global efforts to eradicate the virus have reduced the incidence of the disease by more than 99 percent since 1988, down from an estimated 350,000 cases to 416 in 2013. By 2014, Afghanistan, Nigeria, and Pakistan were the only countries in which polio reached epidemic levels.

During the last polio epidemic, one standard treatment for a person with paralysis of breathing muscles was placement in an iron lung, a machine that pushed and pulled the chest muscles as artificial respiration. Today smaller, more portable ventilators are used when necessary.

Symptoms

Most people who contract the poliovirus have no symptoms and may not realize they are infected. Some people contract abortive polio or nonparalytic polio, and symptoms may be similar to a mild case of the flu or other viral illnesses, such as fever, sore throat, headache, vomiting, or fatigue; pain or stiffness in the neck, back, arms, or legs; muscle weakness; and meningitis. Symptoms may last up to 10 days.

Forms of the rare paralytic polio are based on the affected area of the body: spinal cord (spinal polio), brainstem (bulbar polio), or both (bulbospinal polio). At first, symptoms may be similar to nonparalytic polio, but they usually progress to include loss of reflexes, severe muscle weakness or ache, and limbs that become floppy or loose. The onset of paralysis may occur suddenly.

For those who develop PPS, common symptoms may include problems breathing or swallowing; a decreased tolerance of cold; muscle atrophy; pain, general fatigue, and exhaustion after minimal activity; progressive weakness in muscles or joints; and sleep apnea and other sleep-related breathing disorders.

Causes and Risk Factors

The highly contagious poliovirus lives in humans, usually entering the environment in the feces of an infected person. It spreads in areas where sanitation is inadequate, most often by ingestion of water contaminated by an infected person. The droplets from an infected person's sneezes or coughs may also transmit it. Infected people can also contaminate food and water if they do not wash their hands. Those who are not immunized are highly susceptible to contracting the virus. Additional risk factors may include traveling to places where polio is active, living with an infected person, and working in a laboratory containing live poliovirus.

Diagnosis

A physical examination can establish the presence of polio symptoms. A diagnosis can be confirmed with a sample of throat secretions, stool, or cerebrospinal fluid (fluid surrounding the brain and spinal cord) that shows the presence of the poliovirus.

Treatments

There is no cure for polio or treatment to reverse its effects. Treatments focus on managing symptoms, increasing comfort, and preventing further complications, which may include pain relievers, bed rest, drinking fluids, ventilators to assist breathing, modest exercise to prevent deformity and loss of muscle function, and a nutritious diet.

Although there are no medications that can stop or reverse the effects of PPS, strategies recommended to manage symptoms include exercise to improve muscle strength and reduce fatigue; getting treatment for neuromuscular disorders; utilizing mobility aids, ventilation equipment, and lifestyle changes to avoid rapid muscle tiring and exhaustion; and avoiding activities that cause pain or fatigue lasting for more than 10 minutes.

Prevention

The only effective way to prevent contracting the disease is to receive a polio vaccine, which can protect a child for life. The recommendation for children in the United States is four doses of inactivated polio vaccination (IPV) between the ages of two months and six years old. It is also recommended that adults who travel to countries where polio is active make sure they have completed the recommended vaccine series and have received a single lifetime IPV booster dose. It is not possible to prevent post-polio syndrome, or PPS, after recovering from polio.

Prognosis and Outcomes

Many people with nonparalytic polio can fully recover, but those with paralytic polio usually live with permanent paralysis, as well as deformities of the hips, ankles, and feet. Although many deformities can be corrected with surgery and physical therapy, these treatments may not be options in the countries where polio is still prevalent. As a result, children who survive polio may encounter lifelong disabilities.

An individual's prognosis for PPS depends on the severity of the original illness. Those who had minimal symptoms will likely experience mild PPS; those who have been left with more severe weakness may experience greater muscle deterioration and fatigue, as well as difficulty swallowing.

Future

The Global Polio Eradication Initiative—a public–private partnership led by national governments and the World Health Organization (WHO), Rotary International, the U.S. Centers for Disease Control and Prevention (CDC), and the United Nations Children's Fund (UNICEF)—has set the goal of eradicating polio everywhere in the world. Since its launch in 1988, more than 2.5 billion children have been immunized, and the number of cases has been reduced by more than 99 percent.

To help people with post-polio syndrome, scientists are investigating how motor neurons behave in those affected, as well as working to discover how the brain, nerves, muscles, and the junction of nerve cells and muscles affect fatigue. Researchers have discovered an immunological response, or inflammation, around motor neurons and muscles in those affected by PPS and are examining its causes.

Ray Marks

See also: Neurological Diseases; Neuromuscular Disorders; Swallowing Disorders; Vaccines

Further Reading

Centers for Disease Control and Prevention. (2015, September 2). Global health—polio. Retrieved from http://www.cdc.gov/polio/.

Halstead, L. S. (2015). *Managing Post-Polio: A Guide to Living and Aging Well with Post-Polio Syndrome.* Washington, DC: MedStar NRH Press.

KidsHealth (2014). Polio. (2015). Retrieved from http://kidshealth.org/parent/infections /bacterial_viral/polio.html.

Mayo Clinic. (2015). Polio. Retrieved from http://www.mayoclinic.org/diseases-conditions /polio/basics/definition/con-20030957.

National Institute of Neurological Disorders and Stroke. (2015, February 23). Post-polio syndrome fact sheet. Retrieved from http://www.ninds.nih.gov/disorders/post_polio /detail_post_polio.htm.

World Health Organization. (2015). Poliomyelitis. Retrieved from http://www.who.int /mediacentre/factsheets/fs114/en/.

POLLUTION

Pollution refers to substances in the environment that affect health. Examples are air pollution, including smog and radiation; industrial toxins; and secondhand smoke, which is an important risk factor among children for both acute and chronic respiratory disease, such as asthma, chronic obstructive pulmonary disease, and lung cancer in adults. Other types of air pollution can be caused by

- Industrial exhausts
- Home heating
- Open fires
- Machines
- Chemicals

According to the World Health Organization (2014), indoor air pollution is responsible for 2 million deaths annually. Air pollution can also cause allergies, as can acid rain, and human waste and nuclear radiation can cause cancer. According to Gammon (2012), pollution affects more than 100 million people worldwide. In some of the world's most polluted places, babies are born with birth defects, children lose 30 to 40 IQ points, and life expectancy may be as low as 45 years of age.

Other forms of pollution that affect health are water pollution due to toxic substances or chemicals or other types of harmful pollutants. Noise, pesticides, soil, light, and heat pollutants can also cause health-related issues if a person is excessively or repeatedly exposed. Exposure to lead through the air or from food, paint, water, soil, or dust can affect the kidneys, liver, nervous system, and other organs.

Excessive exposure to lead may cause anemia, reproductive disorders, and neurological impairments such as seizures, mental retardation, or behavioral disorders (U.S. Environmental Protection Agency 2015). A study by the University of Rochester showed that exposure early in life to air pollution may lead to changes in the brain associated with autism and schizophrenia (Allen et al. 2014).

Some other examples of health effects of pollution include

Headache
Fatigue
Nerve damage
Respiratory illness
Cardiovascular illness
Gastroenteritis
Cancer
Nausea
Skin disorders

Maintaining a clean environment and using nontoxic products is key to preventing chronic health problems attributable to pollutants.

Other solutions are

- Community programs
- Improving standards, policies, and laws that enforce these solutions
- Surveillance
- Agency enforcement from the Environmental Protection Agency
- Recycling

Ray Marks

See also: COPD (Chronic Obstructive Pulmonary Disease); Emphysema; Lung Cancer; Lung Diseases; Pneumonia; Secondhand Smoke; Tobacco Addiction

Further Reading

Allen, J. L., Liu, X., Pelkowski, S., Palmer, B., Conrad, K., Oberdörster, G., Weston, D., Mayer-Pröschel, M., & Cory-Slechta, D. A. (2014). Early postnatal exposure to ultrafine particulate matter air pollution: persistent ventriculomegaly, neurochemical disruption, and glial activation preferentially in male mice. *Environ Health Perspectives, 122,* 939–945. doi:http://dx.doi.org/10.1289/ehp.1307984.

Gammon, K. (2012). Types of pollution. *Live Science.* Retrieved from http://www.livescience .com/22728-pollution-facts.html.

Physicians for Social Responsibility. (2012). How air pollution contributes to lung disease. Retrieved from http://www.psr.org/assets/pdfs/air-pollution-effects-respiratory.pdf.

U.S. Environmental Protection Agency (EPA). (2015). Air pollution and health risk. Retrieved from http://www3.epa.gov/airtoxics/3_90_022.html.

World Health Organization. (2014). Air pollution. Retrieved from http://www.who.int/ceh /risks/cehair/en/.

POLYMYOSITIS

Polymyositis is a chronic inflammatory muscle disease with no known cause that causes varying degrees of symmetrical weakness of the muscles located close to the trunk or torso that control movement. The condition begins when white blood cells associated with inflammatory processes start to invade selected muscles, and it is characterized by increased levels of certain muscle enzymes, changes in the electrical responses of the muscle during movements, and periods of flare-up coupled with periods of remission. The term *polymyositis* is derived from several Greek words including *myo*, meaning muscle, *itis*, meaning inflammation, and *poly*, meaning many.

People with polymyositis commonly experience varying degrees of inflammation and degeneration of their muscles, as well as progressive atrophy or wasting of their affected muscles as the disease progresses. The muscles most commonly affected are those of the hips, shoulders, arms, and the front of the throat and neck. The disease is rare, and in the United States, African Americans are more likely to suffer than whites, adults 45 to 60 years of age are more likely to be affected than younger adults or children, and women are more likely to be affected than men. Polymyositis can occur on its own as well as in association with other inflammatory collagen vascular diseases, and it is accompanied by a skin rash it is called *dermatomyositis*. It is referred to as a systemic disease because it can also affect other areas of the body and is associated, on occasion, with cancer. Medically, polymyositis is classified as a chronic inflammatory myopathy, where weakness is the main feature. Older patients have a greater chance of worse outcomes than those who are younger; those who are not on cortisone treatment do worse than those who are; and those with cancer, swallowing difficulties, or lung or heart disease do more poorly than those without these conditions.

Symptoms

The signs and symptoms of polymyositis appear gradually on both sides of the body, and may fluctuate from week to week or month to month. These signs and symptoms differ in each affected person and may include rapid or slowly developing progressive muscle weakness, swallowing difficulties (dysphagia), speaking difficulties, involvement of the heart, inflammation of the covering of the heart or pericardium, inflammation of the heart muscle, mild joint or muscle tenderness, muscle pain, shortness of breath, and fatigue, which worsens over time. Later on, functional activities such as climbing stairs, rising from a seated position, lifting objects, or reaching overhead may be very challenging to carry out. If the skin is involved, the area around the eyes has a violet appearance and looks swollen; there may be reddish scales over the areas of the knuckles, elbows, and knees; and a rash may be located on the face, neck, or upper chest.

Other symptoms may include anorexia, fever, morning stiffness, weight loss, and pharyngeal and esophageal muscle weakness causing aspiration pneumonia.

Health problems that may accompany polymyositis include interstitial lung disease, interstitial pneumonitis, bronchiolitis obliterans organizing pneumonia, pulmonary capillaritis, nasal regurgitation, abdominal bloating, constipation, Raynaud's phenomenon, and inclusion body myositis.

Key Causes and Risk Factors

There is no known cause for polymyositis. A heredity or genetic susceptibility may occur in some cases. An infection by an unknown virus resistant to treatment may be the cause of inclusion body myositis. Other related causes may be the presence of defective cellular immunity associated with other systemic autoimmune diseases, or malignancies, or connective-tissue disorders.

Several drugs—such as D-penicillamine, hydralazine, procainamide, phenytoin, and angiotensin-converting enzyme (ACE) inhibitors—can cause an immune-mediated myopathy or myositis as well. Excess or continuous statin consumption has also been investigated as a possible cause of severe muscle inflammation and other muscle disorders.

Diagnosis

A medical examination plus a clinical history will suggest if more detailed tests are required. Some tests that may be used are measures of strength of the muscles closest to the trunk; blood tests to assess the presence of abnormal amounts of muscle enzymes; inflammation, electromyographic recordings, or electrical muscle recordings; magnetic resonance imaging; and a muscle biopsy. Other routine blood and urine tests can be used to detect internal organ abnormalities.

A blood test that can detect specific autoantibodies associated with different polymyositis symptoms may be helpful.

Treatment

Initially, polymyositis may be treated with high doses of corticosteroids given by mouth or intravenously to decrease the muscle inflammation. These are usually required for years, even though their continued use may increase the patient's appetite and weight, produce facial puffiness, and lead to easy bruising. These medications suppress the immune system, thus limiting the production of antibodies and reducing muscle inflammation, as well as improving muscle strength and function.

They can however, also cause sweating, facial-hair growth, an upset stomach, emotional volatility, leg swelling, acne, severe bone damage, cataracts, osteoporosis, high blood pressure, worsening of diabetes, and an increased infection risk.

If they do not work, immunosuppressive medications such as methotrexate and azathioprine (Imuran) may be considered. Cyclophosphamide (Cytoxan), chlorambucil (Leukeran), and cyclosporine (Sandimmune) have also been used for treating serious disease complications, such as the scarring of the lungs (pulmonary fibrosis). These can also have severe side effects.

Biological therapies for severe cases, speech therapy, diet therapy, and physical therapy with gradual muscle strengthening may be used.

Prognosis and Future

The outcome for patients with polymyositis varies, but patients can do well with the introduction of early medical treatment and with exercise and monitoring for side effects of drugs and the presence of cancer, heart, and/or lung disease, although some weakness may persist. Osteoporosis, a common complication of long-term corticosteroid therapy, may cause significant problems, however.

There is no form of prevention for polymyositis because the precise causes of polymyositis are still unknown.

Ray Marks

See also: Swallowing Disorders; Vascular Disorders

Further Reading

Arthritis Foundation. (2013). Polymyositis. Retrieved from http://www.arthritis.org/about -arthritis/types/myositis/.

Ballard, C. (2012, February 13.) Man in full. *Sports Illustrated, 116*(6), 58–67.

Mayo Clinic. (2015). Polymyositis. Retrieved from http://www.mayoclinic.com/health /polymyositis/DS00334.

Myositis Association. (2015). Myositis. Retrieved from http://www.myositis.org/learn-about -myositis/types-of-myositis/polymyositis.

POVERTY

Poverty is a major risk factor for chronic disease. Studies reveal that people living in poverty are at increased risk for numerous chronic health problems, including both physical and psychological problems. They are also more likely to die prematurely than wealthier people. Chronic diseases are the major cause of death in most countries.

U.S. Data

A wide-ranging, in-depth report about the association between income and health in the United States was published by the renowned Gallup data-analysis organization (Brown 2012). The report was based on 288,000 telephone interviews with adults across the United States during 2011.

Among all the diseases covered in the Gallup report, depression had the greatest gap in prevalence between those in poverty and those not in poverty. About 31 percent of adults in poverty said they had been diagnosed as having clinical depression, compared with about 16 percent of adults not in poverty. Asthma and obesity also showed large gaps, with 17 percent of adults in poverty having asthma and 32 percent being obese, compared with 11 percent and 26 percent, respectively, for adults not in poverty. Other conditions that occurred at significantly higher rates among people in poverty versus people not in poverty included diabetes (15 versus 10 percent), heart attacks (6 versus 4 percent), and high blood pressure (32 versus 29 percent).

Lifestyle and Access to Health Care

There are multiple lifestyle reasons for the discrepancies in health between Americans in poverty and those not in poverty. Poor Americans tend to have unhealthier diets, eating more fatty, sugary foods and fewer fruits and vegetables. Part of the explanation for dietary differences may be differences in education regarding what constitutes a healthy diet. However, another part of the explanation concerns availability. In the Gallup report, 16 percent of people in poverty said that affordable fresh fruits and vegetables were not readily available to them, compared with only 8 percent of people not in poverty.

In addition, poor people smoke at a much higher rate than wealthier people—33 versus 20 percent, according to the Gallup report. Poor people also tend to exercise less frequently than wealthier people. The Gallup report noted that one reason for the exercise difference might be that people living in poverty and in dangerous neighborhoods might not have access to safe, nearby places to exercise.

These lifestyle factors are important contributors to obesity, cardiovascular disease, diabetes, certain cancers, and other chronic health problems.

Regarding the high rates of clinical depression among poor Americans, the authors of the Gallup report noted that depression could be both a consequence of poverty and a contributor to poverty. Moreover, chronic depression is a known contributor to various physical illnesses.

Fewer poor Americans have access to good health care than wealthier Americans. Although the Patient Protection and Affordable Care Act ("Obamacare") of 2010 made it possible for millions of poor people to obtain health insurance, about 30 million Americans remained without health insurance as of 2015. Uninsured rates are highest within the Hispanic and African American populations. The ever-increasing costs of insurance premiums and deductibles make it difficult for many of these people to gain access to adequate health care. Thus, poor people are less likely to receive proper health care to prevent disease, to treat disease when it develops, and to treat complications of disease.

International Issues

The reasons for high rates of chronic disease among poor people in the United States and other wealthy, industrialized, Western nations are not necessarily the same as the reasons for chronic disease among poor people in less-industrialized countries. Dietary issues, in particular, may differ in wealthy Western nations compared with poor nations in Africa, southern Asia, and parts of South America. In wealthy nations, poor people commonly have easy access to fatty fast-food outlets, but they may have trouble finding fresh fruits and vegetables. By contrast, many poor people in poorer nations may have trouble finding any sustainable food on a regular basis. Thus, malnutrition is a common cause of health problems in those countries.

In addition, many poor, developing nations have major problems of environmental pollution and lack of clean, safe drinking water, putting their populations at high risk of exposure to toxic chemicals and microbial contaminants. Furthermore, impoverished people in poor nations typically have extremely limited access to modern health care and medications.

The World Health Organization (WHO) (2016) has described a "cycle of poverty" in which poor people with chronic disease become trapped. In this cycle, chronic disease develops in poor people (as a result of the previously mentioned factors), and as they seek to obtain and pay for treatment, they fall deeper into poverty. For families who are already living near the edge of poverty, one chronic disease may be all it takes to push them over that edge. To highlight this problem, WHO points out that people with diabetes in poor communities in India spend 25 percent of their annual income on medical care, compared with the 4 percent of income spent by wealthier Indians with diabetes.

WHO has recommended substantial increases in international investment in poor, underdeveloped countries, with this money targeted to programs designed to prevent chronic disease and alleviate poverty.

A. J. Smuskiewicz

See also: Access to Health Services; Centers for Disease Control and Prevention (CDC); Diet and Nutrition; Environment; Failure to Thrive; Healthy People 2020; Immune System Disorders; Lead Poisoning; Minorities, Chronic Disease; Rickets; World Health Organization

Further Reading

Brown, A. (2012). With poverty comes depression, more than other illnesses. Gallup. Retrieved from http://www.gallup.com/poll/158417/poverty-comes-depression-illness .aspx.

Centers for Disease Control and Prevention. (2014). Health, United States, 2014. Poverty. Retrieved from http://www.cdc.gov/nchs/hus/poverty.htm.

Kurtzleben, D. (2012, October 30). Americans in poverty at greater risk for chronic health problems. *U.S. News & World Report*. Retrieved from http://www.usnews.com/news/articles/2012/10/30/americans-in-poverty-at-greater-risk-for-chronic-health-problems.

World Health Organization (WHO). (2016). Chronic diseases and health promotion; Part two. The urgent need for action; Chapter two. Chronic diseases and poverty. Retrieved from http://www.who.int/chp/chronic_disease_report/part2_ch2/en.

PREDIABETES

Before people develop Type 2 diabetes, they almost always have prediabetes—blood glucose levels that are higher than normal, but not yet high enough to be diagnosed as diabetes (American Diabetic Association 2011). The American Diabetic Association estimates that 79 million American have prediabetes. Recent research shows that some long-term damage to the body—especially the heart and circulatory system—may already be occurring during prediabetes. Prediabetes has a 50 percent higher risk of heart disease and stroke than someone who does not have prediabetes. *Healthy People 2020* proposes "to reduce the disease and economic burden of diabetes mellitus (DM) and improve the quality of life for all persons who have or are at risk for diabetes."

While diabetes and prediabetes occur in people of all ages and races, some groups have a higher risk for developing the disease than others. Diabetes is more common in African Americans, Latinos, Native Americans, and Asian Americans/Pacific Islanders, as well as the elderly. This means they are also at increased risk for developing prediabetes.

The American Diabetes Association *Type 2 Diabetes Risk Test* can help determine increased risk. A high score may indicate that the individual has prediabetes or is at risk.

Screening

The good news is there are blood tests a doctor can perform to determine whether a person has prediabetes. Measuring blood glucose levels aids in determining normal metabolism, or prediabetes, or diabetes. Each test has established ranges for normal, prediabetes, or diabetes.

Hemoglobin A1C test—a test result between ≥5.7 percent and <6.5 percent is considered prediabetes; a test result of ≥6.5% is considered diabetes.

Fasting plasma glucose (FPG) test—a test result between ≥100 mg/dl and <16 mg/dl is considered prediabetes; a test result >126 mg/dl is considered diabetic.

Oral glucose tolerance test (OGTT)—a test result between ≥149 mg/dl and <200 mg//dl is considered prediabetes; a test result of ≥200 g/dl is considered diabetes.

An abnormal blood glucose level following the FPG indicates impaired fasting glucose (IFG); an abnormal blood glucose level following the OGTT indicates impaired glucose tolerance (IGT). Both conditions are also known as prediabetes. Typically, a physician will repeat a test to confirm an abnormal reading.

Risk Factors

The risk factors for prediabetes cover a range of influence. Nonmodifiable risk factors (also known as primary risk factors) include age, gender, race, and family history. An individual's genetic and familial inheritance can favor the person or place him or her at increased risk. Modifiable risk factors (also known as secondary risk factors) are those risks an individual can choose to change. These include obesity, nutrition, physical exercise, hypertension, cholesterol levels, smoking, and stress management.

Symptoms

Diabetic symptoms vary from individual to individual. The most common symptoms of Type 1 diabetes include frequent urination, unusual thirst, extreme hunger, unusual weight loss, and extreme fatigue and irritability. In Type 2 diabetes, the most common symptoms include any of the Type 1 symptoms plus frequent infections; blurred vision; cuts and bruises that are slow to heal; tingling and numbness in the hand and feet; and recurring skin, gum, or bladder infections.

The American Diabetic Association (2011) reports it is not uncommon for the Type 2 diabetic to be asymptomatic—that is, to have no symptoms. Annual wellness examinations are recommended.

Benefits and Risks of Screening

Every test carries risks and benefits. The risk associated with screening is a false positive result. Because blood glucose levels are affected by food, environment, smoking behaviors, and whether or not the individual has a virus, the doctor often will repeat an abnormal test to confirm the findings.

The benefit of blood glucose screening is early detection of abnormal metabolism. The earlier the condition is identified, the earlier behaviors can be modified to reduce potential damage. Conditions that can be prevented or mediated include eye problems (diabetic retinopathy), renal disease (end-stage kidney disease), foot problems (amputation), heart disease (hypertension, stroke), nerve damage (neuropathy), depression, women's health problems (high-risk pregnancy), and men's health problems (erectile dysfunction).

Preventing, Treating, and Managing Prediabetes

Preventing, treating, and managing prediabetes is doable: Small steps make all the difference. The American Diabetes Association and Choose MyPlate.gov provide simple, commonsense, and easy-to-adopt dietary pointers.

As people plan their goals, they consider how long, how often, and how specifically to modify behavior. The following are examples of *realistic* goals:

1. One fruit serving as an evening snack three times a week.
2. Substituting a baked potato for French fries once a week.
3. Walking up the stairs instead of using the elevator at work (home or subway) at least twice a week.

As people become more confident in their abilities to make change, they can expand their efforts.

Because prediabetes is associated with diabetes, hypertension, obesity, and heart disease, even small changes can have big benefits. Small steps make a difference. Other simple suggestions for people diagnosed with prediabetes include the following:

- Quitting smoking.
- Weight loss, if needed.
- Exercising most days of the week for a brisk 30 minutes, especially doing an enjoyable aerobic activity such as dancing; Zumba class; swimming; or riding a bicycle either outdoors or on an indoor, stationary bicycle.
- Eating healthfully: low-fat, low-cholesterol colorful vegetables and fruits and whole-grain breads and cereals.
- Using herbs and spices instead of salt to flavor foods.
- Using monounsaturated fats (canola oil, olive oil, or avocado).

Linda R. Barley

See also: Cholesterol; Diabetes, Type 1; Diabetes, Type 2; Heart Disease; Hypertension; Kidney Diseases; Obesity; Physical Activity; Stroke

Further Reading

American Diabetes Association. (2016). Making healthy food choices. Retrieved from http://www.diabetes.org/food-and-fitness/food/what-can-i-eat/making-healthy-food-choices.html.

American Diabetes Association. (2016). Diagnosing diabetes and learning about prediabetes. Retrieved from http://www.diabetes.org/are-you-at-risk/prediabetes/.

American Diabetes Association. (2016). Living with diabetes. Retrieved from http://www.diabetes.org/living-with-diabetes/.

Centers for Disease Control and Prevention. (2011). National Diabetes Fact Sheet, 2011. Retrieved from https://www.cdc.gov/diabetes/pubs/pdf/ndfs_2011.pdf.

ChooseMyPlate.gov. (2016). My Plate. Retrieved from http://www.choosemyplate.gov/MyPlate.

Cowie, C., Rust, K., & Ford, E., et al. (2009). Full accounting of diabetes and pre-diabetes in the U.S. population in 1988–1994 and 2005–2006. *Diabetes Care, 32*, 287–294.

HealthyPeople.gov. (2016, June 17). Healthy People 2020. Retrieved from https://www.healthypeople.gov/.

Knowler, W., & Barrett-Connor, E., et al. (2002). Diabetes Prevention Program Research Group: Reduction in the incidence of type 2 diabetes with lifestyle intervention. *New England Journal of Medicine, 346*(6), 393–403.

Knowler, W., Fowle, S., & Hamman, R., et al. (2009). Diabetes Prevention Program Research Group. Ten-year follow up of diabetes incidence and weight loss in the Diabetes Prevention Program Outcomes Study. *Lancet*, 374(9702), 1677–1686.

PROSTATE CANCER

Prostate cancer is the abnormal, uncontrolled multiplication of cells within a man's prostate. This cancer kills large numbers of men every year. However, if diagnosed and treated early, it is one of the most curable forms of cancer.

Prevalence and Mortality

In 2014, 233,000 new cases of prostate cancer were diagnosed in the United States, representing 14 percent of all new cancer cases. That same year, more than 29,000 Americans died of the disease, representing 5 percent of all cancer deaths (National Cancer Institute 2015). Prostate cancer is responsible for more deaths among American men than any other form of cancer except lung cancer.

Men of all ethnic groups can get prostate cancer, but African American men are at the highest risk. This cancer is hardly ever diagnosed before age 45, though African Americans are at risk around age 40. Prostate cancer is most commonly diagnosed in men between the ages of 65 and 74.

Prostate cancer has a lower mortality rate than most cancers. If diagnosed and treated early, men with prostate cancer have a good chance of long-term survival. The average five-year survival rate for patients with prostate cancer is 99 percent. If treatment is begun very early, this rate rises to 100 percent. However, if the cancer is not diagnosed and treated until after it has spread to distant parts of the body, the five-year survival rate drops to 28 percent.

Symptoms

Early stages of prostate cancer produce few if any symptoms. Men with more advanced prostate cancer may experience pain or discomfort in the pelvic area, lower back, ribs, or upper thighs, as well as an abnormally frequent urge to urinate. However, passing urine may be difficult. These symptoms are caused by the abnormal enlargement of the prostate gland, which puts pressure on the bladder and the urethra (the tube through which urine flows).

Causes and Risk Factors

The risk of prostate cancer steadily increases with age, especially after age 45. By age 80, about 80 percent of men have some cancer cells in their prostate.

Prostate cancer runs in families. Men who have relatives who had prostate cancer are at elevated risk for the disease themselves. This risk more than doubles for men who have fathers or brothers with prostate cancer.

Heredity alone cannot explain most cases of prostate cancer. There are other factors that increase risk, though these factors are little understood. A high-fat diet, smoking, and exposure to certain environmental toxins (such as heavy metals) are suspected of increasing risk.

Diagnosis

Physicians perform tests to check for prostate enlargement and to determine if this enlargement is the result of cancer or some other, less serious condition. In a digital rectal examination, the patient's prostate is felt with the physician's finger, which is inserted into the rectum. Abnormal hardness or lumps suggest the presence of cancer. In a test known as prostate-specific antigen (PSA), the blood is analyzed for levels of the PSA protein. Elevated levels of this protein are indicative of cancer.

If cancer is suspected based on these tests, an ultrasound examination is usually conducted to produce a detailed image of the prostate. Using this image, the physician inserts needles through the rectum wall to obtain tissue samples from the prostate. Microscopic examination of these biopsy samples will reveal if the tissue if malignant or benign. If malignant, further tests are performed to determine the stage of cancer development—whether the cancer is confined to the prostate or metastasized to other parts of the body.

Treatment

If the cancer is confined to the prostate, surgical removal of the gland and/or radiation therapy can often cure the patient. These procedures may lead to urinary incontinence and/or sexual impotence in patients. Some advanced surgical procedures may be able to remove the cancerous tissue while preserving nerves necessary for sexual functioning.

If the cancer has spread to tissues and organs beyond the prostate, additional treatments beyond prostate surgery and radiation therapy are necessary. These treatments may include orchiectomy (removal of the testes) and administration of certain hormones or other medications. These treatments lower the levels of the male hormones that "feed" the growth of prostate cancer cells.

Prevention

The earlier treatment for prostate cancer is initiated, the more successful the treatment is likely to be. To catch this cancer in an early, curable stage of development, many doctors recommend that men over age 40 get annual digital rectal examinations and PSA tests. PSA tests are able to detect smaller, earlier growths of cancer than rectal exams. Some doctors recommend routine rectal exams but not routine PSA tests because PSA tests may reveal small cancers that grow so slowly that they will never become life-threatening. Treatment for such small cancers could lead to unnecessary potential complications for patients. Thus, when small cancers are detected in the prostate, some doctors recommend waiting to see if the cancer spreads before beginning treatment.

A. J. Smuskiewicz

See also: Abdominal Diseases; Cancer; Environment; Men's Health

Further Reading

Klein, E. A. (2009). *The Cleveland Clinic guide to prostate cancer.* New York: Kaplan Publications.

MedlinePlus. (2014). Prostate cancer. Retrieved from https://www.nlm.nih.gov/medlineplus /prostatecancer.html.

National Cancer Institute. (2015). SEER stat fact sheets: Prostate cancer. Surveillance, Epidemiology, and End Results Program. Retrieved from http://seer.cancer.gov/statfacts /html/prost.html.

National Cancer Institute. (2016). Prostate cancer—patient version. National Institutes of Health. Retrieved from http://www.cancer.gov/types/prostate.

Roth, A. J. (2015). *Managing Prostate Cancer: A Guide for Living Better.* New York: Oxford University Press.

Walsh, P. C., & Worthington, J. F. (2012). *Dr. Patrick Walsh's Guide to Surviving Prostate Cancer,* 3rd ed. New York: Grand Central Life & Style/Hachette.

PSORIASIS

Psoriasis is a chronic skin disease driven by the immune system. Deep skin cells rise to the surface faster than normal, in days rather than about a month, building up rapidly and causing raised lesions that can appear on different parts of the body. The lesions are often painful and range in severity from a few scaly patches to coverage over large areas.

Doctors recognize five major types of psoriasis. The most common, *plaque psoriasis*, is notable for its raised, inflamed, red lesions covered by silvery white scales found on the elbows, knees, scalp, and lower back. The second most common, *guttate psoriasis*, appears as small dots, often in children or young adults, and can be triggered by a strep infection. *Inverse psoriasis* looks like smooth and shiny red lesions in the armpits, groin, under the breasts, behind the knee, and in other skin folds. Found mostly on the hands and feet in adults, *pustular psoriasis* is noninfectious white blisters surrounded by red skin. Rare, severe, and potentially life-threatening, *erythrodermic psoriasis* can leads to widespread itching and painful redness over much of the body that results in the scales coming off in sheets.

About 5 million adults in the United States have psoriasis, and it affects men and women equally. The disease can affect people of all ages, but most are diagnosed as young adults. Psoriasis often appears between the ages of 15 and 35, but it can develop at any age; about 10 to 15 percent receive a diagnosis before turning 10 years old. Although no cure exists for psoriasis and lifelong management is necessary, medication and other treatments can help control the symptoms.

Symptoms

The symptoms of psoriasis depend on the type, and they vary among individuals, but they commonly include red inflamed lesions; silvery scaly plaques; small red spots, especially in children; dry skin that cracks or bleeds; skin that itches, burns, or feels sore; and pitted or ridged nails that may separate from the nail bed. Lesions can range from a few spots or scales to coverage over large areas of the body.

Most types of psoriasis flare up for a few weeks or months and then subside or go into remission, but the disease does return. Triggers that may cause flares include infections, skin injuries, cold weather, stress, dry skin, smoking, excessive alcohol, and certain medications.

Causes and Risk Factors

Precisely what causes psoriasis is unknown, but an overactive immune system that attacks normal tissues in the body, as well as inherited genes, plays a role. Risk factors that increase the likelihood of developing the disease include family history (an estimated 10 percent of people inherit one of the genes creating a predisposition to psoriasis, but only 2 to 3 percent develop it); viral and bacterial infections, such as HIV/AIDS and strep throat; stress, which affects the immune system; excess weight; and smoking tobacco.

Diagnosis

Because it can look similar to other skin conditions, psoriasis may be hard to diagnose. A doctor can make a diagnosis based on medical history and an examination of the skin, scalp, and nails. A skin biopsy may be taken to determine the form of psoriasis.

Treatment

Treatment options for psoriasis depend on the severity of symptoms, which range from mild to moderate to severe, and the total amount of the body area affected; the goals are stopping the cycle of rapidly forming skin cells and removing the scales and lesions to smooth the skin while minimizing any side effects. Mild cases covering about 3 percent of the skin surface may be treated with topical creams, lotions, or sprays. For moderate cases (covering between 3 and 10 percent of skin area) to severe cases (covering more than 10 percent), phototherapy, alone or with medications, can be effective; the skin is exposed to controlled amounts of natural sunlight or artificial ultraviolet light. Severe psoriasis that has resisted other types of treatment may respond to systemic treatment, or oral or injected medications; a variety of drugs work to suppress skin cell production and inflammation, including biologics, which block the interaction between certain immune system cells and inflammatory pathways.

Prevention

There is no way to prevent psoriasis, but measures to manage or improve symptoms and reduce flare-ups include keeping the skin moist, avoiding scratching, limiting alcohol consumption, and no tobacco smoking. Environmental triggers best to avoid include cold, dry weather; skin injuries; strep and other infections; and some medications, such as lithium, antimalarial drugs, and beta blockers.

Prognosis or Outcome

A prognosis depends on the type of psoriasis, the severity, and what parts of the body are affected. One in three people with psoriasis usually develop psoriatic arthritis, which can be debilitating. Psoriasis requires constant and lifelong care to manage and control the symptoms, which come and go. Mild cases can be bothersome, but severe cases can be painful and disabling and may also cause depression and anxiety that lead to social isolation.

Future

Scientists have identified some 25 genetic variants that make people susceptible to the developing psoriasis. Using genetic sequencing technology, they are looking for the genes that may be the primary causes of psoriasis. This may lead to more effective treatments and methods to control the disease, possibly some that correct skin cell behavior or the genes themselves.

Although more research is needed, the results of a preliminary trial in 2015 of the experimental psoriasis drug guselkumab suggested that it may control the plaque psoriasis better than other standard treatments by blocking a protein that plays a role in the immune system and autoimmune diseases (HealthDay 2015).

Ray Marks

See also: Autoimmune Disease; Cellulitis; Dermatitis; Eczema; Immune System Disorders; Meningitis; Obesity, Morbid; Skin Conditions; Thrombophlebitis

Further Reading

Centers for Disease Control and Prevention. (2015, February 25). Psoriasis. Retrieved from http://www.cdc.gov/psoriasis/.

HealthDay. (2015, July 8). Experimental psoriasis drug shows promise. Retrieved from https://consumer.healthday.com/diseases-and-conditions-information-37/misc-diseases-and-conditions-news-203/new-psoriasis-drug-shows-promise-701155.html.

Mayo Clinic. (2015, June 17). Psoriasis. Retrieved from http://www.mayoclinic.org/diseases-conditions/psoriasis/basics/definition/con-20030838.

National Psoriasis Foundation. (2015). About psoriasis. Retrieved from https://www.psoriasis.org/about-psoriasis.

Psoriasis Speaks. (2015). What is psoriasis? Retrieved from https://www.psoriasis.com/what-is-psoriasis.

PSYCHOTIC DISORDERS

Psychotic disorders (or *pyschoses*) are a component of the schizophrenia spectrum and other psychotic disorders. Often affecting men at younger ages than women, the person's inner world and behavior are notably altered.

Some types of psychotic disorders include the following:

Brief psychotic disorders, such as short, sudden episodes of psychotic behavior.

Delusional disorder is seen in a person who has false strong beliefs involving real-life situations that could be true, such as having a disease or being conspired against. These delusions must have persisted for at least one month.

Substance-induced psychotic disorder is caused by withdrawal from substances like methamphetamines and alcohol and causes delusions and hallucinations.

Psychotic disorder due to a medical condition refers to psychotic disorder symptoms resulting from an illnesses affecting brain function.

Schizophrenia is a disorder referring to changes in behavior, delusions, and hallucinations that last longer than six months and are accompanied by a decline in social, school, and work functions.

Paraphrenia is schizophrenia in elderly patients.

Schizoaffective disorders affect people who have symptoms of two or more mood disorders, such as depression and schizophrenia.

Schizophreniform disorder is diagnosed when people with schizophrenia have symptoms that last fewer than six months.

Bipolar disorder, where people face severe mood swings of depression and mania, can include psychotic disorders.

Symptoms

Symptoms of psychotic disorders vary from person to person and may change over time. The major symptoms are hallucinations and delusions. Other possible symptoms of psychotic illnesses include:

- Confused thinking and/or disorganized or incoherent speech
- Strange, possibly dangerous behavior
- Slow unusual movements
- Poor personal hygiene
- Loss of interest in activities
- School, work, and relationship problems
- Cold demeanor and inability to express emotion or empathize
- Mood swings, depression, or mania

Key Causes and Risk Factors

In each case, psychosis is different, and the exact cause is not always entirely clear. There are, however, certain illnesses that cause psychosis. There are also triggers such as drug use, lack of sleep, and other environmental factors. In addition, certain illnesses can lead to specific types of psychosis, including brain diseases such as Parkinson's disease, brain tumors, and dementia; HIV, syphilis, and other infections that attack the brain; some forms of epilepsy; and stroke. Psychosis can also be triggered by the use of alcohol and illegal drugs, stimulants such as methamphetamine and cocaine, and hallucinogenic drugs like LSD. People who do not get enough sleep for long periods of time can experience symptoms of psychosis, as can usage of prescription drugs such as steroids and stimulants. There are also recent studies that indicate that pollution can cause brain changes leading to mental illness, including schizophrenia (University of Rochester Medical Center 2014).

Risk factors are genetic and having a family history of a psychotic disorder.

Diagnosis

Psychosis is diagnosed through a psychiatric evaluation. Medical tests and x-rays may be used to determine whether there is an underlying illness causing the symptoms.

Treatment

Treating psychosis may involve a combination of medications and therapy such as antipsychotics. Other approaches include cognitive-behavioral therapy with the goal of changing thinking and behaviors.

Prognosis and Prevention

If left untreated, it may be hard for the people with this disorder to take care of themselves, and they could develop other illnesses. Most people who experience psychosis will recover with proper treatment. Even in severe cases, medication and therapy can help people live normal lives.

It is important to prevent or decrease the impact of factors that place people at risk for developing a psychotic disorder.

Ray Marks

See also: Bipolar Disorder; Mental Health Disorders; Schizophrenia; Substance Abuse

Further Reading

Carey, E. (2014). Psychosis. Retrieved from http://www.healthline.com/health/psychosis #Overview1.

MedlinePlus. (2016, May10). Psychotic disorders. Retrieved from https://www.nlm.nih.gov /medlineplus/psychoticdisorders.html.

Psych.guides.com. (2014). Psychotic disorders. Retrieved from http://www.psychguides.com /guides/psychotic-disorders/.

Torrey, E. F. (2006). *Surviving Schizophrenia: A Manual for Families, Patients, and Providers.* New York: Collins.

University of Rochester Medical Center. Newsroom. (2014). New evidence links air pollution to autism, schizophrenia. Retrieved from https://www.urmc.rochester.edu/news /story/4100/new-evidence-links-air-pollution-to-autism-schizophrenia.aspx.

Walker, J. I. (2010). *Complete Mental Health: The Go-to-Guide for Clinicians and Patients.* New York: Norton.

PTSD (POST-TRAUMATIC STRESS DISORDER)

PTSD, or post-traumatic stress disorder, is a serious, potentially debilitating mental health condition. It can occur in people who have experienced or witnessed a traumatic or life-threatening event such as a tornado, hurricane, earthquake, flood, or other natural disaster; serious car accident; plane crash; terrorist attack; sudden death of a loved one; combat; sexual or physical abuse as a child; and rape or another violent personal assault. People with PTSD usually have persistent frightening thoughts and memories of the incident, including flashbacks and nightmares, and they may feel emotionally numb or jumpy and become easily irritated and angered.

Most people who experience terrifying events usually recover with time, but fewer than 10 percent develop PTSD, remaining frightened and anxious for months or years following an event. The disorder often contributes to depression and anxiety disorders, substance abuse, insomnia, chronic pain, and problems with employment and relationships.

Nearly 8 million adults in the United States have PTSD, and it can affect anyone of any age. Women are twice as likely as men to develop it, and those at increased risk include members of the military exposed to combat, children who have suffered physical or sexual abuse, and adolescents and teens who have witnessed gun violence. Treatments include psychotherapy, medications, or a combination of both.

Symptoms

Symptoms may not appear until several months or even years after an event. The disorder is characterized by reexperiencing or reliving the trauma through distressing memories, flashbacks, or nightmares; hyperarousal—or feeling jittery and constantly alert for danger, being easily angered or irritated, and having trouble sleeping and concentrating; emotional numbness and avoiding places, people, situations, and activities that may trigger memories of the event; and negative changes in feelings and beliefs, including guilt, fear, and shame, as well as a lack of interest in activities once enjoyed.

Without treatment, a person may remain hyperaroused, which can further damage the brain; this can contribute to job loss and family instability, as well as a heightened risk of suicide.

Causes and Risk Factors

It is not known why some people develop PTSD and others do not. Like other mental health problems, PTSD is a combination of inherited risks and genes, such as those playing a role in creating memories of fear; lifetime experiences that include frequency and severity of traumas; and individual personality and brain structure, including how the amygdala regulates chemicals and hormones that deal with fear and stress.

People of all ages can develop PTSD, but women are twice as likely, and it often occurs along with depression, substance abuse, and anxiety disorders. Some risk factors increase the likelihood, including long-lasting trauma (neglect or abuse beginning in early childhood); surviving or witnessing dangerous events in which people are hurt or killed; regular exposure to traumatic events, as with members of the military or first responders; losses of loved ones, employment, or a home; little or no support following a traumatic event; and family or personal history of mental illness.

Diagnosis

A mental health provider diagnoses PTSD after a person experiences symptoms for at least one month following a traumatic event: one or more reexperiencing symptoms of intrusive, distressing recollections of the event, flashbacks, or nightmares; three incidents of avoiding situations or activities that are feared to trigger memories; and two or more hyperarousal symptoms, such as problems sleeping or concentrating and being easily irritated and angered.

Treatments

Treatments for PTSD focus on helping people regain control over fear after a traumatic event; they include psychotherapy (also called talk therapy), medications, or a combination of both.

Cognitive-behavioral therapy (CBT) has been highly effective for PTSD, and it may include cognitive-processing therapy, which teaches skills to understand how trauma changes thoughts and feelings, and prolonged exposure, in which people talk repeatedly about a traumatic event until the memories are no longer frightening.

Other forms of psychotherapy include exposure therapy to help people face and control their fear by exposing them to the trauma in a safe way; cognitive restructuring to help people make sense of the bad memories; stress inoculation training that teaches how to reduce anxiety; eye movement desensitization and reprocessing, more commonly called EMDR, which involves focusing on eye movements, hand taps, or sounds while talking about a traumatic memory to change the fearful reaction; and virtual reality treatment, which involves exposing a person with PTSD to a virtual environment of the feared situation while wearing goggles and headphones.

The medications most commonly used to treat PTSD are the selective serotonin reuptake inhibitor (SSRI) antidepressants.

Prevention

After experiencing a traumatic event, getting timely support from family, friends, or a mental health provider may prevent normal fear and stress reactions from developing into PTSD. Antidepressant and other types of medications may also contribute to prevention if given soon after an event.

Prognosis and Outcomes

The severity and duration of suffering from PTSD can affect the prognosis. Factors that improve a person's outcome include a strong social support system; early treatment intervention; having good self-esteem, social skills, problem-solving, and impulse control; and living in a stable environment.

Future

To prevent PTSD from developing, researchers are exploring medications that may target its underlying causes. Others are studying how to minimize risk factors to keep it from developing following trauma, as well as working to identify the factors that will lead to more personalized and effective treatments. Ongoing improvements in genetic research and brain imaging technologies allow greater precision about when and where in the brain PTSD takes place, which may lead to individualized treatments or the prevention of the disorder.

Jean Kaplan Teichroew

See also: Alzheimer's Disease; Anxiety Disorders; Bipolar Disorder; Brain Disorders; Dementia; Depression; Fetal Alcohol Syndrome; Men's Health; Mental Disorders; Schizophrenia; Social Health; Women's Health

Further Reading

Anxiety and Depression Association of America. (2015, August). Posttraumatic stress disorder (PTSD). Retrieved from http://www.adaa.org/understanding-anxiety/posttraumatic-stress-disorder-ptsd.

Mayo Clinic. (2014, April 15). Post-traumatic stress disorder (PTSD). Retrieved from http://www.mayoclinic.org/diseases-conditions/post-traumatic-stress-disorder/basics/definition/con-20022540.

National Institute of Mental Health. (2015). Post-traumatic stress disorder (PTSD). Retrieved from http://www.nimh.nih.gov/health/topics/post-traumatic-stress-disorder-ptsd/index.shtml#part_145371.

PsychCentral. (2015, March 28). Posttraumatic stress disorder. Retrieved from http://psychcentral.com/disorders/ptsd/.

PTSD: National Center for PTSD. (2014, November 10). What is PTSD? Retrieved from http://www.ptsd.va.gov/public/PTSD-overview/basics/what-is-ptsd.asp.

PUBLIC HEALTH

Public health refers to organized public and private efforts of those who work to prevent disease; promote and improve health; and prolong life for individuals, families, communities, and populations from the local level to the global. In general, public health is concerned with protecting the health of populations, which can range from a local neighborhood to a country or region of the world. To promote and protect the health of communities, public health activities aim to provide conditions in which entire populations can be healthy. Public health helps influence policy makers to adopt health policies aimed to advance the well-being of the public and reduce the burdens of chronic diseases.

It involves the application of epidemiological science, as well as laws, to reduce the risk of health-related disability among populations. *Epidemiology* refers to the study of the patterns, causes, and effects of health and diseases among specific populations. Considered the cornerstone of public health, epidemiological research identifies risk factors for disease as well as targets for prevention, which aids policy makers and lawmakers. Epidemiologists monitor the spread of diseases and focus on understanding their causes and developing solutions.

Key public health tools include education and promotion. Public health focuses on protecting and improving the health of communities through promoting of healthful lifestyles, researching disease and injury prevention, and detecting and controlling infectious diseases. With this very broad agenda, it may also include efforts to provide a safe, clean environment, as well as encouraging communities to adopt health behaviors.

Primary public health activities include preventing epidemics and the spread of disease, protecting against environmental hazards, preventing injuries, promoting and encouraging healthful behaviors, responding to disasters and assisting communities in recovery, and assuring the quality and accessibility of health services.

Accomplishments

During the 20th century, public health efforts made a significant impact. Public health efforts are responsible for nearly 25 of the 30 years of improved life expectancy in the United States as a result of the widespread advent of vaccinations, safer workplaces, safer and more healthful food, safety regulations concerning motor vehicles, the control of infectious diseases, a decline in deaths from coronary heart disease and stroke as awareness of the relationship between diet and disease increased, family planning, recognizing tobacco use as a health hazard (the U.S. Surgeon General issued the first report in 1964 on cigarette smoking and its connection with cancer), programs for healthier mothers and babies, and fluoridation of drinking water.

Challenges Past, Present, and Future

Those working in public health always face challenging situations that affect large populations. To be prepared, public health officials create processes to identify and manage episodic events if and when they occur. Current challenges include the reappearance and stronger strains of tuberculosis and other infectious diseases that had been gone for many years; the emergence of newer diseases such as HIV/AIDS, West Nile virus, and SARS (severe acute respiratory syndrome); the anthrax crisis in 2001; the faster and farther traveling and transmission of infectious agents; and the stronghold of diabetes, heart disease, cancer, and other chronic diseases that have become leading causes of death in the United States. Recent health threats have included a measles outbreak in 2015, a salmonella outbreak in peanut butter in 2011, the H1N1 flu epidemic in 2009, Hurricanes Sandy in 2012 and Katrina in 2005, and the 9/11 attacks in 2001.

Public Health Fields

People working in public health usually have a public health degree and also undergo certification. A diverse and growing area of the health field, it includes disaster prevention, emergency preparedness and bioterrorism, environmental health promotion, prevention of epidemics such as polio, and many other health-related activities. Research shows that effective public health programs produce better health outcomes and quality of life for all citizens, while lowering the costs of health care.

Some examples of careers in the many fields of public health are first responders, restaurant inspectors, health educators, scientists and researchers, nutritionists, community planners, social workers, epidemiologists, public health physicians and nurses, occupational health and safety professionals, public policy makers, and those who specialize in sanitary science and public health.

William D. Kernan

See also: Access to Health Services; Centers for Disease Control and Prevention (CDC); Environment; Health; Healthy People 2020; Poverty; Waterborne Diseases; World Health Organization

Further Reading

American Public Health Association. (2015). What is public health? Retrieved from http://www.apha.org/what-is-public-health.

Association of Schools & Programs of Public Health. (2015). Discover. What is public health? Retrieved from http://www.aspph.org/discover/.

CDC Foundation. (2015). What is public health? Retrieved from http://www.cdcfoundation.org/content/what-public-health.

Public Health Online. (2015). A guide to public health careers. Retrieved from http://www.publichealthonline.org/careers/.

World Health Organization. (2015). Public health. Retrieved from http://www.who.int/trade/glossary/story076/en/.

R

RAYNAUD'S PHENOMENON

Raynaud's phenomenon is a condition that produces discolorations of the fingers and/or the toes after exposure to changes in temperature, either hot or cold, as well as emotional situations due to abnormal spasms of the blood vessels and a decreased blood supply to the local tissues. Initially, the fingers or toes turn white, then blue because of the extended lack of oxygen. Finally, the blood vessels reopen, causing a local "flushing" phenomenon, which turns the digit or digits red. This series of events is characteristic of Raynaud's phenomenon.

Raynaud's phenomenon most often occurs in women, especially in the second, third, or fourth decades of life. People can have Raynaud's phenomenon alone or as a part of other rheumatic diseases. Raynaud's phenomenon in children is essentially identical to Raynaud's phenomenon in adults. When it occurs by itself, it is called Raynaud's disease or primary Raynaud's phenomenon. When it occurs in conjunction with other diseases—such as scleroderma, lupus, or rheumatoid arthritis—it is called secondary Raynaud's phenomenon (Shiel 2014). It can also affect the nose, ears, and tongue. Women are more likely to have Raynaud's disease than men, as are people who live in cold countries.

The disease was named after Maurice Raynaud (1834–1881), a French physician who first described the disease in 1862.

Symptoms

Symptoms depend on the severity and duration of the problem. There may be mild tingling and numbness and mild skin discoloration. On occasion, if severe, the tips of the digits can ulcerate and become infected. Sometimes these symptoms only last a few minutes, and sometimes they last for hours. The same digits are not always affected.

Causes and Risk Factors

Primary and secondary Raynaud's phenomenon causes are unknown. Both abnormal nerve control of the blood-vessel diameter and nerve sensitivity to cold exposure have been suspected as being contributing factors, however (Shiel 2014). Gender, age, family history, having certain occupations, where one lives, a history of injuries, smoking, exposure to chemicals, and certain medications are other possible causes or risk factors.

Diagnosis

The doctor can run blood tests, run digital artery pressure tests, and conduct physical tests, as well as a conduct a clinical history. An examination of the nail fold under the microscope may be performed. This is called *nail fold vasculature capillaroscopy*, where a fold of hard skin overlapping the base and sides of a finger/toe nail is examined under a microscope and the tiny blood vessels are observed.

Treatments

Medications, as well as taking precaution with clothing and headwear, is commonly recommended. In severe cases, a form of nerve surgery called a *sympathectomy* may be considered to prevent blood-vessel spasm.

Prognosis

The outlook depends on whether the condition is severe or not. If severe, the condition can lead to deformities of the fingers or toes or even loss of digits due to gangrene.

Prevention

Avoiding emotional stress and extremes of temperature, avoiding smoking, and treating underlying health conditions is recommended. Medications that aggravate symptoms should be avoided. Researchers are investigating the causes of Raynaud's phenomenon and trying to find medications or chemicals that will reduce blood vessel spasm in the digits, such as nitric oxide.

Ray Marks

See also: Gangrene; Rheumatoid Arthritis

Further Reading

Hands don't work like they used to? Help is on the way. (2014, November). *Harvard Women's Health Watch*, 22(3), 4–5.

Mayes, M. D. (2005). *The Scleroderma Book: A Guide for Patients and Families*. New York: Oxford University Press, 2005.

Mayo Clinic. (2014). Raynaud's disease. Retrieved from http://www.mayoclinic.org/diseases -conditions/raynauds-disease/basics/definition/con-20022916.

Medical News Today. (2016, March 9). Raynaud's disease: Causes, symptoms and treatments. Retrieved from http://www.medicalnewstoday.com/articles/176713.php.

Shiel, W. C. (2014). Raynaud's phenomenon. MedicineNet.com. Retrieved from http://www .medicinenet.com/raynauds_phenomenon/article.htm#what_is_raynauds_pheno menon.

REACTIVE ARTHRITIS

Reactive arthritis, formerly termed Reiter syndrome, is a painful form of inflammatory arthritis resulting in joint pain and swelling that is triggered by an infection in another part of the body, most often the intestines, genitals, or urinary tract. It occurs in reaction to an infection by certain bacteria located in the genitals, such as chlamydia trachomatis, or the bowel, such as campylobacter, salmonella, shigella, and yersinia.

Reactive arthritis tends to occur most often in men between the ages of 20 and 50 years. The frequency is estimated to be in the range of about 3.5 to 5 cases per 100,000 people.

Some patients with reactive arthritis carry a gene called HLA-B27, and these patients often have a more sudden and severe onset of symptoms that may be more chronic or long-lasting. However, patients who are HLA-B27 negative can still develop reactive arthritis after exposure to an organism that causes it.

Patients with AIDS virus HIV can also develop reactive arthritis. Risk factors are age, gender, and genetic factors.

According to Shiel (2014), reactive arthritis is a chronic form of arthritis characterized by (1) inflamed joints; (2) eye inflammation; and (3) inflammation of the genital, urinary, or gastrointestinal systems.

Symptoms

One or more of the following symptoms can exist: pain and swelling of certain joints, often the knees and/or ankles; mouth ulcers; conjunctivitis; heel swelling and pain; toe and finger swelling; urinary problems; noninfectious urethritis; malaise; fever; and persistent low back pain, which tends to be worse at night or in the morning.

Some patients with this type of arthritis have irritated red eyes. Still other signs and symptoms include burning with urination and a rash on the palms or the soles of the feet.

Causes and Risk Factors

Reactive arthritis is caused by an infection. Genetic factors may raise the predisposition to reactive arthritis.

Diagnosis

A physical examination may be conducted, as well as a medical history. Blood tests, joint fluid tests, urine tests, and imaging tests may be performed. Although there is no specific test for diagnosing reactive arthritis, the doctor may check the urethral discharge for sexually transmitted diseases, as well as stool samples for signs of infection.

Treatments

The type of treatment depends on the stage of reactive arthritis. In early stages, or acute inflammation; nonsteroidal anti-inflammatory drugs and antibiotics may be used. In the late stage, or when chronic, reactive arthritis may require treatment with a disease-modifying antirheumatic drug such as sulfasalazine or methotrexate. Individual joints may benefit from corticosteroid injections (cortisone shots) and physical therapy. Eye inflammation can be treated with steroids.

Prognosis

The outlook for reactive arthritis varies. Most people recover in three to four months, but about 50 percent may experience recurrences over the years. Some patients may develop complications, including heart muscle inflammation, inflammation and spinal stiffening, glaucoma, progressive blindness, feet abnormalities, or accumulation of lung fluid.

Prevention

Avoiding exposure to bacteria, especially if one is genetically susceptible may be helpful.

Ray Marks

See also: Arthritis; Inflammation

Further Reading

Bykerk, V. (2015). Reactive arthritis. American College of Rheumatology. Retrieved from http://www.rheumatology.org/I-Am-A/Patient-Caregiver/Diseases-Conditions/Reactive
-Arthritis.

Mayo Clinic. (2014). Reactive arthritis. Retrieved from http://www.mayoclinic.org/diseases
-conditions/reactive-arthritis/basics/definition/con-20020872.

National Institute of Arthritis and Musculoskeletal and Skin Diseases. (2014). Questions and answers about reactive arthritis. Retrieved from http://www.niams.nih.gov/Health
_Info/Reactive_Arthritis/.

Shiel, W. C. (2015, December 2). Reactive arthritis [formerly Reiter's syndrome]. Medicine Net.com. Retrieved from http://www.medicinenet.com/reactive_arthritis/article.htm.

REHABILITATION

Rehabilitation is the term used to describe one or more treatment strategies designed to restore a patient to his or her optimal level of function. It is commonly applied in chronic health conditions after a person has had surgery or been hospitalized. It can take place in the hospital, in a clinic, or in the home. The purpose is to restore functioning of the cardiovascular, neurological, pulmonary, and musculoskeletal systems most often. Patients may need various forms of assistance to recover optimally, and qualified therapists will assess what is needed either independently or as part of a therapeutic team. Types of rehabilitation specialists are speech therapists, occupational therapists to address occupational and environmental needs, social workers, and physical therapists. Others are respiratory therapists, health coaches, podiatrists, and nurses. Psychologists; orthotists and prosthetists, who make braces or artificial limbs, respectively; and vocational counselors are others. Family members are often encouraged to actively engage in the patient's rehabilitation program.

Various forms of rehabilitation designed to deter or slow chronic disease progression or aid in recovery after surgery include exercise, aquatic therapy, counseling, vision therapy, chest physical therapy, heat, cold, massage, and ultrasound and electrical therapies. Modifications to the home and worksite, such as rearranging equipment and furniture or adding a wheelchair ramp, as well as making bathing and grooming more accessible, may form part of the rehabilitation strategy.

Inhalation therapists, audiologists, and registered dietitians are other types of therapists who may help patients recover maximally from their health situations. Drug rehabilitation may be needed if a person is addicted to specific drugs or substances.

Specific rehabilitation services, as well as special rehabilitation agencies, are often employed to supplement the health care offered in hospitals. Some nurses and therapists make home visits and provide family and patient advice on what is the best form of self-management therapy for a patient with one or more chronic diseases.

According to Thomas et al. (2002), by carefully examining each patient's medical condition and potential for functional improvement, and by implementing early appropriate rehabilitation, there is an increased likelihood of attaining better self-sufficiency and life quality for the patient, regardless of discharge destination and condition.

Ray Marks

See also: Access to Health Services; Physical Therapy; Wellness

Further Reading

Mayo Clinic. (2016). Physical medicine and rehabilitation. Retrieved from http://www.mayoclinic.org/departments-centers/physical-medicine-rehabilitation/overview.

MedicineNet.com. (2016, May13). Definition of rehabilitation. Retrieved from http://www.medicinenet.com/script/main/art.asp?articlekey=5288.

MedlinePlus. (2016, February 22). Rehabilitation. Retrieved from https://www.nlm.nih.gov/medlineplus/rehabilitation.html.

Thomas, D. C., Kreizman, I. J., Melchiorre, P., & Ragnarsson, K. T. (2002). Rehabilitation of the patient with chronic critical illness. *Critical Care Clinics*, 18(3), 695–715.

REPRODUCTIVE DISORDERS

In human males and females, the reproductive system is comprised of internal and external organs. The organs work together to procreate, or reproduce—a process vital for the survival of the species. The external female reproductive organs, or genitals, include the vaginal opening, clitoris, urethra, and labia minora and majora. The internal organs include the vagina, uterus, and ovaries, which are connected to the uterus by fallopian tubes. The major parts of the male reproductive system are the testes, which produce sperm, and the penis; both are also part of the urinary system. When a sperm enters a fallopian tube and fertilizes an ovum, or egg, it makes its way to the uterus, where eventually it develops into a fetus. About nine months later, a fetus mature enough to survive outside the womb starts life as a baby. It's a simple biological process when all goes well. But many conditions, diseases, and disorders can prevent this from taking place.

Infertility; sexually transmitted and underlying diseases, including cancers; as well as congenital, genetic, and hormonal disorders that affect the reproductive systems of both men and women are examples of some of these conditions. Specific to women are ovarian cysts, endometriosis, uterine fibroids, pelvic inflammatory disease, severe menstrual cramping, yeast infection, chronic vaginal pain, and vaginitis. Those specific to men include impotence, erectile dysfunction, low testosterone, prostatitis and other prostate disorders, and noncancerous and anatomical malformations and disorders that affect fertility.

Symptoms

Common symptoms of many female disorders include pelvic pain, genital itching, vaginal discharge, chronic pain, and abnormal vaginal bleeding. Penile sores, discharge, lumps, and testicular pain are common symptoms in men; a decrease in sex drive or in body hair or muscle mass may indicate low testosterone.

Infertility in men is when they produce too few or no sperm, the sperm are abnormal, or they die before they reach an ovum; symptoms are rarely evident. In women, infertility is when the reproductive system prevents ovulation, conception, or carrying a pregnancy full term.

The cancers that affect reproduction, prostate cancer in men and ovarian cancer in women, often have no symptoms in their early stages.

Causes and Risk Factors

Reproductive hazards, which can affect sperm in men and cause problems for pregnant women, as well as other aspects of reproduction, include radiation; lead, mercury, and other metals; pesticides and other chemicals; cigarette smoking; alcohol consumption; and some viruses. Research suggests that the metals and chemicals that disrupt hormones in the environment are the reason they may pose a threat to human reproductive health (National Institute of Environmental Health Sciences 2015).

Some cancers are specific to reproductive organs: the prostate in men and the uterus, ovaries, and cervix in women.

The causes of some disorders experienced by both men and women are unknown. But gonorrhea and chlamydia are the usual causes of female pelvic inflammatory disease, which can result serious and long-term reproductive problems for women. HPV, or human papillomavirus, is the most common sexually transmitted infection, and it can cause genital warts; in some women, this can lead to cervical cancer, and some men may develop anal or penile cancer. Both men and women can experience the sexually transmitted diseases genital herpes, syphilis, and HIV.

Infertility has many causes: In men, it may be due to previous illnesses and subsequent surgeries or treatments; congenital defects; genetic diseases; structural problems; injuries; or overexposure to chemicals, toxins, or high heat. In women, the causes include ovulation and hormonal disorders; physical abnormalities or damage; endometriosis, pelvic scar tissue; cancer and radiation and chemotherapy treatments; illnesses; and genetic abnormalities. Factors contributing to infertility are age, alcohol and tobacco use, excess weight, and being underweight due to eating disorders.

Diagnosis

Doctors take urine, blood, and other lab tests and conduct physical exams on both men and women with symptoms of reproductive disorders. Fertility tests examine hormones, genetics, and reproductive organs, as well as semen analysis and ovulation. Men may also undergo a digital rectal exam, prostate fluid analysis, or a biopsy. Women may have a pregnancy test, pelvic examination, or ultrasound to diagnose pain or abnormal bleeding.

Treatments

Underlying conditions are the focus of the primary treatment. Medications, including antibiotics and penicillin, are used to treat most infections, including some that are transmitted sexually and erectile dysfunction and low testosterone. Those caused by viruses, such as HPV, have no treatment. Surgery may be indicted to remove genital warts or growths. Cold packs, warm water baths, and other home remedies often help relieve symptoms of vaginal pain. Steroids or antidepressants may be prescribed to lessen chronic pain. Antihistamines and corticosteroid creams may reduce itching.

Infertility is treated with medications, surgery, intrauterine insemination, or other techniques to assist reproduction; often, some treatments are combined.

Prevention

Reproductive disorders that are the result of illnesses, genetic defects, and physical abnormalities are not preventable. But practicing safe sex and regular testing against sexually transmitted diseases reduces the risk of many disorders, although abstinence is the only truly effective preventive measure for these.

Many causes of infertility are not preventable, but doctors recommend avoiding anything that might limit sperm production and limiting exposure to high heat, chemicals, and other harmful substances. Both women and men are advised to avoid excessive alcohol and tobacco and sexually transmitted infections. To increase the possibility of pregnancy, women are advised to eat and exercise moderately and make sure prescription and nonprescription drugs do not affect fertility.

Prognosis and Outcomes

Left untreated, sexually transmitted infections and other treatable disorders can spread and worsen. Medications can clear up infections, which can recur, and some have become resistant to antibiotics.

While not medically serious, some types of vaginal pain are chronic conditions, and although they are treated, they can come and go over months or years. Depending on the cause or causes of infertility, many couples who receive treatment eventually have a baby.

Jean Kaplan Teichroew

See also: Ovarian Cancer; Prostate Cancer; Sexually Transmitted Diseases; Testicular Cancer; Uterine Cancer; Uterine Diseases; Vaginal Diseases; Women's Health

Further Reading

Better Medicine. (2015). Male reproductive system. Retrieved from http://www.localhealth.com/category/male-reproductive-system/NIH.Heffner, L. J., & Schust, D. J. (2014). *The Reproductive System at a Glance*. Hoboken, NJ: Wiley-Blackwell.

LiveScience. (2015, April 30). Reproductive system: Facts, functions and diseases. Retrieved from http://www.livescience.com/26741-reproductive-system.html.

Mayo Clinic. (2014, July 2). Infertility causes. Retrieved from http://www.mayoclinic.org/diseases-conditions/infertility/basics/causes/con-20034770.

Merck Manual. (2015). Introduction to symptoms of gynecologic disorders. Retrieved from http://www.merckmanuals.com/home/women-s-health-issues/symptoms-of-gynecologic-disorders/introduction-to-symptoms-of-gynecologic-disorders.

National Institute of Environmental Health Sciences. (2015, April 10). Reproductive health. Retrieved from http://www.niehs.nih.gov/health/topics/conditions/repro-health/.

RESPIRATORY DISEASES

The organs and tissues that enable breathing comprise the respiratory system: the lungs, airways (nasal passages, mouth, larynx, trachea, bronchial tubes), and respiratory muscles. They take in oxygen and expel carbon dioxide, working together to complete this exchange of gases.

The most common chronic respiratory diseases are asthma and chronic obstructive pulmonary disease (COPD), as well as respiratory allergies and occupational lung diseases. Pneumonia, bronchitis, and other acute infections can also affect the respiratory system. The diseases are treatable, even if irreversible, and most individuals experience significant improvement when they follow a prescribed course of medical treatment.

They affect millions of people worldwide, from children to older adults. In the United States, more than 23 million people have asthma, more than 50 million have allergies, and about 13.6 million adults have COPD (HealthyPeople.gov 2015), which is the third leading cause of death (National Heart, Lung, and Blood Institute 2013). A current worldwide estimate is that currently 235 million people have asthma and 64 million people have COPD (World Health Organization 2015).

Symptoms

Respiratory diseases cause breathing problems, which can range from mild to life-threatening. These are common symptoms: nasal discharge; a cough that grows worse over time; coughing up blood or mucus that is yellow, brown, or green; difficulty breathing, including shortness of breath, rapid or deep breathing, tightness in the chest, or wheezing; the absence of breathing (called apnea); and a loose wet cough that produces a thick, colored phlegm.

Causes and Risk Factors

Researchers have identified these major risk factors for respiratory diseases: smoking tobacco, including secondhand smoke; exposure to environmental pollutants both outdoors and inside, including chemicals, fumes, and dust in the workplace; and allergens such as dust, mold, or animals. For asthma, scientists are investigating additional risk factors: a parent with asthma, acute sensitivity to some irritants, childhood respiratory infections in childhood, and excess weight.

The nasal passage is a common pathway for allergens to enter the respiratory system; an allergy, infection, or inflammation in this passage may cause an asthma attack. For COPD, smoking is a primary cause, although genetic predisposition also plays a role for some people.

Panic attacks may trigger shortness of breath, rapid breathing, or other symptoms of respiratory disease, but these are temporary and leave no permanent physical effects. In some cases, such as congestive heart failure and pulmonary hypertension, cardiac conditions cause respiratory disorders. Obstructions in the airways, traumatic lung injuries, and underlying diseases such as cancer may cause respiratory diseases.

Diagnosis

A doctor takes a medical history to learn about experience with illnesses or family history that may be risk factors for respiratory disorders and conducts a physical exam to listen for abnormal airflow or fluid in the lungs, or if they have collapsed.

Tests include spirometry, a breathing test that measures air passage obstruction; pulse oximetry, which measures oxygen levels; arterial blood gas to check the oxygen-carbon dioxide amounts; and imaging such as x-rays or CT scans, which help pinpoint the cause of a disease. A pulmonologist, or specialist in lung conditions, may diagnose respiratory diseases with a pulmonary function test (also called a lung function test) to measure how well the lungs take in and circulate oxygen or a bronchoscopy to search for abnormalities such as bleeding, tumors, or inflammation.

Treatment

Medications are used to treat diseases of the respiratory system. Bronchodilators relax the muscles and open the airways, making it easier to breathe. Medicines known as steroids or corticosteroids reduce inflammation and the resulting production of mucus. They can be administered as pills or via inhalers or nebulizers. Antihistamines and decongestants may be useful as well to combat the effects of allergens. Occasionally, antibiotics are prescribed for bacterial infections that flare up. Pulmonary rehabilitation teaches individuals how to live with chronic symptoms, including exercises and breathing techniques. If necessary for more severe cases, oxygen therapy and surgery may be employed.

Prevention

Of the many risk factors for respiratory diseases, most can be prevented or minimized. Avoiding exposure is the best way to try to control irritants: wearing a dust mask; avoiding animals, outdoor pollen, and secondhand smoke; and changing air conditioner filters and washing bed linens frequently. Smokers are advised to quit. Daily medication regimens also help prevent symptoms.

Prognosis and Outcomes

The overall prognosis depends on the cause and severity of the respiratory disease. Most people can manage their symptoms successfully, particularly if they get medical care and comply with recommended treatment plans, including smokers who have COPD if they quit smoking.

Future

The global rise of new technologies that use new chemicals and materials, such as engineered nanoparticles, is an area of ongoing research. Scientists also continue to study the impact of climate change on respiratory diseases, as well as indoor air quality for work-related symptoms, including exposure to isocyanates used in "green" building materials.

Jean Kaplan Teichroew

See also: Allergies; Asthma; COPD (Chronic Obstructive Pulmonary Disease); Legionnaires' Disease; Lung Diseases; Nasal Disorders; Pneumonia; Whooping Cough

Further Reading

Adams, F. (2006). *The Asthma Sourcebook*, 3rd ed. New York: McGraw-Hill Education.
American Lung Association. (2015). Understand your medication. Retrieved from http://www.lung.org/lung-disease/asthma/taking-control-of-asthma/understand-your-medication.html.

Healthgrades. (2013, September 6). Respiratory symptoms. Retrieved from http://www
    .healthgrades.com/symptoms/respiratory-symptoms.
HealthyPeople.gov. (2015, June 26). Respiratory disease. Retrieved from http://www
    .healthypeople.gov/2020/topics-objectives/topic/respiratory-diseases.
Mahler, D. A. (2014). *COPD: Answers to Your Questions.* Minneapolis, MN: Two Harbors
    Press.
National Heart, Lung, and Blood Institute. (2013, July 31). What is COPD? Retrieved from
    http://www.nhlbi.nih.gov/health/health-topics/topics/copd.
Varkey, B., & Maier, L. A. (2015). Chronic respiratory diseases: Challenges in diagnosis and
    prevention. *Current Opinion in Pulmonary Medicine, 21*(2), 111–113. doi:10.1097/
    MCP.0000000000000146.
World Health Organization (WHO). (2015). Chronic respiratory diseases. Retrieved from
    http://www.who.int/respiratory/en/.

RETINOPATHY

Retinopathy is a disease of the eye that is indicated by a damaged retina, the tissue at the back of the eye that is light sensitive and sends impulses along the optic nerve to the brain to form visual images. People with retinopathy may have symptoms such as seeing spots or floaters, blurred vision, having a dark spot in the center of one's field of vision, and problems seeing at night. It can be caused by a variety of health conditions, including diabetes, heart disease, and other disorders. It is the leading cause of blindness among American adults.

The most common cause of retinopathy is complications from diabetes, a disease in which a person cannot metabolize blood sugar effectively. High levels of sugar in the blood cause damage to many parts of the body, including the eyes, over a long period of time. In diabetic retinopathy, the tiny blood vessels of the retina weaken and leak blood into the part of the retina called the macula. The macula is the part of the eye that sees color and fine detail. Blood that leaks into it causes swelling and cloudy vision. If untreated, it will lead to blindness.

There are two types of diabetic retinopathy—nonproliferative (NPDR) and proliferative (PDR). NPDR is the early stage of retinopathy. Most people do not even realize they have NPDR because the symptoms are usually mild or nonexistent. In this stage, the weakening in the blood vessels of the retina is beginning, resulting in microanuerysms, or small bulges, on the retinal walls. It is from these bulges that blood leaks into the retina, causing the macula to swell.

The more advanced stage of diabetic retinopathy is PDR, in which the circulation problems have become severe enough to deprive the retina of oxygen. To compensate for this, new blood vessels grow in the retina and into the gel-like fluid at the back of the eye, called vitreous humor. It is these vessels that leak blood into the back of the eye, interfering with vision. The interference with the vitreous humor can also cause scar tissue, causing the retina to detach from the eye. Retinal detachment can only be treated with surgery. In addition, increased pressure on the eye from PDR causes an increased risk of glaucoma, a disease of the optic nerve which also leads to severe vision loss or blindness if untreated.

Retinopathy may also be present in people who do not have diabetes. Cardiovascular disease, particularly hypertension, in nondiabetics can lead to development of problems with the retina. Hypertension causes circulation problems in the retina similar to those caused by diabetes. About 11 percent of those diagnosed with high blood pressure also have retinopathy present. Atherosclerosis (hardening of the arteries) may also be a cause of retinopathy, although studies are not yet conclusive. Research has shown that blockage of more than 90 percent of the carotid artery may often cause problems with the eyes that can develop into retinopathy. Some studies have found a link between the presence of retinopathy and incidence of abdominal obesity, high cholesterol, and thickness of the carotid artery.

In addition to cardiovascular disease, various other disorders may also cause retinopathy. Vasculitis, the inflammation of blood vessels, can damage blood vessels and result in restricted circulation, lack of oxygen to certain areas of the body, and tissue damage. Vasculitis in the vessels of the retina can lead to the development of retinopathy. Severe anemia and infections such as AIDS and endocarditis, tuberculosis, and syphilis also can cause retinopathy. Damage to the retina may also occur as a result of exposure to radiation in the head, usually for a past medical condition.

In most cases, retinopathy is diagnosed with a thorough eye examination that emphasizes analysis of the retina. Risk factors, such as the presence of diabetes or hypertension, are first considered. Then the doctor will measure visual acuity to see how the person's vision is affected and conduct a refraction test to determine if there is a change in vision. The retina is also examined by dilating the pupil, and photographs of the retina may be taken. In addition, any excess pressure in the eye is noted.

Treatment for retinopathy depends on the cause and extent of the damage. If detected early enough in diabetic cases, careful monitoring of blood sugar levels can help slow the progression of damage. In more advanced cases, leaky blood vessels can be sealed with photocoagulation, a laser treatment. If the growth of excess blood vessels is extensive, a pattern of laser burns across the wall of the retina is applied that will shrink the vessels. A side effect of laser treatment is that peripheral vision may be adversely affected. If blood is leaking into the vitreous humor, surgery may be performed to remove the damaged fluid and replace it with a clear saline liquid.

Christina M. Girod

See also: Cardiovascular Disease; Cholesterol; Diabetes, Type 1; Eye Diseases; Heart Disease; Hypertension

Further Reading

American Diabetes Association. (2015). Eye complications. Retrieved from http://www.diabetes.org/living-with-diabetes/complications/eye-complications/.

Boyer, D. S., & Tabandeh, H. (2014). *Diabetic Retinopathy: From Diagnosis to Treatment.* Omaha, NE: Addicus Books.

Kellogg Eye Center. (2015). Eye conditions: Diabetic retinopathy. Retrieved from http://www.kellogg.umich.edu/patientcare/conditions/diabetic.retinopathy.html.

Mayo Clinic. (2016). Diabetic retinopathy. Retrieved from http://www.mayoclinic.org/diseases-conditions/diabetic-retinopathy/basics/definition/con-20023311.

National Eye Institute. (2015). Diabetic retinopathy. Retrieved from https://nei.nih.gov/health/diabetic/.

RHEUMATIC FEVER AND RHEUMATIC HEART DISEASE

Rheumatic fever is an inflammatory autoimmune disease that can develop as a complication of inadequately treated group A strep throat infection or scarlet fever.

It occurs most commonly in children ages 5 to 15, but it can occur in younger children and adults. Rheumatic fever occurs very rarely in the United States and other developed countries, but it is still common in many developing nations.

Although the inflammation caused by rheumatic fever may only last a few weeks or months, in some cases, the inflammation may cause long-term complications such as permanent damage to the heart, which results in rheumatic heart disease. One common result of rheumatic fever is heart valve damage, which can lead to valve disorders.

History

Rheumatic fever has been described since the 1500s but that the association between a throat infection and rheumatic fever symptom development was not described until the 1880s. In the 1900s, it was associated with scarlet fever. Prior to the widespread usage of penicillin, rheumatic fever was a leading cause of death among children and one of the leading causes of acquired heart disease in adults.

Symptoms

Rheumatic fever has many symptoms and can affect different parts of the body, including the heart, joints, skin, and brain, and these variable symptoms include fever and the presence of pain in one joint that migrates to another, most often the ankles, knees, elbows or wrists and less often the shoulders, hips, hands, and feet. Red, hot, or swollen joints and the presence of small, painless nodules beneath the skin are additional symptoms. Others are fatigue; heart murmurs; pain in the chest; having a painless rash; and demonstrating uncontrollable body movements of the hands, feet, and face. Accompanying these movements may be outbursts of unusual behavior, such as crying or inappropriate laughing (Mayo Clinic 2014).

Key Causes and Risk Factors

The key cause of rheumatic fever is an infection of the throat by a bacterium known as Streptococcus pyogenes, or group A streptococcus. Group A streptococcus infections of the throat cause strep throat or, less commonly, scarlet fever. Other factors that put an individual at risk are family history and environmental factors, such as poor sanitation and overcrowding.

Diagnosis

There is no simple diagnostic test for rheumatic fever, so the American Heart Association's modified Jones criteria (first published in 1944 and listed here) are used to assist the physician in making the proper diagnosis.

The major criteria for diagnosis include

Arthritis in several joints
Heart inflammation
Skin nodules
Rapid, jerky movements
Skin rash

The minor criteria include fever, a high erythrocyte sedimentation rate, a laboratory sign of inflammation, joint pain, EKG changes (electrocardiogram), echocardiography, and other laboratory findings (elevated C-reactive protein, elevated or rising streptococcal antigen test).

Diagnosing rheumatic heart disease involves looking for evidence of streptococcal infections, including lab tests; listening to the heart for murmurs; and imaging of the heart, including chest x-rays, echocardiograms, electrocardiograms, and MRI.

Treatments

The first step in treating rheumatic fever focuses on eradicating the bacteria, usually by using penicillin. The doctor may also recommend the use of anti-inflammatory medications such as aspirin or naproxen to reduce inflammation, fever, and pain. If symptoms are severe, the doctor may prescribe a corticosteroid, such as prednisone. Anticonvulsant medication is recommended if the patient exhibits severe involuntary movements.

Treating rheumatic heart disease can include years of antibiotics and, in some cases, valve surgery.

Prognosis

Rheumatic fever can cause permanent damage to the heart, including the heart valves, and this can lead to heart failure. Treatments however, can reduce tissue damage from inflammation, lessen pain and other symptoms, and prevent rheumatic fever from re occurring.

Prevention

The only known way to prevent rheumatic fever is to treat strep throat infections or scarlet fever promptly using the correct form of antibiotic.

Ray Marks

See also: Autoimmune Disease; Heart Failure; Heart Murmur; Heart Valve Disorders; Vaccines

Further Reading

Mayo Clinic. (2014). Rheumatic fever. Retrieved from http://www.mayoclinic.org/diseases
-conditions/rheumatic-fever/basics/definition/CON-20031399.

MedlinePlus. (2014, May 11). Rheumatic fever. Retrieved from https://www.nlm.nih.gov
/medlineplus/ency/article/003940.htm.

MedicineNet.com. (2016, March 18). Rheumatic fever (acute rheumatic fever or ARF).
Retrieved from http://www.onhealth.com/rheumatic_fever/article.htm.

WebMD. (2014, May 28). Rheumatic fever. Retrieved from http://www.webmd.com/a-to-z
-guides/rheumatic-fever.

RHEUMATOID ARTHRITIS

Rheumatoid arthritis is a highly disabling autoimmune disease of the muscles and joints, as well as several body systems, such as the cardiovascular system, the eyes, and the skin. A disease of no known cause, the condition affects everyone in a unique way. In some cases, the disease progresses rapidly; in other cases, it may develop slowly. It may start early on in life or among people in their middle years or in the older age ranges. Sometimes, the disease may cease after a period of activity, which is known as a remission stage. This can be permanent or temporary.

The disease is more common in women than men and affects approximately 1 percent of Americans and other worldwide. Most often, the disease occurs because the immune system attacks the cell membranes lining the joints, called the synovium. When this part of the joint becomes thick and inflamed, it causes immense pain, and destroys the underlying bone and cartilage lining the joint. Gradually, the tendons of the joint weaken, causing the joint to lose its shape or alignment. Usually, the joints of the hands and feet are involved first, and after that, other joints such as the spinal joints, the knee joint and hip joints, and shoulder joints may become involved. Most commonly, affected individuals will experience pain, inflammation or swelling of the affected joints, muscle weakness, joint stiffness, bone erosion, joint deformity, and diminished mobility. Eventually, affected individuals may become highly disabled.

Although the disease has no cure, early diagnosis and treatment may slow the disease progression and reduce the extent of the disability.

Symptoms

Rheumatoid arthritis is commonly a long-standing chronic disease that begins suddenly or over time in the small joints of the fingers and toes. Most cases have at least five involved joints, and these affected sites occur on both sides of the body. Another common symptom is stiffness in the early morning that usually indicates the presence of inflammation. Other common features of rheumatoid arthritis are joint swelling, tenderness and pain, anemia, fatigue, appetite loss, and weight loss. Further problems may include depression; some form of systemic illness such as inflammation of the lungs, tear glands, or salivary glands; and inflammation of the larynx or voice box. The affected person may develop rheumatoid nodules or bumps under the skin.

Key Causes and Risk Factors

There is no known cause for rheumatoid arthritis. Several factors may increase the risk of developing rheumatoid arthritis, including age, being between 40 and 60, being female, and having a family history of rheumatoid arthritis. Other risk factors for developing rheumatoid arthritis include smoking and low testosterone levels in men. Environmental factors including viral and bacterial infections may trigger the disease in susceptible individuals, as may the presence of chronic periodontal disease.

Diagnostic Procedures

Several tests, including medical examination; clinical testing for joint swelling, redness, warmth, changes in muscle strength, and reflex responses; and a history—may be helpful for diagnosing the condition.

Several types of blood tests are commonly conducted, including an erythrocyte sedimentation rate and a C-reactive protein (CRP) test to examine inflammation. A test for anemia and a rheumatoid factor blood test can detect the presence of rheumatoid factor in the patient's blood. Imaging scans and x-rays are used to determine the extent of any joint damage.

Diagnostic Criteria

Since 1987, the American College of Rheumatology has used the presence of several factors to diagnose rheumatoid arthritis, including:

- Morning stiffness longer than an hour most mornings for at least six weeks
- Pain and local swelling of more than 3/14 joints/joint groups for at least six weeks
- Pain of the hand joints for at least six weeks
- Symmetrical joint pain arthritis for at least six weeks
- Nodules below the skin at specific sites
- Rheumatoid factor that exceeds the 95th percentile
- Radiological changes that imply joint erosion

For a classification of rheumatoid arthritis, at least four of the preceding criteria are required. However, it is recommended that the condition be treated as early as possible to prevent bone erosion, even if the criteria are not met.

The diagnosis may also be based on the pattern of symptoms, the distribution of the affected joints, and the blood and x-ray findings, and the doctor may perform a procedure called an arthrocentesis using a sterile needle and syringe to draw joint fluid out of the joint for laboratory study. Several visits may be necessary before the doctor can be certain of the diagnosis, and this may require a rheumatologist or person specialized in treating the condition to examine all the facts.

There are four disease stages or classes for people diagnosed with this progressive disease:

- Class I: Able to perform usual daily activities.
- Class II: Able to perform usual self-care and work activities but performs work and other activities less well.
- Class III: Able to perform usual self-care activities, but work and other activities are limited.
- Class IV: Limited in the ability to perform usual self-care, work, and other activities.

Treatment

Treatment is aimed at reducing inflammation to the joints; relieving pain; minimizing disability, joint damage, or deformity; or slowing down or preventing joint damage. With the help of occupational and physical therapists, patients can learn how to protect their joints. In cases of severe joint damage, medication and/or surgery may be required. Types of drugs used include nonsteroidal anti-inflammatory drugs (NSAIDs) to relieve pain and reduce inflammation, steroids to reduce pain and inflammation and slow joint damage, and disease-modifying antirheumatic drugs (DMARDs) to slow the progression of rheumatoid arthritis and other tissues from permanent damage. Immunosuppressants to stabilize the immune system and tumor necrosis factor-alpha (TNF-alpha) to reduce inflammation, along with several other rheumatoid arthritis drugs, may be used to counter inflammation.

Assistive devices, braces, and taping can be used to prevent or slow joint damage, reduce pain, and correct deformities. Surgical procedures may include joint replacement surgery, tendon repair, and joint fusion. Other therapies include exercise, hydrotherapy, heat or cold, relaxation, and tai chi.

The best treatment may involve a combination of medications, rest, joint-strengthening exercises, joint protection, and patient (and family) education. Treatment is usually tailored in light of disease activity; the joints involved; and the patient's health status, age, and occupation.

Prognosis

Rheumatoid arthritis increases a person's risk of developing osteoporosis, carpal tunnel syndrome, heart conditions, and lung disease.

Early, aggressive treatment results in a better outlook than later intervention where patients have deformity, disability, ongoing uncontrolled joint inflammation, and/or rheumatoid disease of other organs. The condition tends to be more damaging when rheumatoid factor is present.

Prevention

Currently, rheumatoid arthritis cannot be prevented. Because cigarette smoking, exposure to silica minerals, and chronic periodontal disease all increase the risk for rheumatoid arthritis, avoiding these conditions is recommended.

Future

Scientists throughout the world are studying treatments that can block inflammation.

Studies involving various types of the connective tissue collagen are in progress and show encouraging signs of reducing rheumatoid disease activity. Finally, genetic research and engineering may permit earlier diagnosis and more accurate treatments in the future, as may gene profiling to determine which patients will be at more risk for more severe disease.

Ray Marks

See also: Addison's Disease; Alcoholism; Arthritis; Bone Diseases; Celiac Disease; Diabetes, Type 1; Felty Syndrome; Hypothyroidism; Immune System Disorders; Joint Disorders; Kidney Failure; Multiple Myeloma; Musculoskeletal Disorders; Osteoarthritis; Pain, Chronic; Sjögren's Syndrome

Further Reading

Arthritis Foundation. (2016). Types of arthritis. Retrieved from http://www.arthritis.org /conditions-treatments/disease-center/rheumatoid-arthritis/.

Levine, H. (2015, November). Your joints: A user's manual. *Health, 29*(9), 99–104.

Lorig, K., & Fries, J. F. (2006). *The Arthritis Helpbook: A Tested Self-Management Program for Coping with Arthritis and Fibromyalgia,* 6th ed. New York: Da Capo Press.

Mayo Clinic. (2013). Rheumatoid arthritis. Retrieved from http://www.mayoclinic.org /diseases-conditions/rheumatoid-arthritis/basics/definition/con-20014.868.

MedlinePlus. (2014). Rheumatoid arthritis. Retrieved from http://www.nlm.nih.gov/med lineplus/rheumatoidarthritis.html.

National Institute of Arthritis and Musculoskeletal Diseases. (2014). Rheumatoid arthritis. Retrieved from http://www.niams.nih.gov/Health_Info/Rheumatic_Disease/default.asp.

Shlotzhauer, T. L. (2014). *Living with Rheumatoid Arthritis,* 3rd ed. Baltimore, MD: Johns Hopkins University Press.

RICKETS

Rickets is a children's disease involving the softening and weakening of growing bones, usually because of extreme prolonged vitamin D deficiency. The condition is found more frequently among infants and children living in industrialized nations and among those who are more affluent, and it may lead to skeletal deformity and shortness of height, pelvic distortion, and an increased tendency toward fractures.

The term *rickets* stems from an old English term "wrickken," meaning to twist or bend.

Symptoms

Signs and symptoms of rickets include bone pain or tenderness in the spine, pelvis, and legs; dental deformities; muscle weakness; delayed formation of teeth; decreased muscle strength; delayed growth; short stature; and a number of skeletal deformities, including an abnormally shaped skull, bowlegs, rib-cage abnormalities, and thickened wrists and ankles. In severe cases, there may be involuntary muscle contractions and seizures and respiratory problems. There may also be evidence of easy fracturing.

Key Causes and Risk Factors

Key causes include a lack of vitamin D, causing nutritional rickets, or *osteomalacia*, and a lack of calcium or phosphate in the diet that leads to *hypophosphatemic* rickets, where the bones become painfully soft and pliable as a result of a genetic cause.

Factors that may increase a child's risk of rickets include age, poverty, having a dark skin, living in northern latitudes, being subject to exclusive breast feeding or a vegan or lactovegan diet, malnutrition, being a premature baby, wearing sunscreen and playing indoors, and being on anti-seizure medication; other factors include having a malabsorption syndrome, liver disease, or renal disease that produces a condition called *renal rickets*.

Diagnosis

A medical, clinical, and nutritional exam may be conducted. The physician may examine the skull, legs, chest, wrists, and ankles for signs of bone or musculoskeletal abnormalities.

X-rays of the affected bones and bone biopsies may be helpful. As well, blood serum, blood gas tests, and urine tests may be used to confirm the diagnosis of rickets and to evaluate the outcome of treatment.

Treatment

Most cases of rickets can be treated with vitamin D and calcium supplements.

In some cases, bowlegs or spinal deformities may require splinting or surgical intervention.

Prognosis

The outcome depends on severity of the condition and how early it is diagnosed, as well as the cause.

Prevention

Most adolescents and adults receive much of their necessary vitamin D from sunlight exposure. Infants and young children, however, need to experience some sunlight or foods that contain vitamin D, such as fatty fish, fish oil, and egg yolks or foods that have been fortified with vitamin D, such as infant formula, milk, cereals, and orange juice. Parental prenatal education and counseling may be helpful.

Ray Marks

See also: Bone Diseases; Poverty; Vitamin D

Further Reading

Mayo Clinic. (2014). Rickets. Retrieved from http://www.mayoclinic.org/diseases-conditions /rickets/basics/definition/con-20027091.

Medical News Today. (2015, September 10). Rickets: Causes, symptoms and treatments. Retrieved from http://www.medicalnewstoday.com/articles/176941.php.

MedicineNet.com. (2016, March 7). Rickets (calcium, phosphate, or vitamin D deficiency). Retrieved from http://www.medicinenet.com/rickets/article.htm.

MedlinePlus. (2014). Rickets. Retrieved from http://www.nlm.nih.gov/medlineplus/ency /article/000344.htm.

RISK FACTORS

Risk factors heighten the possibility of a person sustaining an injury or contracting a disease. In chronic diseases such as heart disease, stroke, kidney disease, and arthritis, common risk factors are age, family history, gender, low birth weight, poverty, level of education, genetic factors, infectious agents, and obesity.

Other risk factors for promoting the onset or severity of a disease are smoking, excess alcohol usage, untreated depression, lack of exercise, unhealthy diets, hypertension or increased blood pressure, elevated blood sugar and blood lipids, psychological stress, and carrying out risky sexual practices.

It is thought that by reducing or eliminating one or more modifiable risk factors, a person has less chance of contracting an illness, and even if he or she does, the person will be less likely to suffer excess disability compared to those who are not able to modify their modifiable risk factors.

Strategies to help a person reduce their risk of disease include exercise, keeping a healthy weight, nutrition programs, giving up smoking, immunizations, counseling, avoid excess sunlight, and practicing safe sex.

A person at high risk for a disease due to family history may want to receive counseling early on from a health care provider.

Environmental and social conditions that serve as risk factors such as pollution, poor housing, unsafe water, and access to good sanitation are very common in developing countries and require help of policy makers and governments to intervene to reduce these risk factors.

Ray Marks

See also: Alcoholism; Cardiovascular Disease; Diabetes, Type 1; Diabetes, Type 2; Environment; Epidemiology; Etiology; Family Health; Healthy Lifestyles and Risky Behaviors; Hypertension; Obesity; Poverty; Substance Abuse

Further Reading

Centers for Disease Control and Prevention. (2013). Preventing chronic disease and reducing risk factors. Retrieved from http://www.cdc.gov/nccdphp/dch/programs/healthy communitiesprogram/overview/diseasesandrisks.htm.

Public Health Agency of Canada. (2014). Chronic disease risk factors. Retrieved from http://www.phac-aspc.gc.ca/cd-mc/risk_factors-facteurs_risque-eng.php.

World Health Organization. (2014). Chronic diseases and their common risk factors. Retrieved from http://www.who.int/chp/chronic_disease_report/media/Factsheet1.pdf.

ROSACEA

Rosacea is a chronic skin disorder that creates redness and acne-like bumps on the face. Because it can look similar to acne or allergic reactions and can flare up and go into remission sporadically, rosacea is commonly mistaken for other skin conditions. Although the disease most often occurs in adult women under 60, men are not immune to the problem. With his signature red, bulbous nose, the late comedian W. C. Fields has long been the "poster child" for rosacea. A large, red, bumpy nose such as Fields' is indicative of *rhinophyma*, an advanced symptom of rosacea.

The symptoms of rosacea are broken into four different subtypes: erythematotelangiectatic rosacea, papulopustular rosacea, phymatous rosacea, and ocular rosacea. Each subtype typically occurs at a different stage of progression, but this is not always the case, and it is possible for a person to have the symptoms of one subtype without ever being affected by the others. At the earliest stages, rosacea usually presents as erythematotelangiectatic rosacea, which is indicated by redness in the center of the face, including the forehead, nose, and chin. In some cases, the redness will also appear on the neck, ears, and other areas of the head. Flushed red skin may also be accompanied by a burning or itching sensation and mild swelling. Generally, the redness and associated symptoms will come and go at first, growing more persistent over time. As rosacea progresses, the blood vessels under the affected skin grow larger, causing red lines to appear. If left untreated at this stage, small bumps develop on the skin; this is the papulopustular rosacea subtype. These bumps may be painful and can contain debris-filled fluid called pus, much like acne. Over time, the skin can become thicker in affected areas and the nose may swell, much like Fields' did. This is the subtype phymatous rosacea. Additionally, in the progressed stages of rosacea, the eyes and eyelids may grow inflamed (ocular rosacea), causing irritation and redness in the eyes, and sometimes vision problems. Some 50 percent of people with rosacea eventually have eye-related issues.

Some 14 million Americans have rosacea, and millions more are affected by the condition around the world. The exact cause of rosacea is not yet known, but there is some indication that it may occur as a result of a genetic abnormality that allows blood vessels to expand too easily or possibly as a combination of both hereditary and environmental factors. People with fair skin who tend to blush readily seem to be at highest risk for the condition. Other factors recognized as possible triggers for rosacea include emotional or mental stress, menopause (in women), hot or spicy foods and beverages, alcohol consumption, and exposure to extremely cold temperatures. Additionally, it is possible that certain blood pressure medications and other drugs used to dilate blood vessels may also trigger rosacea.

There is no specific test designed to diagnose rosacea. Rather, medical professionals rely on patient history and a physical examination of the skin to pinpoint the condition. Depending on the signs and symptoms, more tests may be conducted to rule out other skin disorders. Even though there is no cure for rosacea, the condition can be treated and managed. Topical antibiotic creams and lotions and oral antibiotic medications may be prescribed to relieve inflammation and skin bumps. In the event that antibiotics are not effective at treating the symptoms, acne-fighting medications may also be recommended. If facial skin has thickened, laser surgery and other types of surgical procedures can be used to remove excess tissue from the nose and face. Such procedures are often followed with dermabrasion, a skin resurfacing technique in which a wire brush or other instrument is used to sand down the rough outer layers of the skin and allow for smooth skin to grow in its place.

Early European literature described characters affected by what may be rosacea, and the first medical professional who was thought to have written about the skin condition was a 14th-century French doctor, Guy de Chauliac. By the 19th century, however, the condition was still thought of as an acne-related issue, and up until the late 20th century it was still considered a rare disorder. So little attention was given to it that the Food and Drug Administration (FDA) only approved the first medicine for use in treating rosacea in 1992. Since that time, rosacea has become one of the most commonly diagnosed skin disorders, and more funding and research has been put into finding both the cause and a cure than ever before. A standard definition and description of the subtypes of rosacea was agreed on in 2002, and standard medical management techniques for the disorder were finally published in 2009.

Tamar Burris

See also: Eye Diseases; Skin Conditions

Further Reading

Brownstein, N. D. Arlen. (2001). *Rosacea: Your Self-Help Guide.* Oakland, CA: New Harbinger Publications.

Mayo Clinic. (2016). Rosacea. Retrieved from http://www.mayoclinic.org/diseases-conditions/rosacea/basics/definition/con-20014478.

National Rosacea Society. (2016). All about rosacea. Retrieved from http://www.rosacea.org/patients/allaboutrosacea.php.

Powell, F. (2008). *Rosacea: Diagnosis and Management.* Boca Raton, FL: CRC Press.

Rosacea Research and Development Institute. (2016). What is rosacea? Retrieved from http://irosacea.org/.

S

SALIVARY GLAND DISORDERS

There are three types of salivary glands, located in the mouth, that produce saliva. There are two *parotid* glands in the upper part of the cheek area, two *submandibular* glands in the floor of the mouth, and two *sublingual* glands located below the tongue. In addition, there are hundreds of very tiny salivary glands throughout the mouth. There are many types of problems that can arise that result in salivary gland blockage and/or infection, and these health conditions cause problems in the functioning of the salivary glands that serve to moisten food and help with chewing and swallowing, speaking, and protecting the teeth. Some of these conditions include salivary gland stones or sialolithiasis; sialadenitis or bacterial infections; parotid gland cysts, which may cause inflammation of the salivary glands; noncancerous tumors; cancerous tumors; and Sjögren's syndrome, an autoimmune disorder of the salivary glands that may be long lasting and cause dry mouth. Other possible symptoms are sores in the mouth, tooth decay, enlarged salivary glands, and repeated infections of the salivary glands. The term *sialadenosis* refers to the nonspecific enlargement of the salivary glands, which may not resolve.

Signs and Symptoms

Among the symptoms of salivary health conditions are dry mouth, difficulty opening the mouth and swallowing, pain in the face or mouth areas, a painful lump in the floor of the mouth, swelling in front of the ears or the face or neck areas, and foul-tasting or abnormally tasting foods. There may headaches, fever, and muscle pain.

Causes and Risk Factors

Some of the problems of the salivary glands arise as a result of other health conditions. Some are due to infections, cysts or tumors, dehydration, malnutrition, and eating disorders. Smoking and exposure to radiation are other possible causes.

Diagnosis

A medical examination, blood tests, and/or x-rays, called *sialograms*, may be helpful in diagnosing a particular salivary gland problem. Other forms of diagnosis include the use of magnetic resonance imaging (MRI) or computed tomography (CT). To ascertain if any tumors are present, the physician might require some cells from the salivary glands to be removed by a fine needle, known as fine-needle aspiration. Blood tests, salivary gland biopsy tests, and salivary function tests may also be used. One test known as *sialography* uses dye injected into the duct of the gland so the salivary pathways of saliva flow can be seen.

Treatment

The treatment will depend on the nature of the problem and may require drinking a lot of water with unsweetened lemon added to promote saliva production, drinking orange juice, or receiving fluids intravenously. The removal of stones either manually by the doctor or through surgery, called *sialolithiasis*, may be needed, and infections can be treated with antibiotics or by actively draining the infected glands. Pain medications and rest may help those who have infections and fever, and if cysts do not resolve, they can be removed surgically using lasers.

Tumors may be treated with surgery alone and/or with radiation after that. Larger tumors may also require chemotherapy to be administered.

For those with Sjögren's syndrome, medication to relieve dry mouth and avoiding caffeinated drinks, alcohol, and spicy or acidic foods may be recommended. Other approaches may aim at correcting any underlying medical condition.

Prognosis or Outcome

Most problems associated with the salivary glands respond well to treatment. Sjögren's syndrome may not resolve and is a chronic health condition.

Prevention

Avoiding smoking; and making sure to drink adequate amounts of water per day, practice good dental care, and eat a healthful diet might help to prevent some forms of salivary gland disturbances. There is some evidence that massaging the affected gland will increase saliva flow and prevent infection. Getting immunized against flu and influenza may be helpful.

Ray Marks

See also: Oral Health; Sjögren's Syndrome

Further Reading

Cedars-Sinai. (2016). Salivary gland disease and tumors. Retrieved from http://www.cedars-sinai.edu/Patients/Health-Conditions/Salivary-Gland-Disease-and-Tumors.aspx.
Harvard Medical School. (2016). Salivary gland disorders. Patient Education Center. Retrieved from http://www.patienteducationcenter.org/articles/salivary-gland-disorders/.
Health Guide/New York Times. (2016). Salivary gland disorders. http://health.nytimes.com/health/guides/disease/salivary-gland-disorders/overview.html.

National Institutes of Health. (2013). Salivary diagnostics. Retrieved from http://report.nih
.gov/NIHfactsheets/ViewFactSheet.aspx?csid=65.

SCHIZOPHRENIA

Schizophrenia is a rare, chronic, highly disabling brain disease affecting about
1 percent of the U.S. population (about 2.2 million people), usually people younger
than 45 years of age, most commonly starting in the teenage years. The person with
this health condition hears voices and may believe things are occurring even when
they are not. People with schizophrenia can be very agitated and can frighten others.
It is a serious brain or mental disorder and usually distorts a person's thinking, behaviors, emotions, perception of reality, and ability to relate to others. It is a psychosis whereby the person cannot tell fantasy from reality.

There are different types of schizophrenia:

Paranoid schizophrenia: The person is preoccupied with false beliefs about being
persecuted or being punished by someone.

Disorganized schizophrenia: The person is frequently confused and incoherent and
has jumbled speech. Her or his outward behavior may be emotionless or flat or
inappropriate, even silly or childlike. The person often has disorganized behavior
that may disrupt her or his ability to perform normal daily activities such as show-
ering or preparing meals.

Catatonic schizophrenia: The person may remain immobile and unresponsive to
the world around him or her. At other times, he or she may adopt peculiar movements or take up strange postures. He or she may go back and forth between more
sedentary behaviors and restless, purposeless behaviors and place him- or herself
at risk for malnutrition, exhaustion, or self-inflicted injury.

Undifferentiated schizophrenia: This term is used when the person's symptoms do
not clearly fall into one of the other three subtypes.

Residual schizophrenia: In this type of schizophrenia, the severity of schizophrenia symptoms is decreased, but hallucinations, delusions, or other symptoms may
still be present.

Symptoms

Hallucinations and delusions are common. There may be thought and movement
disorders and disorganized thinking or speech. The person feels a lack of pleasure
in everyday life. She or he may need help with daily tasks and may start something,
but not finish it. She or he may have difficulty focusing and paying attention, may
have memory problems, and may appear to lack emotions.

Key Causes and Risk Factors

Genetic factors, as well as environmental factors play a role in this disease. Recent
findings show genes that can be identified. Schizophrenia might be linked to a gene

that communicates with the immune system to destroy connections in the brain. Scientists at Harvard University and the Broad Institute studied the genomes of 64,785 people around the world and found that those with schizophrenia were much more likely to possess mutations of a gene (Courage 2016).

Taking mind-altering drugs when young, having an autoimmune disease, having an altered brain structure, and a family history of schizophrenia may increase the risk of acquiring this condition. Pollution has also been identified as a possible cause of gene altering.

Diagnosis

A physical exam, a psychological exam, and blood tests and various scans may be performed to arrive at a diagnosis.

Treatment, Prognosis, and Prevention

Antipsychotic medications and psychotherapy are common methods of treatment. Cognitive-behavioral therapy, family therapy, and specific forms of rehabilitation may be required and helpful.

People with this condition can learn to control their symptoms and lead normal lives, but they may require lifelong treatment.

There is no form of prevention for schizophrenia, but early and continued intervention may reduce the severity of the condition.

Ray Marks

See also: Alzheimer's Disease; Anxiety Disorders; Bipolar Disorder; Brain Disorders; Dementia; Depression; Fetal Alcohol Syndrome; Men's Health; Mental Disorders; Psychotic Disorders; PTSD (Posttraumatic Stress Disorder); Social Health; Women's Health

Further Reading

Chase, R. (2013). *Schizophrenia.* Baltimore, MD: Johns Hopkins University Press.

Courage, K. H. (2016, January 29). Variations in a gene provide clues about schizophrenia. NPR. Retrieved from http://www.npr.org/sections/health-shots/2016/01/29/464703705 /variations-in-a-gene-provide-clues-about-schizophrenia.

Mayo Clinic. (2014). Schizophrenia. Retrieved from http://www.mayoclinic.org/diseases -conditions/schizophrenia/basics/definition/con-20021077.

Mental Health America. (2014). Schizophrenia. Retrieved from http://www.mentalhealtham erica.net/conditions/schizophrenia.

Miller, R., & Mason, S. E., eds. (2011). *Diagnosis: Schizophrenia : A Comprehensive Resource for Consumers, Families, and Helping Professionals.* New York: Columbia University Press.

National Institute of Mental Health. (2014). What is schizophrenia? Retrieved from http:// www.nimh.nih.gov/health/topics/schizophrenia/index.shtml.

Sekar, A., et al. (2016, January 27.) Schizophrenia risk from complex variation of complement component 4. (2016). *Nature.* Published online January 27, 2106. doi:10.1038/nature 16549.

SCHOOL WELLNESS PROGRAMS

School wellness programs are programs administered by school districts to promote the physical and mental health of students. These programs are based on the concept that the academic success of students is positively correlated to the good health of the students. Furthermore, these programs are aimed at preventing chronic illness, both in young people and in later years. School wellness programs are used primarily in elementary school and high school to encourage young people to learn and develop lifelong good habits regarding their health. Besides students and teachers, wellness programs may also include the participation of parents, physicians, nurses, mental health therapists, social workers, and even the occasional celebrity, such as a guest speaker who is a famous athlete.

Meeting Public Health Challenges

School wellness programs are becoming increasingly important as a result of certain public health challenges in the United States. Although the U.S. Centers for Disease Control and Prevention (CDC) recommends that children and adolescents participate in at least 60 minutes of physical activity every day, this recommendation is not widely followed. Many young people fail to get any significant physical exercise because they spend excessive amounts of time indoors on their cells phones, computers, or other electronic devices. Furthermore, many school districts—faced with the challenge of addressing declining academic performance among their students—have reduced the number of hours devoted to physical education.

Statistics suggest that overweight and obesity rates among American children and adolescents continue to increase. That rising rate is clearly associated with both the lack of exercise and fatty food consumption. Bad habits regarding physical activity and nutrition that start in childhood are likely to persist into adulthood. Being overweight or obese substantially increases the risk of numerous chronic diseases, including cardiovascular disease (leading to heart attack or stroke), diabetes mellitus, and certain cancers. Administrators of school wellness programs hope that early education and intervention on this subject matter will eventually lead to a healthier American population.

School wellness programs can also help address various socioeconomic problems among families and within communities. Some families do not have access to health insurance, regular physician care, or healthy foods as a result of financial difficulties, a lack of knowledge, or both. Some neighborhoods may not have safe parks or other outdoor environments for after-school activities. Certain communities tend to have high rates of particular diseases, such as asthma, diabetes, or HIV/AIDS. Although school wellness programs cannot solve these problems, they may be able to provide students and their families with useful information so that they can better tackle the problems themselves. For example, wellness programs usually provide safe places for sports activities, as well as knowledge about common diseases. And some wellness programs teach students and parents about obtaining affordable health insurance and financial assistance.

Federal Guidelines

The U.S. Department of Education (DOE) requires any school district that participates in federally funded student meal programs to implement a wellness policy. Most district wellness policies are based partially on the following DOE guidelines:

- Students should be given opportunities to be physically active on a regular basis.
- Food and beverages served in school must meet nutritional recommendations in the *Dietary Guidelines for Americans* (published by the Department of Health and Human Services).
- School meals should be affordable, nutritious, and appealing—meeting students' nutritional needs while also accommodating their religious, ethnic, and cultural preferences.
- Students must be given adequate time to eat in clean, sanitary settings.
- Students should be provided with nutritional and physical educations that foster life-long habits of healthy eating and physical activity.

One way in which schools are attempting to meet these federal nutritional guidelines is by offering students healthier food options in school cafeterias and vending machines. Instead of soft drinks with high-calorie sweeteners, fruit and vegetable juices containing at least 50 percent real juice are offered. Foods containing no more than 35 percent of their calories from fat are preferred healthy dietary options, as are foods with low levels of sodium. Such low-nutrition snack foods as potato chips, crackers, popcorn, and cookies should be served in small portions only.

Lessons in Curricula

As part of their wellness programs, most school districts incorporate a variety of health and physical education requirements into their standard curricula. Generally, elementary and high school curricula include lessons on physical activity and nutrition; emotional and mental health; violence and injury prevention; consumer health; alcohol, tobacco, and drug use prevention; and sexual health (including prevention of HIV/AIDS and other sexually transmitted diseases). Individual school districts have more specific curricular requirements. For example, health and physical education requirements in the curricular standards of New York City high schools include the following:

- Students are taught that sexual responsibility includes understanding one's sexuality, respecting oneself and others, avoiding physical and emotional harm, and recognizing diversity in sexual beliefs.
- Students learn to recognize qualities of healthy relationships, how to nurture healthy relationships, and how to avoid or discontinue unhealthy and unsafe relationships.
- Students learn to recognize signs of stress within themselves and others and how to use positive means of relieving stress.
- Students obtain necessary knowledge and skills to maintain physical fitness, participate in physical activity, and maintain personal health.

- Students learn why physical activity is important, and how it benefits them, through participation in traditional and nontraditional sports and other health-related activities.
- Students learn to make healthy personal decisions and to develop healthy lifestyles.

In addition to providing education about personal health and fitness, many school wellness programs also incorporate "green" education related to the health of the environment. This education may include such subjects as organic gardening, resource sustainability and conservation, recycling, composting, dangers of environmental toxins, and environmental benefits from walking and bicycling.

Outside-School Activities

Beyond their in-school programs, many school districts also sponsor or participate in events outside school to promote healthy lifestyles. For example, fitness festivals, family walks and runs, sports competitions and clubs, fund-raising for health care issues, and wellness summits are types of outside-school events and activities that students may be encouraged to participate in as part of district wellness programs. To encourage student achievement in these activities, small "rewards" might be given, such as medals for reaching 100 minutes of walking in a walking club.

Some school wellness programs are specifically designed for parent participation, such as the following programs offered as part of the Parent Academy run by the Cherry Creek School District in Colorado:

- Collaborative Problem Solving: coaches parents on how to deal with "chronically inflexible, easily frustrated children" and to reduce "meltdowns and shutdowns."
- Guiding Good Choices: coaches parents on how to teach their children "healthy decision making, impulse control, and peer refusal skills," as well as how to "better understand adolescent brain development and how it affects behaviors."

Other wellness programs for parents cover more basic elements of health, such as teaching parents how to prepare nutritious meals and how to make sure that their children engage in outdoor activities. Such parental instruction may take the form of special seminars for parents or take-home handouts given to students.

A. J. Smuskiewicz

See also: Centers for Disease Control and Prevention (CDC); Health; Healthy Lifestyles and Risky Behaviors; Healthy People 2020; Physical Activity

Further Reading

Centers for Disease Control and Prevention. (2016). School health guidelines. Retrieved from http://www.cdc.gov/healthyschools/npao/strategies.htm.

Hopkins, G. M. (2010, October 28). Principals launch school-wide wellness programs. *Education World*. Retrieved from http://www.educationworld.com/a_admin/admin/admin611.shtml.

Louisiana Public Health Institute. (2015). School wellness toolkit. Retrieved from http://lphi.org/CMSuploads/School-Wellness-Toolkit-82802.pdf.

McCary, J. (2007, March 1). Help to create a wellness program for your local schools. *IDEA Health & Fitness*. Retrieved from http://www.ideafit.com/fitness-library/help-create-wellness-program-your-local-schools.

New York City Department of Education, Office of School Wellness Programs. (2015). School wellness programs. Retrieved from http://schools.nyc.gov/Academics/Fitness andHealth/default.htm.

SEASONAL AFFECTIVE DISORDER

Seasonal affective disorder, known as SAD, is a form of depression that occurs at the same time each year. It frequently starts in the fall and may continue into the winter months; less often, it can occur in the early spring or summer. Between 4 and 6 percent of people in the United States are thought to suffer from this condition. Another 10 to 20 percent may experience a mild form of winter-onset SAD (Familydoctor.org 2012). The condition is most common in adult women 20 years and older. Children and teenagers can acquire the condition, however. The form that develops in winter is more common north of the equator, where the winter is typically long and severe.

The term first appeared in print in 1985. Seasonal affective disorder is also sometimes called winter depression, winter blues, or the hibernation reaction. Now, however, extensive research shows that SAD may not really exist as a seasonal disorder. Researchers could not identify markers of seasonally related depression (Association for Psychological Science 2016).

Symptoms

The winter-onset symptoms include anxiety and depression, energy loss, sleeping excessively, weight gain, loss of interest in usual activities and loss of energy, difficulty concentrating, and social withdrawal.

The type occurring in the summer may include weight loss, loss of appetite, insomnia, changes in sex drive, anxiety, and agitation.

Causes and Risk Factors

As noted earlier, recent research questions whether this condition exists, but it does not mean that people do not feel depressed in winter months. Causes have been thought to include disruptions of the circadian rhythm or biological clock that may lead to feelings of depression, reduced levels of serotonin, and a brain chemical that affects mood; in addition, reduced sunlight or inadequate light can cause a drop in serotonin, which may trigger depression. Another hormone, melatonin, and its level may be disrupted, causing changes in sleep patterns and mood.

Diagnosis

A diagnosis usually involves a medical history, a physical exam, and possibly a mental exam.

Treatment and Prognosis

Because depression can be serious, it should be investigated by a health professional. But for seasonal affective disorder, the main form of treatment is light or photo-therapy, psychotherapy, and medications.

The condition becomes less severe for adults over time.

Ray Marks

See also: Anxiety Disorders; Depression; Mental Disorders; Sleep Disturbances and Sleep Disorders

Further Reading

American Psychiatric Society. (2014). Seasonal affective disorder (SAD). Available at, http://www.psychiatry.org/seasonal-affective-disorder.

Association for Psychological Science. (2016, January 20). No evidence of seasonal differences in depressive symptoms. Retrieved from http://www.psychologicalscience.org/index.php/news/releases/no-evidence-of-seasonal-differences-in-depressive-symptoms.html.

Familydoctor.org. (2012). Seasonal affective disorder (SAD). Retrieved from http://familydoctor.org/familydoctor/en/diseases-conditions/seasonal-affective-disorder.html.

Mayo Clinic. (2011). Seasonal affective disorder (SAD). Retrieved from http://www.mayoclinic.org/diseases-conditions/seasonal-affective-disorder/basics/definition/CON-20021047.

SECONDHAND SMOKE

Secondhand smoke is defined as involuntarily or passively breathing in the smoke released by the burning of a tobacco product. There are two types of secondhand smoke (SHS), also known as environmental tobacco smoke (ETS): *sidestream smoke* and *mainstream smoke*. As defined by the American Cancer Society, "Sidestream smoke is the smoke that comes from the end of a lit cigarette, pipe, or cigar. Mainstream smoke is the smoke that a smoker breathes out" (American Cancer Society 2015). Those who are exposed to secondhand smoke are not smoking themselves. Breathing in the smoke released by someone smoking in the street or in your home is an example of secondhand smoke exposure.

A 2006 report of the Surgeon General noted that "there is no risk-free level of exposure to secondhand smoke" and this continues in the most recent Surgeon General report (Centers for Disease Control and Prevention [CDC] 2015). This means that no matter how much or how little smoke you inhale, you are still at risk of disease due to chemicals entering your body. Each breath of smoke, which contains the toxic chemicals in a cigarette, will result in the transfer of these toxins from the lungs into the bloodstream. This will carry toxins to almost every part of the body. It is these chemicals that can eventually cause damage to the cells in your body and lead to a series of chronic diseases and injuries, further leading to removal of body parts due to poor blood flow (circulation).

It should be noted that those exposed to secondhand smoke have a larger exposure to chemicals in tobacco products because more of the toxins are breathed out than kept in when smoking. As a result, studies show that even brief exposure to secondhand smoke can lead to negative health effects as serious as those seen in people who smoke one pack of cigarettes a day (CDC 2015). The health effects of secondhand exposure differ between children and adults. Adults who are exposed to smoke are more likely to have heart disease, strokes (the interruption or reduced blood supply and oxygen to part of the brain), heart attacks, lung cancer, nasal and eye irritation, and nasal sinus cancer. In women, exposure can result in low birth weight of their children.

Lower birth weight caused by smoke exposure can also lead to underdeveloped lungs in children, which can cause children to be at higher risk for developing asthma due to impaired lung function. Children are also at risk for middle ear diseases, lower respiratory illness, and sudden infant death syndrome (SIDS), a disease of unknown cause in children that results in death while they sleep.

For adults and children with asthma (a chronic disease of the lungs), exposure to smoke through both secondhand and third-hand smoke have been indicated as two of the most common environmental triggers for asthma. As such, exposure can make it hard to manage the symptoms of the disease. Children exposed to second-hand smoke are increasingly at risk of bronchitis, pneumonia, and slow lung growth (CDC 2015). Common symptoms from these diseases are wheezing, coughing, and tightness in the chest.

It is estimated that more than 3,000 nonsmokers die of lung cancer every year. It is also noted by the American Cancer Society that exposure to secondhand smoke can cause women to have spontaneous abortions, still births (the baby is not born alive), and other problems with their pregnancy, as well as problems with fertility because of the damage secondhand exposure can cause to sperm (American Cancer Society 2015).

Even brief exposure to secondhand smoke can lead to an increase in the risk of heart attacks. A 2009 report by the Institute of Medicine provided evidence that smoke is one of the causes for heart attacks (American Lung Association 2012). The Institute of Medicine further confirmed that even short amounts of exposure to smoke can trigger a heart attack (Institute of Medicine 2009).

Data from the Centers for Disease Control and Prevention (CDC) show that more than 126 million Americans who are nonsmokers are still being exposed to smoke in their homes, in their vehicles, near workplaces, and in public places. Most of the smoke exposure occurs in either the home or in the workplace, especially for individuals working in outdoor spaces. U.S. legislation is not consistent in terms of laws prohibiting smoking in public spaces. These laws vary from state to state.

Experts have begun to take a closer look at thirdhand smoke exposure and locations where tobacco-related chemicals can be found. *Thirdhand smoke* can be defined as exposure to chemicals that are left behind on different surfaces after a tobacco product has been burned. There are many way to be exposed to third-hand smoke. Some of these include chemicals absorbed into walls, in the carpet, and on sofas and other cloth furniture; chemicals remaining on paper such as drywall and curtains; and those remaining on a person's body. A person who smokes or has been around a person who was actively smoking will retain chemicals from tobacco products on his or her body. These chemicals will remain on the person's clothes, hair, and skin, as well as under the nails and on the breath.

Even if a person is not actively smoking, chemicals released by the burning of tobacco products often remain on these surfaces. New developments show that thirdhand smoke can be detected months after the smoking of the last cigarette. The sooner smokers stop, the sooner the environment will clear. Additional steps to clear a space of chemicals include stripping and repainting the walls (as paint absorbs the chemicals) and removing carpeting. Vents and electrical panels (behind the covers of outlets, switches, and electrical control boxes) must also be cleaned. It is also important to wash clothing, curtains, and remove or steam-clean any cloth furniture that may have absorbed chemicals released by tobacco products.

It is believed that small children are more affected by thirdhand smoke because they lie, crawl, and play on the floor. These behaviors lead to children taking in twice as much dust as adults; therefore, chemicals released by tobacco (the by-products) are inhaled in larger amounts.

As experts continue to assess the health impacts of secondhand smoke exposure and further their investigation of thirdhand smoke impact, we must consider what is necessary to minimize exposure and health impact on the community.

Health education and health promotion efforts to share information with the community about how to lessen their exposure to both secondhand and thirdhand smoke are necessary.

Definition of secondhand exposure so that people understand risk is essential. Latest studies show that secondhand smoke exposure is still underreported (CDC 2015).

In addition to sharing health messages, smoke-free focused organizations are currently attempting to increase the number of smoke-free housing locations throughout New York State in an effort to further decrease exposure and positively impact health. Other places such as Boston and Detroit are also creating similar policies. Ideally, this will become part of the federal guidelines to reduce secondhand and thirdhand smoke exposure and give smokers a reason to quit as restrictions to where they can live if they smoke provide more challenges and make smoking less desirable.

Tiffany Crystal Rivera

See also: COPD (Chronic Obstructive Pulmonary Disease); Emphysema; Legg-Calve-Perthes Disease; Lung Cancer; Lung Diseases; Occupational Cancer; Occupational Health; Pneumonia; Pollution; Tobacco Addiction

Further Reading

American Lung Association. (2012). Second hand smoke. http://www.lung.org/stop-smoking/about-smoking/health-effects/secondhand-smoke.html.

American Cancer Society. (2015). Second-hand smoke—tobacco and cancer. http://www.cancer.org/cancer/cancercauses/tobaccocancer/secondhand-smoke.

Centers for Disease Control and Prevention (CDC). (2015). 2014 Surgeon General's report: The health consequences of smoking—50 years of progress. Retrieved from http://www.cdc.gov/tobacco/data_statistics/sgr/50th-anniversary/index.htm.

Institute of Medicine (IOM). (2009). Secondhand smoke exposure and cardiovascular effects: Making sense of the evidence. Washington, DC: The National Academies Press.

SELF-MANAGEMENT

Self-management is the term applied to the many types of health-related behaviors and activities that people with one or more chronic diseases are expected to carry out on a regular basis to maximize their health. These activities include exercise, diet, getting enough sleep, and controlling stress, among other behaviors. Most diseases that are not effectively managed by the sufferer will progress more rapidly than if they are carefully managed by the person with the condition—for example, arthritis, diabetes, asthma, HIV/AIDS, and heart disease. To assist in self-management skills development and to help patients make informed decisions and obtain information about their condition(s), various educational strategies have been recommendation, such as attending special group education classes and having individual counseling or a trained facilitator. Educators and clinicians who are involved in this approach commonly try to help the client with goal setting, try to activate skills development and coping strategies, and try to reduce barriers to care as well as providing social support.

Ray Marks

See also: Diet and Nutrition; Fibromyalgia; Food Guides from the USDA

Further Reading

Administration on Aging. (2014). American Recovery and Investment Act—Communities Putting People to Work: Chronic Disease Self-Management Program. Retrieved from http://www.aoa.gov/AoA_programs/HPW/ARRA/index.aspx.

Bodenheimer, T., Lorig, K., Holman, H., & Grumbach, K. (2002). Patient self-management of chronic disease in primary care. *JAMA, 288*(19), 2469–2475. doi:10.1001/jama.288.19.2469.

Center for Managing Chronic Disease. (2015). What is chronic disease? Retrieved from http://cmcd.sph.umich.edu/what-is-chronic-disease.html.

Chronic disease self-management. A fact sheet for primary care partnerships. (2014). Retrieved from http://www.health.vic.gov.au/pch/downloads/factsheet07.pdf.

National Council on Aging. (2015). Chronic disease self-management program. Retrieved from http://www.ncoa.org/improve-health/center-for-healthy-aging/chronic-disease.html.

SEXUALLY TRANSMITTED DISEASES

Sexually transmitted diseases (STDs), or sexually transmitted infections (STIs), are generally acquired by sexual contact. The organisms that cause sexually transmitted diseases may pass from person to person in blood, semen, or vaginal and other bodily fluids. Infections can also be transmitted nonsexually, such as from mother to infant during pregnancy or childbirth or through blood transfusions or shared needles.

Symptoms

Sexually transmitted infections have a range of signs and symptoms. Signs and symptoms that might indicate STI include:

- Sores or bumps on the genitals or in the oral or rectal area
- Painful or burning urination
- Discharge from the penis
- Vaginal discharge
- Unusual vaginal bleeding
- Sore, swollen lymph nodes, particularly in the groin but sometimes more widespread
- Lower abdominal pain
- Rash over the trunk, hands or feet

Signs and symptoms may appear a few days to years after exposure, depending on the organism.

A doctor should be consulted immediately if a person is

- Sexually active and believes he or she has been exposed to an STI
- Showing signs and symptoms of an STI

Causes and Risk Factors

Sexually transmitted infections can be caused by:

- Bacteria (gonorrhea, syphilis, chlamydia)
- Parasites (trichomoniasis)
- Viruses (human papillomavirus, genital herpes, HIV/AIDS)

Sexual activity plays a role in spreading many other infectious agents, but there are also nonsexual agents.

Anyone who is sexually active risks exposure to a sexually transmitted infection to some degree. Factors that may increase that risk include:

- Having unprotected sex
- Having sexual contact with multiple partners
- Having a history of STIs
- Abusing alcohol or using recreational drugs
- Injecting drugs

Transmission from Mother to Infant

Certain STIs such as gonorrhea, chlamydia, HIV/AIDS, and syphilis can be passed from an infected mother to her child during pregnancy or delivery. STIs in infants can cause serious problems and may be fatal. All pregnant women should be screened for these infections and treated.

Diagnosis

If a person's sexual history and current signs and symptoms suggest that he or she has an STI, laboratory tests can identify the cause and detect infections he or she might also have contracted.

- *Blood tests* can confirm the diagnosis of HIV/AIDS or later stages of syphilis.
- Some STIs can be confirmed with a *urine sample*.
- Fluid samples may be used to test for active genital sores to diagnose the type of infection.

Screening is recommended for:

- Everyone
- Pregnant women
- Women under age 25 who are sexually active
- Men who have sex with men
- People with HIV/AIDS

Complications

Prompt treatment can help prevent the complications of some STIs. Complications can range from mild to severe and life-threatening and may include sores or bumps anywhere on the body; recurrent genital sores; generalized skin rash; pain during intercourse; scrotal pain, redness, and swelling; pelvic pain; groin abscess; eye inflammation; arthritis; pelvic inflammatory disease; infertility; cervical cancer; other cancers, including HIV-associated lymphoma and HPV-associated cervical, rectal, and anal cancers; opportunistic infections occurring in advanced HIV; and maternal-fetal transmission, which causes severe birth defects. Hepatitis, especially hepatitis B, can also be transmitted sexually.

Treatments and Drugs

STIs caused by bacteria are generally easier to treat. Viral infections can be managed but not always cured. For pregnant women who have an STI, prompt treatment can prevent or reduce the risk of infection of their babies. Treatment usually consists of one of the following, depending on the infection:

- *Antibiotics.* Often given in a single dose, antibiotics can cure many sexually transmitted bacterial and parasitic infections.
- *Antiviral drugs.* Those infected will have fewer herpes recurrences if they take daily suppressive therapy with a prescription antiviral drug, but they can still give their partner herpes at any time.

It is important for those who have been diagnosed with an infection to notify their partner or potential partners.

Prevention

There are several ways to avoid or reduce the risk of sexually transmitted infections, including abstaining from sexual activity; staying with one uninfected partner; waiting and verifying partners' health; using condoms and dental dams consistently and correctly; not drinking alcohol excessively or using drugs; avoiding anonymous, casual sex; communicating; and teaching young people about sexually transmitted diseases.

A common misconception is that nonvaginal intercourse, such as oral sex, and anal sex is safer. Although nonvaginal intercourse will not result in pregnancy, oral sex and anal sex can lead to severe STDs, including life-threatening cancer.

There are now vaccines that can prevent cancer caused by HPV. The Centers for Disease Control and Prevention (CDC) recommends that all boys and girls ages 11 or 12 years be vaccinated. And catch-up vaccines are recommended for males through age 21 and for females through age 26 if they did not receive vaccinations when they were younger (CDC 2015). In July 2012, the Food and Drug Administration (FDA) approved the use of the drug Truvada to reduce the risk of sexually transmitted HIV infection and in those who are at high risk.

David Ajuluchukwu

See also: AIDS; Cervical Cancer; Hepatitis; HPV (Human Papillomavirus); Men's Health; Oral Cancer; Ovarian Cancer; Pelvic Inflammatory Disease; Squamous Cell Carcinoma; Women's Health

Further Reading

Centers for Disease Control and Prevention. (2010). Sexually transmitted diseases treatment guidelines, 2010. Retrieved from http://www.cdc.gov/mmwr/preview/mmwrhtml/rr5912a1.htm.

Centers for Disease Control and Prevention. (2015). Genital HPV infection—fact sheet. Retrieved from http://www.cdc.gov/std/hpv/stdfact-hpv.htm.

French, S. E., & Holland, K. J. (2013, January). Condom negotiation strategies as a mediator of the relationship between self-efficacy and condom use. *Journal of Sex Research*, *50*(1), 48+.

Grimes, J. A., Smith, L. A., & Fagerberg, K., eds. (2013). *Sexually transmitted Disease: An Encyclopedia of Diseases, Prevention, Treatment, and Issues.* Santa Barbara, CA: Greenwood.

Gustafson, R., Montaner, J., & Sibbald, B. (2012, December 11). Seek and treat to optimize HIV and AIDS prevention. *CMAJ: Canadian Medical Association Journal*, *184*(18), 1971. Retrieved from http://www.mayoclinic.com/health/sexually-transmitted-diseases-stds/DS01123.

Kondro, W. (2013, February 19). Die young in America. *CMAJ: Canadian Medical Association Journal*, *185*(3), E153+.

Mayo Clinic. (2016, February 2). Sexually transmitted diseases (STDs). Retrieved from http://www.mayoclinic.org/diseases-conditions/sexually-transmitted-diseases-stds/home/ovc-20180594.

Stock, M. L., Peterson, L. M., Houlihan, A. E., & Walsh, L. A. (2013, January). Influence of oral sex and oral cancer information on young adults' oral sexual-risk cognitions and likelihood of HPV vaccination. *The Journal of Sex Research*, 50(1), 95+.

SHINGLES

Shingles, also known as *herpes zoster*, is a painful, blistering skin rash due to the varicella-zoster virus, the virus that causes chickenpox. Shingles can occur all over the body appearing as a rash or blister. Shingles isn't a life-threatening condition, but it is very painful and not very pleasant to see on the skin. It can also lead to complications, including vision problems if the eyes become involved, and neurological complications. In some cases, it can be chronic because the virus lies dormant in the body and may reoccur and cause an outbreak if the immune system is weakened.

Causes

Shingles are caused by the chickenpox virus, which is a common childhood disease, but it can be prevented by vaccination. Although some who are vaccinated may still contract chickenpox, it will be a milder case. If the chickenpox virus becomes active again, it will cause shingles, not the chickenpox. Stress, disease, or aging may weaken the immune system, making the body prone to awakening this virus.

Shingles commonly occur in the elderly and individuals with a weakened immune system. There is a 20 to 30 percent chance that people will get shingles in their lifetime.

Symptoms

When there is an outbreak, shingles may appear on one area of the body, especially around the trunk. Symptoms of the outbreak include:

- Pain
- Burning
- Numbness
- Red rash
- Fluid-filled blisters
- Itching
- Fever, fatigue, and headaches

People who have these symptoms should see a doctor immediately, and people who are 65 years or older are especially at risk for other complications.

Diagnosis

Shingles is diagnosed by a physician after carefully looking at a person's skin. Tests are rarely needed. Sometimes, a skin test is performed to confirm if the skin is contaminated with the virus that causes shingles. Although it may seem like there is an increase of white blood cells when a person has shingles, it cannot be diagnosed as shingles. Based on the history of pain, rashes, or blisters, shingles can be diagnosed based on this. In testing for shingles, the physician may take a tissue sample for examination.

Treatments

Although there is no cure for shingles, immediate treatment with prescription antiviral drugs can speed healing and reduce your risks of complications. These medications include acyclovir (Zovirax), valacyclovir (Valtrex), and famiclovir (Famvir).

However, if the individual experiences a lot of pain, prescribed pain medications such as anticonvulsants, antidepressants, and numbing agents will help relieve the pain. Taking a cool bath can relieve skin irritation, and wet compresses can relieve the itchiness of a rash. Medications should be started within 72 hours of pain. It takes two to four weeks for blisters to heal. Those with shingles should keep their skin clean and not reuse contaminated items.

Prevention

The chickenpox vaccine and the shingles vaccine can help prevent shingles. The chickenpox (varicella) vaccine is a routine immunization children are given in the first few years. The shingles (varicella-zoster) vaccine is given to adults 50 years and older. Individuals with a weakened immune system cannot be given these vaccines (Mayo Clinic 2014)

Ray Marks

See also: Immune System Disorders; Skin Conditions; Vaccines

Further Reading

Centers for Disease Control and Prevention. (2014). Shingles. Retrieved from http://www.cdc.gov/shingles/.

Healthline. (2015). Shingles. Retrieved from http://www.healthline.com/health/shingles#Overview1.

Mayo Clinic. (2014). Shingles. Retrieved from http://www.mayoclinic.com/health/shingles/DS00098.

National Library of Medicine. (2015, December). Shingles information page. Retrieved from http://www.ninds.nih.gov/disorders/shingles/shingles.htm.

The Children's Hospital of Philadelphia. (2014, August 21). A look at each vaccine: Shingles vaccine. Retrieved from http://www.chop.edu/service/vaccine-education-center/a-look-at-each-vaccine/shingles-vaccine.html.

WebMD. (2016). Shingles: Topic overview. Retrieved from http://www.webmd.com/skin-problems-and-treatments/shingles/shingles-topic-overview.

SICKLE-CELL DISEASE

Sickle-cell disease (also known as sickle-cell anemia) is the most common inherited blood disorder in the United States and affects about 100,000 Americans. About 1 of 13 African American babies is born with sickle-cell trait (Centers for Disease Control and Prevention 2016). Newborn screening (testing all newborn babies) and recent therapies for sickle cell disease have prolonged life expectancy from 14 years in 1974 to more than 50 years today. Each year, life expectancy gets higher as doctors and scientists discover new ways to manage or prevent symptoms of sickle-cell disease.

In 1910, James Herrick, a Chicago physician, was treating a patient from the West Indies. The patient was quite ill and showed all the signs and symptoms of anemia. When Herrick studied a blood sample, he found unusually shaped red blood cells. He described the cells as appearing like a sickle. The name stuck, and the disorder became known as sickle-cell disease.

Sickle-cell disease, the most common of the inherited blood disorders, refers to a group of blood disorders that affect the red blood cells of the body. Normally, red blood cells under the microscope look like a disc or like a doughnut without holes. The shape helps them move smoothly through the tube-like structures of the blood vessels. The red coloring of the cell comes from an iron-carrying protein called hemoglobin. Red blood cells of someone with sickle-cell disease have a distorted shape. Instead of having the efficient disc shape, they look like a sickle or crescent. The hemoglobin is known as sickle hemoglobin or hemoglobin S and cannot carry the regular load of oxygen. In addition to their unusual shape, sickle cells are sticky and stiff. They block the flow of blood into tissues and organs and cause pain, infections, and serious damage to organs.

In sickle-cell disease, the cells live only about 10 to 20 days, instead of the normal 120. The bone marrow, where red blood cells are produced, cannot work fast enough to keep up with the demand for new red blood cells. In addition, when the cells are shaped like a sickle, they break down prematurely, causing anemia.

Symptoms

The signs of sickle-cell disease begin early in childhood. Symptoms include fatigue, numerous infections, shortness of breath, delayed growth, yellowing of eyes and skin (jaundice), pain, organ damage, high blood pressure, and heart failure. These symptoms can vary with the individual. For some, the signs are mild; others may have to be hospitalized.

Causes

Mutations in the *HBB* gene cause sickle-cell disease. The condition is recessive, meaning that a person must have two copies of the mutated gene (one from each parent) in order to have the condition. Those who have only one copy of the mutated genes are considered carriers. Interestingly, those with one copy of the mutated gene have heightened immunity to malaria (although those with both copies do not). Researchers believe that such immunity created an evolutionary advantage that encouraged the continued transmission of the gene from one generation to another, even if having both copies of the gene proved to be very disadvantageous.

Treatment

Treatment may include the following:

Oral penicillin and pneumococcal vaccine: To help decrease the risk of infections in young children with sickle cell disease, they are often given pneumococcal vaccines and daily oral penicillin.

Pain medications: For mild to moderate pain, acetaminophen (i.e., Tylenol) and nonsteroidal anti-inflammatory drugs (NSAIDS) such as ibuprofen can be used, but moderate or severe sickle cell-related pain should be treated with stronger pain medications such as opioids (e.g., morphine, oxycodone, etc.).

Blood transfusions: Red blood cell transfusions are used to help improve blood flow and the oxygen-carrying capacity of blood.

Hydroxyurea: In 1995, hydroxyurea became the first drug shown to prevent many of the complications of sickle-cell disease. It is the only drug approved for sickle-cell disease that changes the process of the disease, rather than treating the symptoms. It prevents crisis and reduces the frequency of crisis. Hydroxyurea stimulates the production of hemoglobin F, and in so doing, lowers the levels of the abnormal hemoglobin S (HbS). Regular use of hydroxyurea leads to fewer painful episodes, fewer episodes of acute chest syndrome, and a decreased need for red blood cell blood transfusions.

Possible Cure

A bone marrow transplant is currently the only potential cure for sickle-cell disease. It is usually recommended only for children with sickle-cell disease who suffer from many sickle-cell-related problems because approximately 10 percent of children receiving a transplant can die as a result of complications. Recently, however, advances have been made to improve the survival rates for patients with sickle-cell disease who receive bone marrow transplantation. In 1984, a child with sickle-cell disease received the first bone marrow transplant. The actual transplantation was done to treat acute leukemia, and the sickle-cell cure was unexpected.

Evelyn B. Kelly

See also: Blood Diseases; Genetics and Genomics

Further Reading

Center for Disease Control and Prevention. (2016). Sickle cell disease: Data and statistics. Retrieved from http://www.cdc.gov/ncbddd/sicklecell/data.html.

National Heart, Lung, and Blood Institute. (2015). Who is at risk for sickle cell anemia? Retrieved from http://www.nhlbi.nih.gov/health/health-topics/topics/sca/atrisk.

Platt, A. F., Jr., Eckman, J., & Hsu, L. (2011). *Hope and Destiny: The Patient and Parent's Guide to Sickle Cell Disease and Sickle Cell Trait*, revised 3rd ed. Indianapolis, IN: Hilton Publishing Co.

Wailoo, K., & Pemberton, S. (2006). *The Troubled Dream of Genetic Medicine: Ethnicity and Innovation in Tay-Sachs, Cystic Fibrosis, and Sickle Cell Disease*. Baltimore: Johns Hopkins University Press.

World Health Organization. (2010). Sickle-cell disease and other haemoglobin disorders. http://www.who.int/mediacentre/factsheets/fs308/en. Accessed November 1, 2014.

SINUSITIS

Sinusitis, or a sinus infection, occurs when mucus in the upper nose becomes infected by bacteria. This infection always comes after a period of ordinary congestion caused by cold viruses or allergies. Although, technically, sinusitis can be caused by allergy, bacteria, viruses, or other infections, most doctors use this term only for bacterial infections of the sinuses. Sinus infections may be considered chronic if they last for eight weeks or more. Some people tend to get frequent sinus infections, which may be caused by a deviated septum or polyps.

Symptoms

Ordinarily, the sinus cavities themselves are sterile—no germs are supposed to live in them. In the nose, however, all sorts of bacteria and viruses may be present. These are ordinarily kept out of the sinuses by several overlapping and very effective mechanisms, including mucus; immune cells; and small, hair-like structures called cilia. Sinus infections always begin with some condition leading to excessive sticky mucus, like a viral cold or allergy. Once the nose is stuffed up, the sinuses cannot drain properly and the mucus stagnates. This mucus, originally designed to trap pathogens and move them out of the area, becomes an ideal breeding ground for bacteria. The result is a sinus infection.

Diagnosis

When diagnosing a sinus infection, the doctor must determine if the nasal congestion is caused by an actual bacterial infection or the lingering effects of a viral cold or allergy. To really know what is causing sinus congestion, a doctor would need to put a needle into a sinus cavity to collect the mucus for study. This is rarely done in ordinary practice, however. Usually a doctor will examine the patient and look for certain features that indicate a bacterial sinus infection is likely. These include facial pain and pressure, length of congestion (more than 10 days), and lack of other common cold symptoms such as coughing and sneezing.

Treatment and Prevention

Standard treatment for sinusitis is a course of oral antibiotics. In fact, sinus infections are one of the most common reasons for antibiotic prescriptions. However, such prescriptions are controversial because, in some cases, doctors may prescribe antibiotics when the patient does not actually have a bacterial sinus infection. Other treatments include nasal corticosteroids, which help prevent and treat inflammation, and oral or injected corticosteroids, which reduce inflammation from severe sinusitis, including for those who have polyps in their sinus cavity. Examples of this kind of treatment are prednisone and methylprednisolone.

In cases that continue to resist treatment or medication, sinus surgery may be an option. For this procedure, the doctor uses an endoscope—a thin, flexible tube with an attached light—to examine the sinus passages and then possibly remove tissue or polyps with various instruments.

The most effective way to prevent sinus infections is to prevent the viral infections that trigger them. Washing hands frequently and avoiding sick people are the best strategies. Also, avoid and treat allergies that cause chronic nasal congestion. When an individual does have a cold, simple and effective measures can be used to help clear the mucus. This includes proper hydration and keeping air humid through the use of steam humidifiers. This prevents mucus from getting thick and sticky. Nasal saline drops or spray can also be used to help clear out the nose. Using decongestants, antihistamines, expectorants, or any combination of these does not reduce an individual's chance of developing a sinus infection from a cold.

Roy Benaroch

See also: Allergies

Further Reading

Mayo Clinic. (2013). Chronic sinusitis. Retrieved from http://www.mayoclinic.org/diseases-conditions/chronic-sinusitis/basics/definition/con-20022039.
National Institute of Allergy and Infectious Disease. (2015, May 15). Sinusitis (sinus infection). Retrieved from https://www.niaid.nih.gov/topics/sinusitis/Pages/index.aspx.

SJÖGREN'S SYNDROME

Overview

Sjögren's syndrome is classified as a chronic inflammatory autoimmune disorder. It is named after the Swedish opthalmologist Henrik Sjögren (1899–1986), who identified the disorder in writings in the 1930s, although other physicians had also identified it earlier. When the disease occurs independently of other diseases, it is called primary Sjögren's syndrome. When it occurs in conjunction with other disorders such as rheumatoid arthritis, it is called secondary Sjögren's syndrome. The condition is technically one that affects the mouth and eyes, which become dry, mainly because the moisture-producing glands are damaged. Other parts of the body that can be affected are the lungs, brain, liver, kidneys, vagina, and thyroid gland. Affecting men and women of all races, the majority of cases are women, usually in their 40s or older. Approximately 4 million Americans suffer from Sjögren's syndrome. Babies born to mothers with Sjögren's syndrome may develop heart problems.

Symptoms

The symptoms of Sjögren's syndrome may vary depending on the cause. Some typical symptoms are dryness of the eyes and mouth, swollen eyelids, swollen salivary glands, burning eyes, itchy eyes, prolonged fatigue, problems chewing or swallowing, weight loss, hoarseness of the voice, skin rashes or dry skin, and a persistent dry cough. Other symptoms include joint swelling, pain, and stiffness; vaginal dryness; tooth decay; decreased tear production; and possible eye infections due to dryness. Gum disease; sores or swelling in the mouth; night sweats; inflammation of the blood vessels, which can damage other tissue areas of the body; and tingling, burning, or numbness of the arms or legs or coldness or numbness of the hands may prevail.

Key Causes and Risk Factors

Sjögren's syndrome is an autoimmune disease, meaning the body attacks its own tissues and cells, usually the tear glands and the salivary glands. Factors that specifically cause this problem in the immune system are not known, but heredity, nervous system explanations, and possible viral or bacterial infections may play a role. Often found in families, most of these family members have a form of autoimmune disease. Some forms of medication result in similar symptoms and signs to that of Sjögren's syndrome.

Diagnostic Procedures

A medical diagnosis is usually based on the presence of dryness of the eyes and mouth. Other tests that may be carried out are blood tests to check for inflammation and immune system problems and eye tests that measure tear production, known as the Rose Bengal and Schirmer tests. Imaging tests of the salivary glands or a parotid gland flow test to measure saliva production rates may also be conducted. Another related test is called salivary scintigraphy, which measures salivary function, and a special x-ray called a *sialogram*, which can determine how much saliva flows into the mouth. Biopsies of the salivary glands—specifically of the glands of the lower lip—also prove helpful, as may a slit-lamp exam of the eye to detect inflammation. To detect if kidneys are affected, a urine test may be carried out.

Treatment

Treatment is directed to the affected areas of the body and is designed to reduce the harmful effects of the condition and reduce discomfort. For the eyes, artificial tears and eye lubricants and ointments may be helpful, as well as eye drops that reduce inflammation and moisture chamber glasses (goggles designed to keep eyes moist). Permanently closing the tear ducts with collagen or silicone, as well as surgically sealing the ducts with the use of a laser may help keep the eyes moist. For dry mouth, taking in plenty of fluids is suggested, as are medications that stimulate saliva production and artificial saliva preparations to moisten the mouth. Nasal sprays and vaginal lubricants may also prove helpful. For those in pain, or with eye inflammation, nonsteroidal anti-inflammatory drugs, as well as corticosteroid drugs in severe cases, may be applied. Other immunosuppressants may be recommended if the individual develops lung, kidney, nerve, or blood vessel problems. Guided exercise programs may reduce fatigue or joint problems frequently associated with Sjögren's syndrome.

Prognosis

There is no cure for Sjögren's syndrome; however, the symptoms can usually be managed medically. In rare cases, primary biliary cirrhosis, associated with Sjögren's syndrome, can lead to scarring of the tissues of the liver. Some patients with Sjögren's syndrome may develop lymph node cancer after many years or lymph node enlargement; lung inflammation; nerve, kidney, and muscle disease; and joint inflammation. Others may develop vision problems, such as blurred vision, corneal ulcers, and light sensitivity.

Prevention

Avoiding smoking or exposure to secondhand smoke or air conditioning may reduce dryness problems. Protecting oral health through good oral hygiene and using appropriate lubricants and keeping hydrated may reduce discomfort in affected sites. Increasing indoor humidity may also prove helpful.

Future

An injectable medication called Rituxan has been found to improve symptoms of Sjögren's syndrome, but more research is needed in this area. Drops produced by a person's own serum located in his or her blood may prove beneficial for treating severe eye dryness. Another drug being tested is Epratuzumab.

Ray Marks

See also: Addison's Disease; Autoimmune Disease; Celiac Disease; Diabetes, Type 1; Eye Diseases; Immune System Disorders; Oral Health; Rheumatoid Arthritis; Salivary Gland Disorders

Further Reading

American College of Rheumatology. (2015). Sjogren's syndrome. Retrieved from http://www.rheumatology.org/I-Am-A/Patient-Caregiver/Diseases-Conditions/Sjogrens-Syndrome.

Mayo Clinic. (2011). Sjogren's syndrome. Retrieved from http://www.mayoclinic.com/health/Sjogrens-syndrome/DS00147.

Medical News Today. (2014, September 10). What is Sjogren's syndrome? What causes Sjogren's syndrome? Retrieved from http://www.medicalnewstoday.com/articles/233747.php.

Sjogren's Syndrome Foundation. (2016). Conquering Sjogren's syndrome. Retrieved from http://www.Sjogrens.org.

SKIN CANCER

Skin cancer is the uncontrolled multiplication of damaged, abnormal cells in the skin. Worldwide, it is the most common form of cancer. Approximately 75 percent of all cancer cases throughout the world are skin cancers.

Types

There are two main types of skin cancer—*melanoma* and *nonmelanoma*. Melanoma is the much more deadly type. Melanoma originates in the skin's *melanocytes*, the cells that produce the pigment that gives the skin its color. This type of cancer often grows aggressively, rapidly spreading to other parts of the body if not detected and removed early. The most common sites of melanoma include the face, arms, legs, chest, and back, though it can occur anywhere on the body. Sites to which the cancer can spread include internal organs, the bones, and the brain.

Nonmelanoma skin cancer may occur as basal cell carcinoma or squamous cell carcinoma, each named after the types of cells it affects. These forms of cancer rarely spread beyond the skin, and they are generally easy to cure. However, some nonmelanoma skin cancers do spread, especially new nonmelanomas that occur in people who previously had a nonmelanoma that was removed.

Prevalence and Mortality

About 1 million people in the United States are diagnosed as having some form of skin cancer every year. The vast majority of these cancers are nonmelanoma skin cancers, which are seldom life-threatening.

Approximately 76,000 new cases of the much more serious melanomas are diagnosed each year in the United States, accounting for almost 5 percent of all new cancers. Melanomas kill approximately 10,000 Americans every year—about 2 percent of all cancer deaths.

Melanoma prevalence increases with age, up to the early 60s, after which the prevalence decreases. This cancer is most frequently diagnosed between the ages of 45 and 64. Among ethnic groups, melanoma is, by far, most common in whites. It is least common in blacks and Asians/Pacific Islanders.

The average five-year survival rate for patients diagnosed as having melanoma is 91 percent. If the cancer is diagnosed when still confined to the primary skin site, the five-year survival rate increases to 98 percent. If the cancer is diagnosed after it has metastasized to distant parts of the body, the five-year survival rate falls to 16 percent. Deaths from melanoma are most common in people aged from 75 to 84.

Risk Factors

The main cause of skin cancer is long-term, excessive exposure of the skin to the ultraviolet (UV) rays of the sun, which damages the DNA in the cells, causing them to divide out of control in a malignant manner. The potential for this cellular damage is especially high for individuals who have certain physical characteristics, such as light-colored skin, green or blue eyes, and existing moles (in which some mela-nomas begin to develop). The risk is greatest for fair-skinned people who live in warm, sunny places, such as Arizona and Hawaii.

To reduce the risk from the sun, people who spend a lot of time outside should wear clothing that covers most of the skin, and they should use sunscreen on ex-posed skin. These measures will help protect the skin cells from UV damage and sunburn. (Sunburn substantially raises the risk of skin cancer.) The use of tanning beds and sun laps should also be avoided or minimized because these products expose the user to the same kind of damaging UV rays as the sun. Frequent expo-sure to x-rays is another risk.

Symptoms and Diagnosis

Physicians recommend that people regularly examine their skin for early signs of cancer—especially those people who are at heightened risk. The primary signs of melanoma are unusual pigmented areas that develop on the skin. Basal cell car-cinoma usually appears as a smooth pearly bump. Squamous cell carcinoma looks like a red, scaly, thickened bump. Melanoma typically occurs as brownish or black-ish lesions. A new mole or a change in an existing mole may also indicate cancer.

To recognize the signs of skin cancer, a four-letter memory aid can be used: ABCD. A doctor should be consulted if any of the following characteristics are observed:

A=asymmetry. The shape of one side of the pigmented area is different than the shape of the other side.
B=border. The pigmented area has an irregularly shaped border.
C=color. The pigmented area changes in color over time.
D=diameter. The diameter of the pigmented area is more than six millimeters (roughly the diameter of a pencil eraser).

A doctor typically makes a diagnosis based on results of a skin scan and biopsy. The scan is made with a handheld, computerized imaging device that evaluates the malignant or benign nature of the lesion. A biopsy tissue sample is examined under a microscope to look for malignant cells. Blood tests, x-rays, and other tests may be conducted to determine the stage of cancer development.

Treatment

Treatment for skin cancer has a high success rate if cancerous growths—and sur-rounding nearby tissues—are surgically removed early in the disease process. Such early removal usually results in a cure.

However, advanced skin cancers that have spread to other tissues or organs will require additional, more complex treatment approaches. Surgery may be needed to remove the tissues to which the cancer has metastasized. Chemotherapy and ra-diation therapy may also be necessary. Various medications can be used in the treatment of patients with skin cancer. Some drugs kill the cancer cells directly. Other drugs inhibit the growth of the cancer cells. Still other drugs stimulate the body's immune system to attack the cancer.

To check for signs of recurring cancer, physicians recommend that patients who have had skin cancer get regular physical examinations and blood tests.

A. J. Smuskiewicz

See also: Basal Cell Carcinoma; Cancer; Melanoma; Squamous Cell Carcinoma

Further Reading

American Cancer Society. (2016). What are basal and squamous cell skin cancers? Retrieved from http://www.cancer.org/cancer/skincancer-basalandsquamouscell/detailedguide/skin-cancer-basal-and-squamous-cell-what-is-basal-and-squamous-cell.

Centers for Disease Control and Prevention. (2015). Basic information about skin cancer. Retrieved from http://www.cdc.gov/cancer/skin/basic_info/index.htm.

Mayo Clinic. (2016). Skin cancer. Retrieved from http://www.mayoclinic.org/diseases-conditions/skin-cancer/basics/definition/con-20031606.

National Cancer Institute. (2015). SEER stat fact sheets: Melanoma of the skin. Retrieved from http://seer.cancer.gov/statfacts/html/melan.html.

National Cancer Institute. (2016). Skin cancer overview. Retrieved from http://www.cancer.gov/cancertopics/types/skin.

World Health Organization. (2015). Skin cancers: How common is skin cancer? Ultraviolet Radiation and the INTERSUN Program. Retrieved from http://www.who.int/uv/faq/skincancer/en/index1.html.

SLEEP DISORDERS

In the earliest years of childhood, humans spend more than half their lives asleep. From about age five onward, approximately one-third of the time is spent asleep. Sleep is universal among animals and necessary for survival—as critical as food, water, and oxygen—yet why this is so is incompletely understood. Much, however, is known about the mechanics of sleep: its patterns, how the brain and body behave during sleep, the negative consequences of inadequate sleep, and physiological problems that can affect sleep duration and quality. Poor sleep can worsen chronic diseases as well as weaken the immune system and lead to memory problems.

The Sleep Cycle

Normal, healthy human sleep follows a specific pattern. While the amount of time spent at each stage varies with age and life events (such as pregnancy), the specific stages, or phases, consistently appear in a particular order called the sleep cycle. Each phase of the sleep cycle is associated with characteristic brain-wave patterns and physiological effects, and each phase appears to be associated with different aspects of physical and psychological health and well-being.

A natural sleep cycle passes through several phases in sequence. The first several phases are nonrapid eye movement stages, or NREM sleep. The final, characterized by observable, back-and-forth motions of the eyes, is rapid eye movement, or REM, sleep. Many researchers divide NREM into four stages, but some divide it into three, combining traditional stages three and four into a single stage called slow-wave sleep, or SWS.

Stage 1 is light sleep. It typically initiates the sleep cycle and may also reappear between deep NREM and REM. It is characterized by drowsiness and reduction in speed of eye movements, reaction time, and muscular response. Individuals in stage 1 may drift in and out of consciousness and be unaware they have entered sleep. Stage 1 is associated with the phenomena of hypnagogic trance (a semi-lucid, dream-like state), hypnagogic hallucination ("waking dreams"), and hypnic myoclonia (random, involuntary muscle movements). Stage 1 is associated with alpha brain waves, and alpha-like mu brain waves. Alpha and mu waves are also associated with meditative states.

Stage 2 sleep is the transitional period between falling asleep and entering deep sleep. It is characterized by theta brain waves. Sudden spikes or dips in brain activity, known as sleep spindles and K-complexes, periodically interrupt theta waves during stage 2 sleep.

Slow-wave, or deep sleep may be considered a single phase (stage 3) or be divided into two phases (stages 3 and 4). Delta waves characterize SWS. In the initial period of SWS, delta waves are punctuated by brief surges of rapid waves, while in later SWS, brain activity is almost entirely delta waves. Muscular movement and environmental response are suppressed in SWS, and individuals in this phase can be extremely difficult to rouse. A person roused from SWS is likely to be extremely disoriented and may rapidly reenter deep sleep with no memory of being awakened. Slow-wave sleep is particularly associated with parasomnias (sleep disorders).

In well-rested individuals past early childhood, REM follows SWS, sometimes after a brief transitional phase of stage 1 activity. Rapid-eye-movement sleep is most powerfully associated with dreaming, though dreams can occur during any phase of the sleep cycle. This stage is also called paradoxical sleep because brain activity is higher than at any other time—even wakefulness. Atonia, or muscular inhibition, as well as rapid, observable eye movements characterize REM. Individuals in REM are more rousable than during SWS, but they may be disoriented upon waking. During natural sleep, most individuals drop from periods of REM back into stages 1, 2, and SWS, to finally wake from a period of light, post-REM stage 1 sleep at the end of a complete sleep period. From a physiological and psychological standpoint, REM appears to be the most critical sleep phase, and the body will go to great lengths to "make up" missed REM during subsequent sleep periods.

The amount of time spent in each type of sleep shifts dramatically throughout an individual's life. Late-term fetuses spend more than 90 percent of their time asleep, about half in REM and half in SWS, with the rest of their hours in an indeterminate state. Newborns sleep between 75 and 90 percent of each day. Babies spend between one-half and two-thirds of the day asleep. Until around the age of three years, when the brain begins to produce alpha waves, children alternate rapidly between wakefulness, deep sleep, and REM, with very little evidence of transitional states. The amount of time an individual spends in each stage of sleep changes over the course of life and with life events. Amount of time spent in REM gradually diminishes with age. Pregnant women experience a dramatic increase in REM and may report unusually vivid dreams. Children's sleep cycles last approximately 50 minutes, while most healthy, nonpregnant adults transition through three to four sleep cycles of approximately 90 minutes each during a night of sleep.

Sleep and Health

Sleep is the period when animals consolidate memory and learning. It is also the time of greatest immune activity, cellular repair, and tissue generation. How and why sleep initially evolved is unknown. Yet we do know that the body requires sleep for multiple functions. Sleep is when the brain removes most waste products from its tissues and extracellular spaces. It appears to "reset" neural functions. It is also the time when the body devotes the greatest amount of energy to wound healing and production of white blood cells.

Deep sleep, or SWS, appears to be the time of greatest release of growth hormone as well as other hormones related to growth and development. Adequate sleep is associated with normalizing blood pressure and the ability to regulate body temperature.

Different forms of memory depend on adequate amounts of deep and REM sleep. Working memory (the ability to retain and draw upon information while proceeding through a task) requires adequate overall sleep. Declarative memory (the ability to remember facts) seems to require deep sleep, while procedural memory (the ability to remember how to do things) is dependent on REM sleep.

Sleep Deprivation

Inadequate sleep impairs multiple body and cognitive functions and is a risk factor for a multitude of physical and psychological impairments. Prolonged periods of inadequate sleep can cause inability to regulate heart rate, blood pressure, metabolism, and hormone levels, as well as inability to gauge tiredness and inaccurate perceptions of one's own need for sleep and time spent asleep. Chronic sleep deprivation elevates incidence and seriousness of infections, suppresses normal growth, slows tissue repair, and causes body aches and involuntary tremors. Total loss of sleep will eventually lead to death. Lack of adequate sleep is a risk factor for hypertension, obesity, Type 2 diabetes, and attention deficit hyperactivity disorder (ADHD). Both too little and too much sleep are risk factors for cardiovascular disease. Sleep deprivation is a major contributor to industrial and motor vehicle accidents, accounting for an estimated 20 percent of automobile crashes.

Sleep deprivation severely inhibits learning and impairs cognitive function. Persons suffering sleep deprivation demonstrate inability to regulate emotions and manage emotional reactions; impaired judgment, perception, and critical thought; inability to concentrate; memory lapses and inability to recall information and learned processes; and irritability and anxiety. Severe, chronic sleep deprivation can cause hallucinations, extreme paranoia, depression, mania, psychosis, and seizure.

Sleep Disorders

Healthy sleep requires passage through each stage of sleep, in the appropriate order, for an adequate number of times before waking, and during an appropriate point in an individual's circadian rhythm. Sleep disorders can affect onset, quality, phases, or duration of sleep. Primary care physicians may diagnose sleep disorders based on observation and patient history, or a patient with a suspected disorder may be referred to a sleep laboratory for *polysomnography*. This type of test records breathing, heart rate, and brain waves during sleep.

Insomnia—inability to easily fall or stay asleep—is the most common sleep disorder. Its causes are many and may include lifestyle choices or underlying physiological issues. Diagnosis is by observation and patient history. Treatment depends on the underlying cause and may include lifestyle changes, treatment for other conditions, or treatment with hypnotic or hormonal drugs.

Sleep apnea is a common breathing disorder typically caused by the collapse of muscles surrounding the airway during sleep. Diagnosis is by polysomnography and treatment may include supplemental oxygen delivered under continuous pressure (CPAP) during sleep, lifestyle changes to reduce weight and improve respiration, propping up the body during sleep, and breathing coordination exercises to strengthen airway muscles.

Other sleep disorders that affect duration and quality of sleep include restless leg syndrome and periodic limb movement disorder, REM sleep disorder, upper airway resistance syndrome, and phenomena such as night sweats and night terrors. Narcolepsy is a condition that causes uncontrollable, seizure-like bouts of sudden, deep sleep during daytime, while hypersomnia is an inability to wake up and stay awake during the day. Fatal familial insomnia is a rare genetic disorder that causes gradual, progressive loss of the ability to sleep.

Recommendations for Better Sleep

Sleep hygiene refers to activities and environmental factors that help or hinder a good night's sleep, including falling asleep and staying asleep throughout the night.

Medical professionals maintain lists of sleep hygiene guidelines to educate their patients about best practices for sleeping soundly. Sleep hygiene education emphasizes health practices or habits that assist or interfere with sleep. These factors are within the individual's control and do not involve prescription drugs. The goal is to optimize one's habits to bring about better sleep. Although there is no universal agreement about what specific behaviors and environmental considerations make up sleep hygiene, most sleep researchers advise within these categories:

- Creating a calming routine before bedtime
- Maintaining a regular sleep routine
- Refraining from staying in bed while awake
- Avoiding naps
- Avoiding watching TV or using the computer in bed
- Avoiding caffeine at certain times and other substances that interfere with sleep

- Maintaining a regular exercise routine
- Creating a quiet, comfortable bedroom environment

Practicing healthy sleep hygiene is generally a good idea for preventing sleep problems. If these practices do not work, consulting a qualified clinician is suggested because certain sleep disorders require specific treatments, and another chronic health issue might be present that should be treated.

Angela Libal and Nelda Street

See also: Attention Deficit Hyperactivity Disorder (ADHD); Cardiovascular Disease; Diabetes, Type 2; Hypertension; Obesity; Obesity, Morbid; Seasonal Affective Disorder

Further Reading

American Sleep Association. (2007). How many hours of sleep do I need: Sleep hygiene tips. Retrieved from https://www.sleepassociation.org/patients-general-public/what-is -sleep/.

Centers for Disease Control and Prevention. (2015). Insufficient sleep is a public health problem. Retrieved from http://www.cdc.gov/features/dssleep/.

Fryer, B. (2006, October). Sleep deficit: The performance killer. *Harvard Business Review.* Retrieved from https://hbr.org/2006/10/sleep-deficit-the-performance-killer.

Hobson, J. A. (2002). *Dreaming: An Introduction to the Science of Sleep.* New York: Oxford University Press.

Lombardo, G. T. (2005). *Sleep to Save Your Life: The Complete Guide to Living Longer and Healthier Through Restorative Sleep.* New York: Collins.

Ohayon, M. M. (2002). Epidemiology of insomnia: What we know and what we still need to learn. *Sleep Medicine Reviews, 6*(2), 97–111.

Standards of Practice Committee of the American Academy of Sleep Medicine. (2006). Practice parameters for the psychological and behavioral treatment of insomnia: An update— an American Academy of Sleep Medicine report. *Sleep, 29*(11), 1415–1419.

Webster, M. (2008, May 6). Can you catch up on lost sleep? *Scientific American.* Retrieved from http://www.scientificamerican.com/article/fact-or-fiction-can-you-catch-up-on -sleep/.

SPINAL DISEASES

Spinal diseases refer to health problems that originate in the spine. These diseases can affect the spinal cord or nerve pathway from the brain that travels through the vertebrae of bones of the spine or through the bones themselves. An example of a disease that can affect the spinal cord is multiple sclerosis. An example of a disease that can affect the vertebrae and the tissues surrounding them is ankylosing spondylitis. Others are osteoporosis, or thinning of the bones, which can lead to vertebral fractures. Another is degenerative disc disease. Some conditions affect posture detrimentally, such as the presence of a kyphosis or abnormally rounded spine; another is scoliosis, which is an abnormally curved spine.

Symptoms

The symptoms associated with spinal disorders will vary dependent on the health condition and what tissue or tissues are affected. Usually, these disorders are long-standing and become chronic and lead to considerable disability. Pain problems and lack of mobility, stiffness, and aching may be common symptoms indicating the presence of a spinal disorder. Others are reflex changes, nerve-related changes (such as numbness), and tingling in one or more areas of the body. Some result in muscle weakness, or complete paralysis, such as in the case of a complete spinal cord lesion or spinal tumor.

Diagnosis

Spinal disorders are diagnosed on the basis of a history, a physical examination, and x-rays or scans.

Neurological tests may also be conducted.

Treatments

Treatments may include medications; exercise therapy; spinal injections; various forms of electrical therapy, heat, or ice to relieve pain; acupuncture; and possible surgery. Braces to support the spine and, if necessary, assistive devices and a wheelchair may be needed if the condition becomes disabling. The outlook for a spinal disease or disorder is not always positive, but early treatment and adherence to treatment recommendations may reduce the cause of the condition.

Prevention

Most spinal conditions are hard to prevent. The symptoms may be lessened by careful use of the body and preventing excess stress and maintain a healthy body weight. Exercise is usually beneficial if applied in an appropriate manner.

Ray Marks

See also: Bone Diseases; Multiple Sclerosis; Osteoporosis

Further Reading

Lyons, B., Boachie-Adjei, O., Podzius, J., & Podzius, C. (1999). *Scoliosis: Ascending the Curve*. New York: M. Evans and Co.
MedlinePlus. (2014). Spine injuries and disorders. Retrieved from http://www.nlm.nih.gov/medlineplus/spineinjuriesanddisorders.html.

SPIRITUALITY

The word *spirituality* is derived from *spirit*, and the Latin *spirare*, which means "to breathe." Spirituality, as one of the most ill-defined words in the English language, means something different to everyone. For some, it is about participating in organized religion, such as going to a church, synagogue, mosque, etc. For others, it is more personal and includes such activities as private prayer, yoga, meditation, quiet reflection, or even long walks. Spirituality is more frequently described than defined, and there is no one, clear comprehensive definition of spirituality in the literature (Testerman 1997). The term originated in the Christian tradition, where it has a long history of religious practice and theology. In modern usage, it includes a dimension of the human experience from traditional religions, New Age teachings, personal mystical experience, a relationship with a supreme being, and the quest for meaning in life. In examining many of the world's religions, King found that the term spirituality has become a universal code word to indicate the human search for direction and meaning; for wholeness and transcendence; and as an attempt to grow in sensitivity, to self, to others, and to nonhuman creations (King 2010). This is reflected in writings by recognized spiritual leaders.

The Dalai Lama, seen as one of the world's greatest spiritual leaders, refers to spirituality as the full blossoming of human values that is essential for the good of all (Dalai Lama & Stril-Rever 2011). The recognized antonym of spirituality is *physical* or *material*. Relating spirituality to the physical is significant in this writing when considering the imbalance of the physical, which is often referred to as disease.

Spirituality and Disease

Because spirituality cannot be scientifically measured, researchers have not been able to agree on a universal definition, yet even skeptics report a sense that there is something greater than the concrete world we see. As the brain processes sensory experiences, we naturally look for patterns and then seek out meaning in those patterns. The phenomenon known as *cognitive dissonance* shows that once we believe in something, we will try to explain away anything that conflicts with it.

Researchers at Harvard Medical School have studied mind-body interactions since the early 1970s. Their research suggests that when a person engages in a repetitive prayer, word, sound, or phrase, a specific set of physiologic changes does follow. These changes include decreased metabolism, heart rate, blood pressure, and rate of breathing, which are the opposite of those induced by stress, and such changes have been called the *relaxation response*. Surveys indicate that more than 60 percent of visits to health care professionals are for conditions caused or exacerbated by stress and that the relaxation response is an effective therapy for stress-related conditions. Many people who elicit the relaxation response also note increased spirituality, expressed as experiencing the presence of a power, a force, an energy, or what was perceived of as God, and this presence is close to the person. This finding opened the door to questions about the healing effects of spirituality and was one of the first to relate medicine with spirituality and healing (Harvard Medical School 2015).

Severe stress and depressive symptoms are associated with decrease in the function of the immune system. In his work, Testerman (1997) found that spiritual individuals—having an underlying sense of meaning and purpose for their lives and access to spiritual methods of coping with stress, including prayer—may have greater resistance to stress-related health breakdown and heightened resistance to diseases-causing agents and environments and were able to offset possible depression from stressful life events.

Karen Jeanne Coleman

See also: Stress

Further Reading

Benson, H. (2000). *The Relaxation Response*. New York: HarperTorch.

Dalai Lama, & Stril-Rever, S. (2011). *My Spiritual Journey*. New York: HarperOne.

Diamond, S. A. (2011, May 4). Clinical despair: Science, psychotherapy and spirituality in the treatment of depression. *Psychology Today*. Retrieved from https://www.psycholo gytoday.com/blog/evil-deeds/201103/clinical-despair-science-psychotherapy-and -spirituality-in-the-treatment.

Foglio, J. P., & Brody, H. (1988). Religion, faith and family medicine. *Journal of Family Practice*, 27(5), 473–474. Retrieved from http://www.ncbi.nlm.nih.gov/pmc/articles/PMC 1305900/?log$=activity.

Harvard Medical School. (2015, January 14). Spirituality and healing. Retrieved from http:// hms.harvard.edu/news/spirituality-and-healing.

King, U. (2010). Spirituality. In *The Penguin Handbook of the World's Living Religions*, edited by John Hinnells. New York: Penguin Books, 669–683.

Puchalski, C. M. (2001). The role of spirituality in health care. Retrieved from http://www .ncbi.nlm.nih.gov/pmc/articles/PMC1305900.

Testerman, J. K. (1997). Spirituality vs religion: Implications for healthcare. Prepared for the 20th Annual Faith and Learning Seminar, at Loma Linda, CA. Retrieved from http:// ict.adventist.org/vol_19/19cc_283-297.pdf.

SQUAMOUS CELL CARCINOMA

Squamous cell carcinoma (SCC) is a common form of skin cancer that develops in the outer layer of the skin. Every year, some 700,000 people in the United States are diagnosed with SCC. Although SCC usually grows slowly and is generally not life-threatening, in an estimated 2 to 10 percent of cases, the cancer will spread to different tissues and organs throughout the body; in the United States, around 2,500 people a year die from the condition. It has been found to occur twice as frequently in men as in women and is most often found in older adults.

SCC often appears as scaly or rough patches of slightly raised skin. It occurs when abnormal squamous cells begin developing in the outer layers of the skin called the epidermis. The condition is typically caused by damages to the DNA in the skin cells, which is usually created through chronic overexposure to ultraviolet (UV) radiation either from sunlight or tanning bed lamps. In some cases, the damaged DNA that creates SCC may also be caused by such things as xeroderma pigmentosum (a rare genetic disorder that causes a person to be extremely sensitive to sunlight), immune deficiency disorders, chronic infections, or burns or other skin injuries that may have been exposed to x-rays or cancer-causing chemicals. Although anyone who has prolonged exposure to the sun over a lengthy period of time or who has suffered from multiple sunburns during their lifetime may develop SCC, people with fair skin and light eyes are at greatest risk for the disease.

Although SCC most often appears in areas of the body that are commonly exposed to the sun—including the face, back of the hands, or the scalp—cancerous lesions may appear inside the mouth, on the genitals, or elsewhere on the body. SCC may appear in several different forms. It can show up as a flat sore with crusty, irregular skin that bleeds often, a red or rough skin patch, a raised area similar to a wart, or even a firm, reddish bump. If such a symptom arises and does not disappear on its own within a few months, there is a good possibility that it is SCC rather than another skin disorder.

There are five stages of SCC: stages 0, I, II, III, and IV. In stage 0, the tumor has not spread below the surface of the skin. In stage I, the cancer may have grown to nearly an inch across but has not spread to other organs or tissues. In stage II, the cancer may be larger than an inch across but has still not spread to other areas of the body. In stage III, the cancer may have spread into the bones of the face or a single nearby lymph node but has not gone beyond this. In stage IV, the original SCC tumor may be any size or shape, and the cancer has spread throughout the body. To properly diagnose SCC, a medical professional will conduct a physical exam and take a biopsy of any suspicious skin growth. This sample is then tested in a laboratory to determine the presence of abnormal cancerous cells. Once SCC has been confirmed, it can be treated in several different ways, depending on such factors as the size, location, and growth pattern of the tumor. Most cases of SCC are treatable with a relatively minor outpatient surgical procedure or topical medicated creams and lotions. In some instances, radiation treatments may be administered to destroy the cancerous cells without surgical intervention. If the SCC is only superficial, the use of liquid nitrogen to freeze the tumor off rather than cutting it out via surgery may be recommended. If a person has had SCC before, he or she is at greater risk of developing another tumor. Because of this, it is recommended to use sunscreen and stay out of direct sunlight from 10 a.m. to 4 p.m., when the sun is strongest.

Different types of SCC have been studied as far back as the mid-18th century, when research was being conducted on the connection between toxins in coal and the development of SCC. In 2003, doctors were able to begin pinpointing potential genes that cause SCC through the use of the human genome project. Less than a decade later, in 2011, researchers made a breakthrough discovery in determining that SCC might originate in hair follicle cells. This discovery has led to much more research into new ways to prevent and treat SCC.

Tamar Burris

See also: Basal Cell Carcinoma; Cervical Cancer; HPV (Human Papillomavirus); Esophageal Cancer; Head and Neck Cancer; Melanoma; Sexually Transmitted Diseases; Skin Cancer; Skin Conditions; Urethral Cancer

Further Reading

Kwabi-Addo, B., & Lindstrom, T. L. (2011). *Cancer Causes and Controversies: Understanding Risk Reduction and Prevention.* Westport, CT: Praeger.

Mayo Clinic. (2016). Squamous cell carcinoma of the skin. Retrieved from http://www .mayoclinic.org/diseases-conditions/squamous-cell-carcinoma/basics/definition/con -20037813.

Memorial Sloan Kettering Cancer Center. (2016). About squamous cell carcinoma. Retrieved from https://www.mskcc.org/cancer-care/types/squamous-cell-carcinoma/about-squa mous-cell-carcinoma.

Pories, Susan E., et al. (2009). *Cancer: Biographies of Disease.* Westport, CT: Greenwood.

Skin Cancer Foundation. (2015). The second most common form of skin cancer. Retrieved from http://www.skincancer.org/skin-cancer-information/squamous-cell-carcinoma.

Stanford Health Care. (2015). What is squamous cell carcinoma? Retrieved from https:// stanfordhealthcare.org/medical-conditions/cancer/squamous-cell-carcinoma.html.

STRESS

Stress is the natural response of the brain and body to certain challenging demands. Various experiences and events can trigger stress, especially any sort of change. Such change might be unexpected and unwelcomed, or it might be welcomed but nevertheless difficult to deal with. Examples of stress-causing events are diverse, including a difficult test, the start of a new school year, starting a new job, being in a car accident, participating in a football game, being diagnosed with a serious illness, planning for a marriage, going through a divorce, getting ready for a date, going on a vacation with family, and being the victim of a crime. Some stress may be part of one's everyday routine—such as school or work—but it continues to be stressful anyway. As these examples suggest, stress is either always with us or just around the corner.

All people experience stress, at least occasionally. It is a normal part of living. The top causes of stress in the United States include job pressures, money worries, health problems, relationship issues, poor nutrition, media overload (too much Internet, cell phones, or television), and sleep deprivation. Many people learn to accept stress and to deal with it the best they can. Stress, depending on the cause, can be good, by psychologically gearing a person up to confront the challenges of the day, or it can be bad, by paralyzing a person into a state of inaction.

Some people do not cope well with stress. For those people, stress can lead to additional problems, such as alcohol or drug abuse or violent outbursts, or serious physical problems, leading to chronic diseases such as cardiovascular disease and chronic mental illness (such as depression and anxiety disorders).

Physiological Processes

The brain and body respond in characteristic ways to stressful situations. One of the most common physiological reactions to stress is the so-called "fight-or-flight response," also called the *acute stress response*. This is a basic biological reaction that evolved in most animal species as a way of increasing the chances of survival in life-threatening situations, such as the attack of a predator. The expression *fight or flight* refers to the individual's possible actions—either put up a fight or run away. Although few humans have to worry about getting attacked by animal predators today, we experience the same genetically ingrained responses to other stressful situations.

In response to a stressful situation, the brain gears up to cause certain biochemical changes that get the body ready to respond to the stress. For example, the hypothalamus of the brain secretes corticotropic-releasing hormone, which stimulates the brain's pituitary gland to secrete other hormones, including adrenocorticotropic hormone, which activates the sympathetic nervous system. As part of this activation, the adrenal glands, located on top of the kidneys, release still other hormones, most notably adrenaline and noradrenaline (also called epinephrine and norepinephrine). These hormones flow through the bloodstream to other parts of the body, where they increase heart rate, blood pressure, breathing rate, muscle tension, and brain activity. The activity of the immune system may also be temporarily enhanced during stress.

This ramped-up physiological state prepares the body to aggressively confront the threat (whatever it is) or to quickly flee the scene (should that be the better option). Whether the threat is real (such as an attacker on a dark city street) or imagined (such as believing in such an attacker, who really isn't there), the body has the same fight-or-flight biochemical response. This is the response experienced during stress. After the threat—real or imagined—disappears, the body requires from 20 to 60 minutes for its aroused biochemical state to return to its usual state.

These changes are the normal physiological responses to stress. However, people who experience chronic stress can experience other, problematic physiological responses. Their immune system can weaken, leaving them susceptible to infectious diseases, such as influenza and colds. Their digestive system, endocrine system, reproductive system, and other body systems can also develop problems. In short, too much stress can make one sick. In fact, continued, chronic stress and strain on the body can lead to heart disease, hypertension, diabetes, depression, suicide attempts, and several other serious conditions.

Coping with Stress

People cope with stress in different ways. But before one can cope with stress, the person has to recognize its signs. Signs that one is having trouble coping with stress may include difficulties in sleeping, frequent stomachaches, increased alcohol or drug use, feelings of depression, increased irritability and anger, inability to concentrate on the task at hand, and diminished energy. Individuals also need to figure out what exactly is causing their symptoms of stress.

After understanding the causes of stress, an individual is ready to address it. Many people find that reaching out to friends and family for support is useful in times of stress. It is also important to prioritize worries and responsibilities so as not to become overwhelmed. Decide what needs to be done first, and be open to saying "no" to new things that one may not be able to handle. Lots of people find that physical exercise—or such relaxing activities as yoga or meditation—helps to relieve stress.

Psychotherapy and Medications

If self-coping strategies don't help the individual effectively manage his or her stress, professional mental health therapy (psychotherapy) may be needed. A therapist will help the individual pinpoint behaviors or situations that are contributing to his or her stress, and then develop a plan for addressing the problem. Millions of Americans receive psychotherapy for stress.

For approximately 40 million Americans, their stress is so severe that it is classified as an anxiety disorder. Unlike most cases of stress, which are relatively manageable and associated with specific, temporary experiences or worries, anxiety disorders may persist for several months or years, with feelings of worry, tension, and impending doom filling each and every day. People with these disorders are typically prescribed antianxiety medications and antidepressants to lessen their sensations of fear, panic, and doom. They also are typically advised to receive psychotherapy.

A. J. Smuskiewicz

See also: Anxiety Disorders; Health; Irritable Bowel Syndrome; Mental Disorders; Physical Activity; Self-Management

Further Reading

American Heart Association. (2015). How does stress affect you? Retrieved from http://www.heart.org/HEARTORG/HealthyLiving/StressManagement/HowDoesStressAffectYou/How-Does-Stress-Affect-You_UCM_307985_Article.jsp#.Vro4tWfrvcs.

American Psychological Association. (2016). How stress affects your health. Retrieved from http://www.apa.org/helpcenter/stress.aspx.

Anxiety and Depression Association of America. (2015). Stress. Retrieved from http://www.adaa.org/understanding-anxiety/related-illnesses/stress.

Carnegie, D. (1990). *How to Stop Worrying and Start Living: Time-Tested Methods for Conquering Worry.* New York: Pocketbooks.

Harvard University, Center of the Developing Child. (2016). Toxic stress. Retrieved from http://developingchild.harvard.edu/science/key-concepts/toxic-stress/.

Mayo Clinic. (2016). Stress management. Retrieved from http://www.mayoclinic.org/healthy-lifestyle/stress-management/in-depth/stress-symptoms/art-20050987.

STROKE

A stroke occurs when the blood flow to the brain is cut off, depriving brain cells of oxygen and causing them to die very quickly. When that happens, the abilities controlled by the affected area of the brain such as such as memory, speech, or muscle control are lost. The most common type is an ischemic stroke, caused by a blood clot in a blood vessel in the brain. A hemorrhagic stroke takes place when a blood vessel breaks and bleeds into the brain. Transient ischemic attacks, or TIAs, occur when the brain's blood supply is temporarily interrupted for a short time.

Stroke symptoms happen very quickly and they require immediate medical attention. The most common are numbness or weakness of the face, arm, or leg (mainly on one side); trouble seeing (in one or both eyes); difficulty walking, dizziness, or loss of balance; confusion or trouble talking or understanding speech; and severe headache with no known cause. The risk of stroke increases with age, but they occur at any age. It is the leading cause of disability among adults and the fifth leading cause of death in the United States. Nearly 800,000 people experience a new or recurrent stroke each year. About 60 percent of stroke deaths occur in women and 40 percent in men. African Americans face nearly twice the risk for a stroke as other populations, as well as a much higher death rate. Depending on the type of stroke, emergency treatment involves medications to break up blood clots or control the bleeding and reducing pressure inside the brain. Follow-up treatment focuses on recovering as much function as possible.

Symptoms

Stroke symptoms happen very quickly and they require immediate medical attention. They may last more than a few minutes, or start, go away, and return. The most common stroke symptoms are paralysis, numbness, or weakness of the face, arm, or leg (usually on one side); trouble seeing (in one or both eyes); difficulty walking, dizziness, or loss of balance; confusion or trouble speaking and understanding; and a severe headache with no evident cause.

The effects of a stroke depend on how quickly it is diagnosed and treated, as well as where it occurs in the brain and the amount of damage. A small stroke may cause only temporary weakness of an arm, while a larger stroke may cause permanent paralysis on one side of the body or the loss of speech. Some people recover completely, but most experience some negative long-term effects or disability, such as bladder or bowel control problems; depression; pain in the hands and feet that worsens with movement or changes in temperature; paralysis or weakness on one or both sides of the body; and difficulty controlling or expressing emotions.

Causes and Risk Factors

Stroke can be caused either by a blood clot in the brain, as in an ischemic stroke; by a ruptured blood vessel called a hemorrhagic stroke; or a temporary disruption of blood to the brain in a transient ischemic attack. Regardless of the type of stroke, the affected area of the brain cannot function normally because it has been deprived of oxygen and nutrients and the brain cells begin to die.

Lifestyle risk factors that increase the chance of having a stroke also increase the chance of having a heart attack, including obesity or overweight; physical inactivity; excessive alcohol consumption; and use of cocaine and methamphetamines. Medical risk factors include high blood pressure; high cholesterol; cardiovascular disease; atrial fibrillation (an irregular heartbeat that can cause blood to collect in the heart and potentially form a clot, travel to the brain, and cause a stroke); diabetes; obstructive sleep apnea; and smoking or exposure to secondhand smoke. Risk factors that cannot be controlled include personal or family history of stroke, heart attack, or TIA; being African American; and age (55 or older). Men also face a higher risk, but women have a higher death rate because most are older when they have a stroke; they may face slight risk from estrogen, pregnancy, and childbirth.

Diagnosis

To minimize brain damage, a stroke should be diagnosed as quickly as possible, and treatment at a hospital should occur within three hours of the symptoms' first appearance. To determine the type of stroke and appropriate treatment, diagnostic tools include a physical exam of the symptoms and medical history; blood tests to discover how quickly the blood is clotting; CT scan, which can show hemorrhages, strokes, and other abnormalities inside the brain (one of the few ways to determine the type of stroke); MRI scan to detect any damaged brain tissue; ultrasound of the carotid arteries' blood flow; cerebral angiogram for a detailed view of the brain and neck arteries; and an echocardiogram, or image of the heart, that may indicate sources of blood clots that may have reached the brain.

Treatments

The chances of survival and fewer complications increase with prompt emergency treatment, usually within three hours. Ischemic and hemorrhagic strokes require different treatments, and a CT scan is the only positive method to diagnose the type of stroke. For an ischemic stroke, medications can quickly dissolve the blood clot to stop a stroke while it is happening. Procedures to decrease the risk of having another stroke or TIA include opening an artery narrowed by plaques, or fatty deposits, and preventing the artery from narrowing in the future. Treatment of a hemorrhagic stroke includes medications to stop the bleeding and reduce pressure on the brain, which may be followed by surgical repair of blood vessels.

Following a stroke and emergency treatment, rehabilitation helps people recover from the complications and disabilities. Depending on the area of the brain damaged, it may include speech, physical, occupational therapy, or a combination.

Prevention

As many as 80 percent of strokes can be prevented, usually by making lifestyle changes such as avoiding illicit drugs, quitting smoking, getting regular exercise, maintaining a healthy body weight, eating a healthful diet, and avoiding alcohol or consuming a moderate amount. Prevention measures for a first or recurrent stroke also include treating high blood pressure, atrial fibrillation, diabetes, heart disease, high cholesterol, and other underlying medical risk factors. Anticoagulant and antiplatelet medications, as well as arterial surgery, may also be recommended to reduce the risk of future strokes.

Prognosis and Outcomes

Strokes affect the whole body, commonly causing paralysis or weakness on one side of the body. Stroke survivors often experience long-term problems with thinking, awareness, attention, learning, judgment, emotion, and memory. They may also have numbness or pain in the hands and feet that feels worse by movement and cold temperatures. About 25 percent of those who recover from a stroke will have another one within five years.

Future

A recent clinical trial suggests promising evidence that the selective serotonin reuptake inhibitor (SSRI) class of antidepressants and norepinephrine reuptake inhibitor (NRI) can help patients recover from strokes in addition their effect on mood by improving dependence, disability, neurological impairment, anxiety, and depression. Another trial suggests that the acetylcholinesterase inhibitor drugs for Alzheimer's disease can improve aphasia, or the loss of ability to understand or express speech, caused by stroke-related brain damage.

Ray Marks

See also: Arrhythmias/Dysrhythmias; Atherosclerosis; Cardiovascular Disease; Cerebral Vascular Disease; Cholesterol; Congenital Heart Disease; Coronary Artery Disease; Diabetes, Type 2; Diet and Nutrition; Food Guides from the USDA; Heart Diseases; Obesity; Physical Therapy; Prediabetes; Tachycardia

Further Reading

American Stroke Association. (2015). About stroke. Retrieved from http://www.stroke association.org/STROKEORG/AboutStroke/About-Stroke_UCM_308529_SubHome Page.jsp.

Brazier, Y. (2015, October 23). Could Alzheimer's drugs or antidepressants help stroke patients? *Medical News Today.* Retrieved from http://www.medicalnewstoday.com/articles /301439.php.

Centers for Disease Control and Prevention. (2015, April 30). Preventing stroke: What you can do. Retrieved from http://www.cdc.gov/stroke/prevention.htm.

Mayo Clinic. (2015). Stroke. Retrieved from http://www.mayoclinic.org/diseases-conditions /stroke/home/ovc-20117264.

National Institute of Neurological Disorders and Stroke. (2015, October 18). NINDS stroke information page. Retrieved from http://www.ninds.nih.gov/disorders/stroke/stroke .htm.

National Stroke Association. (2015). What is stroke? Retrieved from http://www.stroke.org /understand-stroke/what-stroke.

SUBSTANCE ABUSE

Substance abuse continues to be a problem in the United States. According to the latest research, the United States has the highest substance abuse rate of any developed nation. It is estimated that 22.7 million Americans, aged 12 or older, have tried an illicit drug at least once in their lifetime (National Institute on Drug Abuse 2015).

The first step in describing substance abuse begins with the types of substances that can be abused. Abused substances can be considered either illegal or legal. Legal substances may include any products that are approved by law to be available to consumers in an over-the-counter format. Examples of substances that fall into this category include all over-the-counter medications, caffeine, alcoholic beverages, nicotine (found in all tobacco products) and inhalants (gasoline, nail polish, glue, etc). Another category of legal substances involves those that are legally obtained by a prescription from a licensed health care professional and include prescriptions drugs such as amphetamines, barbiturates, benzodiazepines, steroids, and tranquilizers. Either of these two groups of drugs is considered illegal when used in improper ways, other than what it was intended to treat. There are also illegal substances that, no matter the reason you are using them, they are still considered illegal. Examples of substances that are included in this area are cocaine, marijuana, heroin, designer drugs such as MDMA (ecstasy or E), or party drugs such as GHB (gamma-hydroxybutyrate), among others. Other substances that are starting to get a closer look are herbs or other natural products.

Often times, *substance abuse* is used interchangeably with *drug abuse*. These can be defined as the chronic or habitual use of any chemical substance to alter states of the mind or body for reasons other than medical purposes. However, substance abuse is also dependent on how the rest of society looks at that particular substance. For example, chewing cocoa leaves in the Andes doesn't have the same reaction as someone who is using crack cocaine in an urban, inner-city setting.

History

Few drugs have been considered illegal from the moment they are discovered or created. Most substances become illegal as evidence begins to appear that demonstrates the abuse of that particular substance. For example, many drugs that are now used for recreational purposes were used to relieve a variety of ailments such as coughs, physical pain, and diarrhea and even as cures for dependence on other drugs. After World War 1, the Harrison Act made the first attempt to make psychoactive drugs illegal by allowing the selling of specific narcotics to be done only by registered physicians, which resulted in a decline of its use among the middle class (Musto 1999). Shortly after, the temperance movement led to the prohibition of alcohol by the Eighteenth Amendment to the Constitution but was eventually repealed in 1933. Use of substances became centered on "outside groups." Since World War II, substance abuse had become more widespread and has continued into today's society.

Effects of Substance Abuse

The effects of substance abuse can be seen on many levels from individual, family, and friends to society. Individuals who use drugs on a chronic basis are more likely to incur negative health effects as a result. Acute health effects of substance abuse include drug overdose or death. Many users also experience withdrawal symptoms, which can range from mild flu-like symptoms such as fatigue, vomiting, or muscle cramps to severe life-threatening symptoms such as seizures, convulsions, or delirium. In addition, individuals who share needles with others also run the risk of contracting AIDS and hepatitis.

Drug abuse can also negatively affect family life by causing marital problems or by creating destructive patterns of codependency, such as allowing the person to continue to use drugs by denying there is a problem. Finally, drug abuse has a significant impact on society, primarily financially. There can be lost work time and inefficiency due to drug abuse. Individuals under the influence of drugs are more likely to be involved in occupational accidents, causing injuries to themselves as well as those around them.

Treatment

Treatment for substance abuse varies from state to state. It can be in the form of behavioral or pharmacological treatment or a combination of both. The treatment is dependent on many factors, such as severity of abuse, motivation of the abuser, and the availability of services. Some treatments require short-term hospitalization to deal with the life-threatening effects of the withdrawal, while others can be treated in an outpatient clinic. Treatment is also dependent on the goal of the treatment—for some, the goal is complete withdrawal from the substance; to others, it may be to receive drug replacement therapy where they are provided with a less dangerous version of the drug. Some opponents do not consider this a viable treatment option; however, for some individuals, it allows that person to rejoin society in a productive manner.

Fighting Substance Abuse

Throughout the years, the perception of substance abuse has fluctuated based on society's attitudes and perceptions of a particular substance. Looking at history demonstrates this. Efforts to fight substance abuse also follow this cycle, with an increased focus on treatment prevention occurring when a substance abuse problem becomes dangerous to the users themselves or to society in general. Most drug enforcement efforts are localized with the cooperation of international, interstate, and federal agencies. Efforts to combat substance abuse generally focus on two areas: reducing supply and demand of illegal substances. Reducing the supply makes the existing supply more expensive because there is less available to purchase. This effort assumes that individuals will be less likely to spend more money on supporting their drug habit if it became more expensive. An example of this strategy can be seen in states that are increasing the taxes on cigarettes. Fewer individuals are buying cigarettes as the price becomes prohibitively high.

Another effort for combating substance abuse is focusing on the demand for drugs. Attempts to do this are generally focused on education and treatment. The education aspect traditionally falls to schools to complete, and the treatment falls to local hospitals and public and private treatment centers. While the federal government does providing some funding for both these initiatives, the reality is that the actual implementation falls to local organizations with limited budgets.

In addition to funding, the federal government also tracks the issues regarding substance abuse and provides statistics for both public and private organizations. The federal government also has enacted several laws regarding specific substance abuse and its potential issues. Some of the laws are attempts to educate the public (like the mandate that all cigarette cartons and alcohol beverages have warning labels), while others impose stiff penalties for drug possession, manufacturing, and trafficking.

Legalization and Decriminalization

Throughout history, there have been numerous efforts—both successful and unsuccessful—to legalize different substances. Prohibition was an attempt to make the consumption of alcoholic beverages illegal, but it was repealed after 13 years. States also experimented with the drinking age—ranging from 18 to 21 at times and finally settling at 21—in large part to the efforts of the group MADD (Mothers Against Drunk Driving). Currently, there are 17 states that allow for the use of medical marijuana. Some people argue that legalizing drugs would prevent some of the problems associated with current illegal drugs, such as violence, crime, and drug trafficking. They also argue that drugs would be safer because there could be more drug regulations regarding the dosage of certain chemicals and the elimination of contaminants that can be potentially life-threatening. Similar arguments surround the decriminalization of drugs. By eliminating the penalties for using or dealing in small amounts, it would again decrease the dangers associated with illegal drug use.

Rachel Torres

See also: Alcoholism; Fetal Alcohol Syndrome; Head and Neck Cancer; Healthy Lifestyles and Risky Behaviors; Hemochromatosis; Psychotic Disorders; Sexually Transmitted Diseases

Further Reading

Beattie, M. (1986). *Codependent No More: How to Stop Controlling Others and Start Caring for Yourself.* Center City, MN: Hazelden Publishing.

Musto, D. F. (1999). *The American Disease: Origins of Narcotic Control,* 3rd ed. Oxford: Oxford University Press.

National Institute on Drug Abuse (NIDA). (2015, June). Drug Facts: Nationwide trends. Retrieved from https://www.drugabuse.gov/publications/drugfacts/nationwide-trends.

Substance Abuse and Mental Health Services Administration (SAMHSA). (2015). *Drug facts: Nationwide trends—National Household Survey on Drug Abuse.* Washington, DC: National Institute on Drug Abuse.

SUGAR DIABETES

Sugar diabetes, also known as *diabetes insipidus* ("lacks flavor"), is an uncommon disorder characterized by intense thirst and the excretion of large amounts of urine that is free from sugar and other abnormal constituents. In most cases, it is the result of the body not properly producing, storing or releasing a key hormone. Miller and Keane (1972) describe it as a metabolic disorder involving decreased activity in the posterior lobe of the pituitary gland. Diabetes insipidus can also occur when the kidneys are unable to respond properly to the antidiuretic hormone, vasopressin. While rare, diabetes insipidus can occur during pregnancy (gestational diabetes insipidus).

Diabetes insipidus is caused by a defect in secretion of vasopressin (antidiuretic hormone), which is secreted from pituitary gland present in hypothalamus. Its function is to reabsorb water from distal tubules in the kidney and control the concentration of urine. But its deficiency causes increased water excretion through urine even when there is low intake of water.

According to the Mayo Clinic (2016), diabetes insipidus is assumed to be related to what's commonly known as diabetes mellitus. Both disorders share a name and have some common signs: extreme thirst and excessive urination. However, diabetes mellitus (Type 1 and Type 2) and diabetes insipidus are unrelated.

Causes

The hypothalamus is responsible for producing an antidiuretic hormone (ADH); this hormone is stored in the pituitary gland. When needed, ADH (or vasopressin) is released into the blood stream and acts to concentrate urine by causing the tubules in the kidney to reabsorb water into the blood rather than excreting as much water into the urine. There are four types of disrupted ADH production and effect.

Dipsogenic diabetes insipidus. The term *dipsogenic* means "induces thirst and promotes ingestion of fluids." Dipsogenic diabetes insipidus is diagnosed as a metabolic disorder in which excessive fluid intake leads to suppression of ADH. In other words, drinking excess liquids results from the abnormal thirst caused by damage to the thirst-regulating mechanism of the hypothalamus.

Central diabetes insipidus. This type is usually caused by damage to the pituitary gland or hypothalamus resulting from surgery, a tumor, an illness (such as meningitis), inflammation or a head injury that acts to disrupt normal production and storages of ADH. Often, the etiology of central diabetes insipidus is unknown.

Nephrogenic diabetes insipidus. This type is the result of congenital failure of renal tubules to reabsorb water and is notable in that the kidneys are unable to properly respond to the ADH. This condition can be the result of an inherited (genetic) disorder or a chronic kidney disorder, or caused by certain drugs, such as lithium and tetracycline.

Gestational diabetes insipidus. Kollamparambil et al. (2011) report that gestational diabetes insipidus occurs only during pregnancy and when an enzyme made by the placenta—the system of blood vessels and other tissue that allows the exchange of nutrients and waste products between a mother and her baby—destroys the antidiuretic hormone in the mother.

Risk Factors

According to the National Institute of Diabetes and Digestive and Kidney Diseases (2015), the risk factors for diabetes insipidus vary according to how the individual's system is affected. Dipsogenic diabetes insipidus is associated with damage to the hypothalamus and can be the results of certain medications used in mental illness. In central diabetes insipidus, the condition can be caused by caused by surgery, illness, tumor, or head injury. Nephrogenic diabetes insipidus that is present at or shortly after birth usually has a genetic cause that permanently alters the kidneys' ability to concentrate the urine. Hague (2009) reports that mostly nephrogenic diabetes insipidus affects males, though women can pass the gene on to their children.

Complications

Except for dipsogenic diabetes insipidus, which causes water retention, diabetes insipidus causes the body to retain too little water to function properly, thus causing dehydration. Dehydration can lead to dry mouth, muscle weakness, low blood pressure (hypotension), elevated blood sodium (hypernatremia), a sunken appearance to the eyes, fever, headache, rapid heart rate, and an unhealthy weight loss. While not life-threatening, these physical responses leave the individual feeling un-well.

Screening for Diabetes Insipidus

To diagnose diabetes insipidus, physicians screen their patients to determine the type of diabetes insipidus they suffer. The diagnosis is based on a series of tests, including a urine osmolality and water deprivation test.

Water deprivation test. In this test, the patient stops drinking fluids two to three hours before the test so that the doctor can measure changes in body weight, urine output, urine composition, and ADH blood levels when fluids are withheld. The water deprivation test is a complicated procedure that should be done in a controlled setting where the patient can be closely monitored.

Urinalysis. This is the physical and chemical examination of urine. If the urine is less concentrated (meaning the amount of water excreted is high and the salt and waste concentrations are low), it could be due to diabetes insipidus.

Magnetic resonance imaging (MRI). Some physicians may want an MRI to look for abnormalities in or near the pituitary gland. The MRI alone is not diagnostic of diabetes insipidus. However, at diagnosis, it is estimated that 71 percent of patients show an abnormally thickened pituitary stalk on MRI (Mayo Clinic 2011).

Treatment

Depending upon the type of diabetes insipidus, the doctor may prescribe medication. The types of medication vary from a synthetic hormone (desmopressin) to prevent urine excretion, to diuretics or "water pills" (hydrochlorothiazide, amiloride) to treat fluid retention, ridding body of unneeded fluid and salt, or a combination diuretic to prevent the loss of too much potassium.

Points to remember about diabetes insipidus:

- It is a rare disease that causes frequent urination and excessive thirst.
- It is not related to diabetes mellitus (DM).
- Central diabetes insipidus is caused by damage to the pituitary gland and is treated with medication.
- Nephrogenic diabetes insipidus is caused by drugs or kidney disease and is treated with medication.
- Scientists have not yet discovered an effective treatment for dipsogenic diabetes insipidus, which is caused by a defect in the thirst mechanism.
- Most forms of gestational diabetes insipidus can be treated with medication.
- A doctor must determine which type of diabetes insipidus is involved before proper treatment can begin.

Linda R. Barley

See also: Kidney Diseases; Metabolic Diseases

Further Reading

Arima, H., & Oiso, Y. (2010). Mechanisms underlying progressive polyuria in familial neurohypophysial Diabetes Insipidus. *Journal of Neuroendocrinology, 22*(7), 754–757. doi: 10.1111/j.1365-2826.2010.02028.x.

Bockenhauer, D., van't Hoff, W., Dattani, M., Lehnhardt, A., Subtirelu, M., Hildebrandt, F., & Bichet, B. (2010). Secondary nephrogenic diabetes insipidus as a complication of inherited renal diseases. *Nephron Physiology, 116*(4), 23–29. doi: 10.1159/000320117.

Hague, W. (2009). Diabetes insipidus in pregnancy. *Obstetric Medicine*, 2, 4: 138–141. doi:10.1258/om.2009.090027.

Histiocytosis Association. (n.d.). Diabetes insipidus. Retrieved from http://histio.org/page.aspx?pid=409&gclid=CPKTrcKI6LsCFSUOOgodVBEAOw.

Kollamparambil, T., Mohan, P., Gunasuntharam, K., Jani, B., & Penma, D. (2011). Prenatal presentation of transient central diabetes insipidus. *European Journal of Pediatrics, 170*(5), 653–656. doi:10.1007/s00431-010-1340-2.

Mayo Clinic. (2016, March 19). Diabetes insipidus. Retrieved from http://www.mayoclinic.org/diseases-conditions/diabetes-insipidus/home/ovc-20182403.

Miller, B., & Keane, C. (1972). *Encyclopedia and Dictionary of Medicine and Nursing*. New York: W. B. Saunders, 267.

National Institute of Diabetes and Digestive and Kidney Diseases (NIDDK). (2015). Diabetes insipidus. Retrieved from http://www.niddk.nih.gov/health-information/health-topics/kidney-disease/diabetes-insipidus/Pages/facts.aspx.

SWALLOWING DISORDERS

Swallowing is a very important function of the body and can be disrupted by a variety of health conditions. Disturbances in swallowing or dysphagia can arise due to problems in the brain or in the esophagus, or swallowing tube, itself. Swallowing problems can result in choking, or pain when swallowing, plus a variety of problems from malnutrition to speaking difficulties. There are three main types of swallowing disorder, categorized according to where the problem originates, namely, the esophagus, pharynx, and oral cavity. Swallowing problems can occur at any age but are more common among older adults.

Signs and Symptoms

Signs and symptoms of swallowing disorders other than pain and choking may include being unable to swallow, unanticipated weight loss, regurgitation of food, drooling, coughing when swallowing, and frequent heartburn.

Causes and Risk Factors

Various forms of structural problems that lead to swallowing difficulties may include problems in the muscle walls of esophagus, known as diffuse spasm. The esophagus can narrow, a condition called esophageal stricture. Problems in the lower esophageal muscle can cause food regurgitation, and this condition is called achalasia.

Other problems include the presence of esophageal tumors, or foreign bodies in the esophagus, and the narrowing of the lower end of the esophagus called esophageal ring.

Radiation therapy, a condition called scleroderma that causes tissues to scar and harden, and various neurological problems of the throat area can cause swallowing problems.

A condition called gastroesophageal reflux disease (GERD), which can damage esophageal tissues from due to acid refluxing from the stomach into the esophagus, can lead to spasm or scarring and narrowing of the lower esophagus, making swallowing difficult (WebMD 2016).

Key risk factors are aging and the presence of a neurological or nervous system problem.

Diagnostic Tests

Cineradiography is a form of imaging that videotapes the act of swallowing using x-rays. Another test is known as an impendence and pH test; it examines whether acid reflux is the cause of a swallowing problem. Manometry is a special test that can record both the strength and timing of the contraction and relaxation phases of the esophagus. Finally, upper endoscopy is a method of examination that uses a thin narrow tube and passes this into the esophagus where it can project images of what is happening inside this region onto a screen.

Doctors who may be involve in examining and treating swallowing disorders are primary care physicians; otolaryngologists; speech pathologists; physical therapists; ear, nose, and throat surgeons; and oncologists.

Treatments

Treatment may depend on the type of condition and its severity. These can include various forms of exercise, the use of special liquid diets, the use of a feeding tube in severe cases, medications, esophageal dilation procedures, and surgery

Ray Marks

See also: Gastroesophageal Reflux Disease (GERD); Laryngeal Cancer; Oral Pharyngeal Disorders; Throat Disorders

Further Reading

Garbin, S. G. (2013). *Swallowing Disorders: Managing Dysphagia in the Elderly*. Amazon: CreateSpace Independent Publishing Platform.

Groher, M. E. (1997). *Dysphagia: Diagnosis and Management*, 3rd ed. Waltham, MA: Butterworth-Heinemann.

Groher, M. E. (2009). *Dysphagia: Clinical Management in Adults and Children*. Maryland Heights, MO: Mosby Publishing.

Mayo Clinic. (2014). Dysphagia. Retrieved from http://www.mayoclinic.org/diseases-conditions/dysphagia/basics/definition/con-20033444.

McMahon, M. (2014). What are the different types of swallowing disorders? *Wisegeek*. Retrieved from http://www.wisegeek.net/what-are-the-different-types-of-swallowing-disorders.htm#didyouknowout.

National Institute of Neurological Disorders and Stroke. (2015). NINDS swallowing disorders information page. Retrieved from http://www.ninds.nih.gov/disorders/swallowing_disorders/swallowing_disorders.htm.

Sayadi, R., & Herskowitz, J. (2010). *Swallow Safely: How Swallowing Problems Threaten the Elderly and Others—A Caregiver's Guide to Recognition, Treatment, and Prevention*. Natwick, MA: Inside/Outside Press.

WebMD. (2016). Difficulty swallowing (dysphagia)—overview. Retrieved from http://www.webmd.com/digestive-disorders/tc/difficulty-swallowing-dysphagia-overview.

TACHYCARDIA

The term *tachycardia* refers to having a faster than normal heart rate when at rest. That is the heart rate exceeds the normal heart rate of healthy person, which is 60 to 100 times per minute. A person with tachycardia is at increased risk for stroke, a sudden cardiac arrest, or death.

Types

The most common types of tachycardia include:

Atrial or supraventricular fibrillation
Atrial flutter
Paroxysmal atrial or supraventricular tachycardia
Ventricular tachycardia

Signs and Symptoms

The signs and symptoms of tachycardia include having a rapid pulse rate; light-headedness, dizziness, or fainting; experiencing shortness of breath; palpitations; or chest pain.

Causes and Risk Factors

The most common causes of tachycardia are the presence of a heart disease, the presence of any congenital abnormality in the person's neural system and heart-beat rate, the presence of anemia, high blood pressure or the presence of a fever. Risk factors for tachycardia include smoking, being over age 60, the presence of anxiety, genetics, a history of excess alcohol or caffeine use, recreational drug abuse, and the presence of certain medications. Having an overactive thyroid, high blood pressure, mental stress, or an imbalance of electrolytes needed to conduct electrical impulses effectively are other factors that may cause a faster than normal heartbeat rate. In some cases, the exact cause of tachycardia cannot be determined.

Diagnostic Tests

Diagnostic tests may include a physical examination, plus the use of an electrocardiogram (ECG or EKG) to record electrical signals as they travel through the heart or a holster monitor, or portable EKG. An event recorder or portable ECG device to monitor heart activity over an extended period can also be used. Electrophysi-ological tests using flexible tubes placed in the groin, neck, or arm can used to con-firm the diagnosis or pinpoint the location of related problems in the heart's circuitry. A tilt table test is sometimes used to monitor how the heart and nervous system respond to changes in position.

Additional Tests

The cardiologist may order additional tests, if desirable, in order to diagnose any underlying condition that may be contributing to tachycardia or to examine the status of the heart.

Treatments

Treatments for tachycardia include the use of:

- Vagal maneuvers such as coughing, bearing down as if you're having a bowel move-ment, and putting an ice pack on your face.
- Medications in the form of pills or injections of anti-arrhythmic medications to re-store a normal heart rate.
- Cardioversion, a procedure involving the use of an electric shock delivered to the heart through paddles or patches placed on the chest in order to restore a normal heart rhythm. As well, an implantable cardioverter-defibrillator can also be surgically im-planted in the chest to deliver precisely calibrated electrical shocks, if needed, to re-store a normal heart rhythm.
- In some cases open-heart surgery may be needed to destroy an extra electrical path-way, but this is usually only done if all other treatment options fail.

Prognosis

The risk of complications from the condition depends on the severity of the prob-lem, the duration of the problem, the type of tachycardia, the extent of the tachycar-dia, the person's age, and whether or not there is another heart condition present.
Common complications of tachycardia include:

Blood clots
Fainting spells
Heart failure
Sudden death

Prevention

It may be possible to prevent or manage episodes of tachycardia by using a process called catheter ablation, where a doctor inserts catheters into the groin, arm, or neck and guides them through the blood vessels to the heart. Electrodes at the top of the catheter use heat, extreme cold, or radiofrequency energy to damage the extra electrical pathway and prevent it from sending electrical signals.

As well, anti-arrhythmic medications may be given to prevent a fast heart rate. A pacemaker or small device implanted surgically under the skin can also help to regulate a person's rapid heartbeat.

Ray Marks

See also: Arrhythmias/Dysrhythmias; Chest Conditions; Heart Diseases; Stroke

Further Reading

American Heart Association. (2015). Tachycardia—fast heart rate. Retrieved from http://www.heart.org/HEARTORG/Conditions/Arrhythmia/AboutArrhythmia/Tachycardia_UCM_302018_Article.jsp.

Cohen, T. J. (2010). *A Patient's Guide to Heart Rhythm Problems*. Baltimore, MD: Johns Hopkins University Press.

Mayo Clinic. (2014). Tachycardia. Retrieved from http://www.mayoclinic.org/diseases-conditions/tachycardia/basics/definition/con-20043012.

Natale, A. (2009). *Ventricular Tachycardia/Fibrillation Ablation: The State of the Art Based on the Venice Chart International Consensus Document*. Hoboken, NJ: Wiley-Blackwell.

Nordqvist, C. (2015). Tachycardia: Causes, symptoms, and treatments. *Medical News Today*. Retrieved from http://www.medicalnewstoday.com/articles/175241.php.

Wang, P. J., & Estes, M. (2015). Supraventricular tachycardia. *American Heart Association Journals*. Retrieved from http://circ.ahajournals.org/content/106/25/e206.full.

TAY-SACHS DISEASE

Tay-Sachs is a rare disease passed from parents to child. According to the Mayo Clinic (2014), which diagnoses and supports families of children affected with Tay-Sachs, this disease is caused by a defective gene on chromosome 15. It occurs when the body lacks hexosaminidase A, a protein that helps break down a chemical found in nerve tissue called *gangliosides*. Without this protein, gangliosides, particularly ganglioside GM2, build up in cells, especially nerve cells in the brain.

Tay-Sachs most often appears in families with no prior history of the disease and can be carried without being expressed through several generations. In fact, anyone can be a Tay-Sachs carrier. The carrier rate for Tay-Sachs in the general population is 1 in 250. Some evidence suggests people of Irish and/or British Isle descent have an increased risk—over the general population—of between 1 in 50 and 1 in 150. French Canadians, Louisiana Cajuns, and Ashkenazi Jews are considered at highest risk with a carrier rate of 1 in 27. When both parents carry the defective Tay-Sachs gene, a child has a 25 percent chance of developing the disease. The child must receive two copies of the defective gene—one from each parent—in order to become ill. If only one parent passes the defective gene to the child, the child is called a carrier. He or she won't be sick but will have the potential to pass the disease to his or her own children.

Tay-Sachs has been classified into infantile, juvenile, and adult forms, depending on the symptoms and when they first appear. Most people with Tay-Sachs have the infantile form. In this form, the nerve damage usually begins while the baby is still in the womb. Symptoms usually appear when the child is three to six months old.

In infantile Tay-Sachs, the most common form, an affected baby will begin to show symptoms at about six months old. As the disease progresses, the child's body loses function, leading to blindness, deafness, paralysis, and death. These losses happen because a fatty substance in the child's brain builds up to toxic levels and affects the child's neurologic system. The disease worsens quickly, and the child usually dies by age four or five. Late-onset Tay-Sachs disease, which affects adults, is very rare.

Symptoms

The symptoms of infantile Tay-Sachs include deafness, decreased eye contact due to blindness, decreased muscle tone leading to paralysis, delayed mental and social skills, increased startle reaction, irritability, listlessness, loss of motor skills, seizures, and slow growth. In the rare case of late-onset Tay-Sachs, dementia may be observed.

Diagnosis

Tests to diagnosis Tay-Sachs disease include a physical examination, with a detailed family history, an enzyme analysis of blood or body tissue for hexosaminidase levels, and an eye examination (to reveal a cherry-red spot in the macula).

Complications

In infantile Tay-Sachs, symptoms generally appear during the first 3 to 10 months of life and progress to spasticity (a muscle control disorder), seizures, and the loss of all voluntary movement.

Prevention

There is no known way to prevent this disorder. Genetic testing can detect if you are a carrier of the gene for this disorder. If you or your partner is from an at-risk population, it is recommended that you undergo testing before starting a family. Testing the amniotic fluid can diagnose Tay-Sachs disease in the womb.

Linda R. Barley

See also: Genetics and Genomics; Neurological Diseases

Further Reading

Desnick, R. J., & Kaback, M. M. (2001). *Tay-Sachs Disease*. Cambridge, MA: Academic Press.

Freedman, J. (2009). *Genes & Disease: Tay-Sachs Disease*. New York: Chelsea House Publishers.

Johnson, M. (2007). Neurodegenerative disorders of childhood. In *Textbook of Pediatrics*. Philadelphia, PA: Saunders Elsevier.

Mayo Clinic. (2014, October 21). Tay-Sachs disease. Retrieved from http://www.mayoclinic.org/diseases-conditions/tay-sachs-disease/basics/definition/con-20036799.

National Tay-Sachs and Allied Diseases Association (NTSAD). (n.d.). Leading the Fight to treat and cure Tay-Sachs, Canavan, Sandhoff, GM1 and related diseases. Retrieved from http://www.ntsad.org.

TESTICULAR CANCER

Testicular cancer is a disease in which cells of one or both testicles become cancerous. These tumors can spread to other organs such as the lymph glands, lungs, and brain, causing serious illness or death.

The disease is rare and constitutes approximately 1 percent of all male cancers; it is the most common form of male cancers in men between the ages of 15 to 35, especially those who are white and of Scandinavian descent. Men of other races may, however, develop this health condition.

An estimated 8,500 men, or 1 in 250 men, are diagnosed annually in the United States with testicular cancer and of this number, 350 will die prematurely from the disease.

Testicular cancer is highly treatable if diagnosed early on, before it has spread, or even if it has spread, and the survival rate is almost 100 percent. Later, the survival rate drops to 80 percent.

Based on the characteristics of the cells in the tumor, testicular cancers may be classified as *seminomas*, which are less aggressive, or *nonseminomas* that are more aggressive. Seminoma cancers can present as one of three types: classic, anaplastic, or spermatocytic. Nonseminoma cancers include choriocarcinomas, embryonal carcinomas, teratomas, and yolk sac tumors. Testicular tumors may contain both seminoma and nonseminoma cells.

Symptoms

Signs and symptoms of testicular cancer include having:

- A painless lump, swelling, or enlargement in either testicle
- A feeling of heaviness in the scrotum
- A dull ache in the lower abdomen, back, or groin
- A sudden fluid collection in the scrotum
- Pain or discomfort in a testicle or the scrotum
- Enlarged or tender breasts

Key Causes and Risk Factors

Although there may be no risk factors, having certain conditions such as undescended testicle(s), congenital abnormalities of the testicles, having other forms of cancer, and a family history of testicular cancer may increase the risk of developing testicular cancer.

The exact causes of testicular cancer are not known, however.

Diagnosis

To help find the cause of symptoms, the doctor may carry out a physical exam and order laboratory and diagnostic tests including blood tests, ultrasound tests, and biopsies.

Treatment

Most cases of testicular cancer can be cured using radiation therapy, surgery, or chemotherapy.

Prevention

Monthly testicular self-exams are important. Regular testicular self-exams can help identify growths early on when the chance for successful treatment of testicular cancer is highest.

Prognosis

Prognosis is good if the cancer is diagnosed and treated early on.

Ray Marks

See also: Cancer; Men's Health

Further Reading

American Cancer Society. (2014). Testicular cancer index. Retrieved from http://www.cancer
.org/cancer/testicularcancer/index.

Gilbaugh, J. (2008). *Men's Private Parts: A Pocket Reference to Prostate, Urologic and Sexual Health*. New York: Simon and Schuster.

Mayo Clinic. (2014). Testicular cancer. Retrieved from http://www.mayoclinic.org/diseases
-conditions/testicular-cancer/basics/definition/con-20043068

McWhirt, K. A. (2010). *Together We Will Win: What Happens When We Don't Talk About Testicular Cancer*. Denver, CO: Outskirts Press.

Testicular Cancer Society. (2014). Testicular cancer 101. Retrieved from http://www
.testicularcancersociety.org/tc_101.html?gclid=CIL7jZnFiLwCFawB4god_ycAOA.

Verville, K. (2009). *Testicular Cancer: The Biology of Cancer*. New York: Chelsea House.

THORACIC OUTLET SYNDROME

The term *thoracic outlet syndrome* refers to a series of conditions that involve the compression of nerves and blood vessels in a region of the body known as the thoracic outlet. This is located in the region between the first rib and the collar bone, where there is very little space for associated muscles, nerves, and blood vessels to pass through.

The condition is rare and occurs more frequently in women than men.

There are three types of thoracic outlet syndrome, depending on which structure is being compressed: neurogenic, venous, and arteriole.

Symptoms

Among the symptoms of thoracic outlet syndrome are pain, finger numbness, and tingling in the arm or fingers of the affected side. The person's ability to grip an object may be decreased, and his or her muscles near the thumb area may appear wasted.

Depending on what structures are compressed, the hand may become discolored, and the hand and fingers may feel cold.

The affected person may experience weakness of the arm and neck muscles, swelling or redness of the arm, clumsiness of the hand, limited hand range of motion, or coolness and ready fatigue of the affected arm.

Key Causes and Risk Factors

The causes of thoracic outlet syndrome are unclear, but poor muscle function, posture, and obesity may be involved.

There may also be an anatomical defect from birth in the neck and rib areas, such as an abnormal first rib, or trauma that causes the nerves in the thoracic outlet region to be compressed.

A further possible cause is repetitive strain or movements that influence the thoracic outlet negatively.

Diagnosis

To diagnose the condition, a physical exam, and medical history may be helpful. Other tests used to help identify thoracic outlet syndrome are imaging tests; nerve conduction tests; and tests that assess the viability of arteries and veins or circulation, called *arteriography* and *venography*.

Another test involves assessing muscle signals and their strength using electromyography.

Nerve conduction tests can examine if the nerve in the region of the first rib and collar bone region is functioning or is damaged or compressed; an elevated arm stress test in which the patient raises his or her arms upwards for three minutes and opens and closes his or her fists can be used.

Treatment

The treatment will depend on the type of condition that prevails, as well as the severity of condition.

Common forms of treatment include physical therapy and exercise, medications, and steps to minimize or remove any blood clots that may occur.

Surgery can be used if the preceding approaches do not work, using a procedure called thoracic outlet decompression.

Sometimes, the first rib is removed or the artery in this region is replaced with another intact artery or artificial graft, sometimes a portion of the first rib is removed. And sometimes, clots from veins or arteries in the area are removed surgically.

Prognosis

If treated, the symptoms and complications are less likely to occur for a prolonged time period.

Prevention

Reducing stress on the area of the body, reducing repetitive motions that stress the structures in the thoracic outlet area, maintaining a good posture, and avoiding heavy lifting and carrying heavy items may be helpful.

Keeping a healthy weight and getting professional help might be helpful for minimizing this problem.

Ray Marks

See also: Neuromuscular Disorders; Venous Disorders

Further Reading

Glaser, D. L., & Widmer, B. (2011). Thoracic outlet syndrome. American Academy of Orthopedic Surgeons. Retrieved from http://orthoinfo.aaos.org/topic.cfm?topic=a00336.

Illig, K. A., et al. (2013). *Thoracic Outlet Syndrome*. New York: Springer.

Mayo Clinic. (2013). Thoracic outlet syndrome. Retrieved from http://www.mayoclinic.org/diseases-conditions/thoracic-outlet-syndrome/basics/definition/con-20040509.

Medifocus. (2016). *Thoracic Outlet Syndrome: A Comprehensive Guide to Symptoms, Treatment, Research, and Support*. Online: Medifocus.com, Inc.

Molina, J. E. (2012). *New Techniques for Thoracic Outlet Syndromes*. New York: Springer.

Sanders, R. J., Haug, C. E., & Raymer, S. (1991). *Thoracic Outlet Syndrome: A Common Sequela of Neck Injuries*. New York: Lippincott Williams & Williams.

THROAT CANCER

Overview

Cancer that develops in the region of the throat, the voice box, or the tonsils is a health condition known as throat cancer. As with other cancers, the cells in this region start to grow and multiply, and these can form cancerous tumors in the surrounding tissues. The early stages of throat cancer may not be easy to detect because the symptoms may be similar to those of the common cold or sore throat. Other areas that may be affected by cancer in the area of the mouth are the lips, the gums, the tongue, the roof and floor of the mouth, and the salivary glands. While throat or mouth tumors may not be malignant, it is also possible for cancer of the throat or mouth areas to spread to other areas of the body and cause cancer in those areas. Throat cancer is also termed *laryngeal cancer* and *pharyngeal cancer*.

Symptoms

The key symptoms associated with throat or mouth cancer include having a sore throat, experiencing voice changes, having swallowing difficulties, and having a cough that does not resolve. Other problems are weight loss that is not easily explained; bleeding of the nose and/or mouth areas; and jaw, throat, neck, or eye swelling. Sores that don't heal and pain in the region of the ear are other possible symptoms.

Key Causes and Risk Factors

The cause of throat or mouth cancers is not clear and may be genetic or due to excess tobacco or alcohol use. Some throat cancers are due to transmission of the human papillomavirus (HPV).

Diagnosis

Doctors will examine the area of the throat and mouth after taking a careful history. They may order x-rays, as well as tissue biopsies to examine cells of the throat or mouth microscopically. The doctor can also use a scope with a special lighting system and magnification applied to the throat or larynx that captures a picture of the tissues that can be transmitted to a screen by a camera for viewing. Other tests include ultrasound imaging, computerized tomography, position emission tomography, and magnetic resonance imaging.

Treatment

Like other forms of cancer, chemotherapy or radiation therapy are used for treatment. Surgery may also be used depending on the stage of the cancer. In other cases, a procedure known as targeted drug therapy may be employed. Foods that cause irritation may need to be avoided.

Prognosis

The outcome of the condition is fair for a sizable number of cases. Early detection and treatment will help to produce a more optimistic outcome.

Prevention

Avoiding tobacco usage, excess alcohol usage, and eating health foods may be helpful for preventing throat or mouth cancer. Protective actions during sexual encounters can also be helpful.

Ray Marks

See also: Oral Cancer; Oral Health; Oral Pharyngeal Disorders; Swallowing Disorders; Throat Disorders

Further Reading

Cancer Treatment Centers of America. (2014). Throat cancer. Retrieved from http://www.cancercenter.com/throat-cancer/.

Gourin, C. G. (2010). *Johns Hopkisn Patients' Guide to Head and Neck Cancer*. Burlington, MA: Jones & Bartlett Learning.

Mayo Clinic. (2014). Throat cancer. Retrieved from http://www.mayoclinic.org/diseases-conditions/oral-and-throat-cancer/basics/definition/con-20042850.

National Cancer Institute. (2015). Head and neck cancer: Patient version. Retrieved from http://www.cancer.gov/cancertopics/types/throat.

Wenig, B. M. (2016). *Atlas of Head and Neck Pathology*. Philadelphia, PA: Elsevier.

THROAT DISORDERS

The throat, known medically as the *pharynx*, is a muscular tubal passage that extends from the back of the nasal cavity down into the esophagus. Its primary organs are the larynx, or voice box; trachea, or windpipe; and esophagus, which transports food and liquids to the stomach. Made of soft tissues, the throat can be easily irritated, leading to the common problem of a sore throat and other conditions.

Viral and bacterial infections and allergies are the most common causes of throat disorders. More serious causes include stomach acids moving into the esophagus (gastroesophageal reflux disease, or GERD), abnormal growths, ulcers and paralysis of the larynx, cancers, and secondary infections of HIV. Throat infections, such as tonsillitis, and those caused by streptococcus bacteria and some growths are most common in children. Adults experience laryngitis and other throat disorders, which can change the voice and impair swallowing, particularly in older adults. In most cases, if the causes and symptoms are similar, so are treatments. Except in cases of viral infections and allergies, where medical intervention may not be necessary, treatment depends on the specific condition and its underlying cause.

Types of Throat Disorders

Some of the most common disorders associated with the throat are tonsillitis, pharyngitis, epiglottitis, hoarseness, laryngitis, laryngoceles, and strep throat, as well as vocal cord nodules, polyps, and granulomas (noncancerous growths). Less common are vocal cord contact ulcers and vocal cord paralysis, a serious condition that can close the trachea.

Symptoms

Depending on the cause, the severity of the symptoms can vary, but the most common are the following:

- Painful or difficult swallowing
- A dry throat
- Hoarseness or a change in voice (muffled or altered speech)
- Persistent irritation, pain, or scratchy sensation
- Sore or swollen lymph nodes in the neck or jaw
- Red swollen tonsils
- Phlegm or mucus buildup

Infections causing a throat disorder can lead to additional symptoms: high fever with chills and body aches; coughing, sneezing, and nasal congestion; and nausea, often with vomiting. The most serious infection is *epiglottitis*, which swells the larynx enough to close off the trachea. Symptoms include drooling, muffled speech, and shortness of breath and difficulty breathing. Symptoms due to GERD include a chronic cough, heartburn, pain the midsection of the chest, and a sour taste.

Causes and Risk Factors

The most common causes of throat disorders are viral infections from bronchitis, pneumonia, colds and influenza, and other respiratory illnesses; mononucleosis; measles; chickenpox and croup; and bacterial infections, including strep throat (group A streptococcus), whooping cough, and diphtheria, which is uncommon in developed countries. Other causes include dry air and allergies to dust, mold, pollen, and pet dander; irritants from air pollution, smoking, and exposure to chemicals; rare throat abscesses and epiglottitis, which blocks the trachea and is a medical emergency; and straining the vocal cords.

Throat disorders can affect anyone, but children and teens are more susceptible, particularly for strep throat. Individuals of all ages may be at risk if they live in close conditions (such as dormitories) or frequently spend time in environments with many others (in offices, classrooms, day care centers, military posts, on public transportation). Those who have chronic sinus infections, a compromised immune system, allergies, or are often exposed to tobacco (including secondhand) or chemical irritants are at increased risk of throat disorders. Singers, teachers, preachers, and others people who are required to use their voices a lot are at risk of vocal cord contact ulcers.

Diagnosis

Minor sore throat symptoms usually disappear after about one week without medical care. For those that last longer, a doctor will determine the cause and severity, asking about symptoms, risk factors, and medical history; palpating for swollen lymph nodes; and listening for breathing. Further tests may include laryngoscopy, or a thin, flexible viewing tube inserted through the nose; neck x-rays; and a rapid strep test for children and a throat culture for adults. Test is the only way to distinguish viral from bacterial causes. If necessary, a doctor may take a biopsy sample or a blood test if mononucleosis or HIV infections are suspected.

Treatment

Treatment depends on the diagnosis of the underlying cause of a throat disorder. Viral infections usually do not require treatment, but bacterial infections respond to penicillin or other antibiotics. Most nodules caused by vocal strain usually go away with voice therapy in which the patient learns how to sing or speak without damaging the vocal cords. Surgical intervention is necessary for vocal cord paralysis; epiglottitis; and the removal of polyps, abscesses, and some other growths. Pain-relief medication (prescription and over-the-counter) is key so people can swallow food and liquids comfortably; for GERD, treatment includes antacids. Home remedies provide temporary relief: warm liquids, ice chips or popsicles, saltwater gargles, and lozenges or throat sprays, humidified air, and rest.

Prevention

Frequent hand-washing, the avoidance of shared eating and drinking utensils, as well as covering mouth and nose, and other good hygiene practices help prevent many throat disorders, especially those caused by infections. Reducing exposure to allergens and other irritants, avoiding cigarette smoke, using a humidifier, resting or retraining vocal cords, and keeping a distance or avoiding other people with upper respiratory infections can prevent throat problems for those who are susceptible.

Prognosis

If not due to a separate, serious underlying cause, most throat disorders go away with or without treatment; although if caused by infections, they may reappear.

Jean Kaplan Teichroew

See also: Gastroesophageal Reflux Disease (GERD); Laryngeal Cancer; Oral Cancer; Oral Health; Oral Pharyngeal Disorders; Swallowing Disorders; Throat Cancer

Further Reading

American Academy of Otolaryngology: Head and Neck Surgery. (2011, January). Patient health information. Retrieved from http://www.entnet.org/content/patient-health.

Healthgrades. (2013, September 20). Throat symptoms. Retrieved from http://www.healthgrades.com/symptoms/throat-symptoms.

Judd, S. J. (2006). *Ear, Nose, and Throat Disorders Sourcebook*. Detroit: Omnigraphics.

Mayo Clinic. (2013, May 7). Diseases and conditions: Sore throat. Retrieved from http://www.mayoclinic.org/diseases-conditions/sore-throat/basics/definition/con-20027360.

Sasaki, C. T. (2015). *Introduction to Mouth and Throat Disorders*. Merck Manual. Retrieved from http://www.merckmanuals.com/home/ear-nose-and-throat-disorders/mouth-and-throat-disorders/introduction-to-mouth-and-throat-disorders.

THROMBOPHLEBITIS

Introduction

Thrombophlebitis, sometimes referred to as phlebitis, is swelling in vein due to inflammation. The term is derived from the *thrombo*, meaning clot, and *phlebitis*, meaning inflammation of a vein. Most often, the inflammation is caused by a blood clot in a leg vein, but on rare occasions, the condition can occur in the arm or neck areas. If an affected vein is near the skin surface, it is called superficial thrombophlebitis. If it is located deep in a muscle, it is called deep vein thrombosis (DVT).

Superficial thrombophlebitis is quite common and can occur spontaneously. It can also occur as a complication of medical or surgical interventions. The risk is increased by prolonged sitting or being in a prolonged post-operative recuperation state. It is rarely life-threatening but should be investigated because it may be associated with the presence of a DVT, which can be life-threatening. It can also increase the risk of serious health problems such as having a dislodged blood clot that may travel to the lungs and block the artery to that organ causing a condition known as pulmonary embolism.

If superficial phlebitis occurs together with an infection, this condition is referred to as septic thrombophlebitis. This situation requires special attention and treatment procedures to reduce the infection. Although not common, the superficial form of thrombophlebitis can progress by perforating veins to involve adjacent deep veins.

Signs and Symptoms

The condition is accompanied by signs of redness, warmth, pain, swelling, and tenderness in the affected area.

Diagnosis

There are several tests used to diagnose superficial thrombophlebitis, including blood tests such as coagulation studies, Doppler ultrasound, CT or MRI scans, and venography to diagnose blockages. Clinically, the physician might be able to find tender and inflamed superficial veins through palpation techniques. However, further testing is required to evaluate for a DVT.

Treatment

Treatment is aimed at improving patient comfort and preventing any superficial phlebitis from progressing to DVT. Self-care methods can ease pain and reduce the risk of clots. Various treatments, including blood-thinning or clot-reducing medications and surgery, compression stockings, and varicose vein stripping procedures, are also used for treating thrombophlebitis.

Prognosis

The outcome is normally good, but if superficial phlebitis is not treated and spreads to the veins, it can cause damage to deep vein valves, which can lead to chronic deep venous insufficiency or postphlebitic syndrome. Varicose veins, leg swelling, and skin discoloration are other complications that may arise.

The risk of thrombophlebitis increases with having on or more of the following risk factors:

- An injury to a vein
- Prolonged inactivity
- Being confined to bed for a prolonged period
- The presence of pancreatic cancer
- A stroke history followed by arm or leg paralysis
- Having a pacemaker
- Being pregnant or have just given birth
- The use birth control pills or hormone replacement therapy
- Having a family history of a blood-clotting disorder
- The presence of being overweight or obese
- Being older than 60 or having a genetic disposition to the condition

Prevention

Avoiding prolonged sitting or lying; using compression stockings; elevating the affected limb; and, if necessary, using medications to reduce the chance of clotting or to decrease pain and inflammation may be helpful.

Linda R. Barley

See also: Cellulitis; Deep Vein Thrombosis; Physical Activity; Psoriasis; Venous Disorders

Further Reading

Holm, G., & Roth, E. (2012). Thrombophlebitis. HealthLine.com. Retrieved from http://www.healthline.com/health/thrombophlebitis#Overview1.

Mayo Clinic. (2014). Thrombophlebitis. Retrieved from http://www.mayoclinic.com/health/thrombophlebitis/DS00223/DSECTION=complications.

Rosh, A. J. (2014). Superficial thrombophlebitis. Medscape. Retrieved from http://emedicine.medscape.com/article/463256-overview.

THYROID CANCER

Overview

Thyroid cancer is a rare health condition in which cells of the thyroid gland, which lies in the front of the throat and produces hormones that enable the body to generate energy and function successfully, multiply abnormally to form a tumor. It is more common in women than men and has a good outcome, in general.

The four main types are called, anaplastic (which is rare), medullary, follicular, and papillary—the most common form. A fifth type is called thyroid lymphoma, which starts in the immune system cells of the thyroid gland and grows rapidly (Mayo Clinic 2014).

Symptoms

The symptoms of thyroid cancer include neck pain, the presence of a lump or swelling in the region of the neck, swollen neck glands, and swallowing problems. As well, breathing may be affected, there may be a cough, the voice may become hoarse, and the affected person may wheeze constantly. Sometimes, there may be no symptoms.

Key Causes and Risk Factors

The causes of thyroid cancer are unknown but, like other cancers, may involve DNA damage to the thyroid cells. This can occur especially if the thyroid gland is exposed to radiation.

On occasion, having a family history can lead to medullary thyroid cancer.

Diagnosis

The physical examination of the neck may be followed by a needle or surgical biopsy if a lump is found or if the physician wants to establish a definite diagnosis. Other tests are blood tests, ultrasound tests, CT scans, genetic testing, and MRIs.

Treatment

Treatment procedures may involve targeted drug therapy in cases of advanced disease, surgery, treatment with radioactive iodine to destroy thyroid tissues, and on occasion, radiation therapy or chemotherapy, but this is rare.

Surgery can involve removal of most of the thyroid gland, removing neck lymph nodes, or removing a portion of the thyroid gland. After surgery, a patient may be put on thyroid medication containing hormones to replace those missing, and this will be for life and involve frequent blood testing to make sure levels of the hormone are optimal.

A procedure called *thyroid ablation*, involving the injection of alcohol into the cancerous tissue, may be recommended for recurrent thyroid cancers restricted to small areas of the gland.

Prognosis

The outlook for this type of cancer is good and varies with age, severity of condition, type of condition, and duration of condition, among other factors. Even if apparently successful after treatment, thyroid cancer can reoccur.

Prevention

Prevention is not currently possible, but people who have had exposure to neck radiation should be followed up every two years.

Ray Marks

See also: Cancer; Head and Neck Cancer; Swallowing Disorders; Thyroid Disease

Further Reading

Ain, K. (2010). *The Complete Thyroid Book.* New York: McGraw-Hill Education.

Mazzaferri, E. L., Amdur, R. J., & Kirwan, J. (2006). *Essentials of Thyroid Cancer Management.* New York: Springer Science & Business Media.

Mayo Clinic. (2014). Thyroid cancer. Retrieved from http://www.mayoclinic.org/diseases -conditions/thyroid-cancer/basics/definition/con-20043551.

MedicineNet.com. (2015, May 13). Thyroid Cancer. Retrieved from http://www.medicinenet .com/script/main/art.asp?articlekey=8693.

National Cancer Institute. (2014). Thyroid cancer. Retrieved from http://www.cancer.gov /cancertopics/types/thyroid.

Rosenthal, M. S. (2003). *The Thyroid Cancer Book.* Charleston, SC: CreateSpace.

Van Nostrand, D. (2010). *Thyroid Cancer: A Guide for Patients.* Manchester, NH: Keystone Press.

Wartofsky, L. (2015). *Thyroid Cancer: A Comprehensive Guide to Clinical Management.* New York: Springer-Verlag.

THYROID DISEASE

Thyroid disease is a condition that affects the thyroid, and the disease has several types. Most are signaled by one of two changes to the thyroid function: either *hypothyroidism* (an underactive thyroid) or *hyperthyroidism* (an overactive thyroid). Some 200 million people around the world and about 30 million people in the United States alone have some type of thyroid disease, with many of these disorders going undiagnosed. Although anyone can have a thyroid disorder, women are about four to seven times more likely to suffer from one.

The thyroid gland is an endocrine gland at the base of the neck that produces thyroid hormones used to regulate many of the organs in the body, including the heart, liver, and skin. Thyroid hormones are also essential to the metabolism and growth functions of the body. When the thyroid is not producing enough hormones—or is producing too many hormones—this is an indicator of an underlying thyroid disease. Other symptoms can include changes to the heartbeat (a weak or slow beat in hypothyroidism and a rapid beat in hyperthyroidism), weakness in the muscles, constipation (hypothyroidism) or diarrhea (hyperthyroidism), unusual levels of fatigue or depression, near-constant feelings of irritability or nervousness, and a structural change to the thyroid known as a nodule or a goiter (a nodule is a lump in the thyroid, while a goiter is the actual enlargement of the thyroid itself, which may include several nodules).

Thyroid disease itself includes different types of thyroid cancers and all the versions of thyroiditis, including Hashimoto's thyroiditis, which is a chronic inflammation of the thyroid gland caused by abnormal blood antibodies. Hashimoto's thyroiditis causes white blood cells to attack and destroy the cells of the thyroid, resulting in hypothyroidism if not addressed. Other types of thyroiditis include silent thyroiditis, which gives off no symptoms or signs of thyroid inflammation; postpartum thyroiditis, which is a temporary attack of thyroiditis that occurs after giving birth; and subacute thyroiditis, which is usually caused by a viral infection. There are four main types of thyroid cancer known to science: papillary thyroid cancer, which is the most frequent type and often spreads to the lymph nodes in the neck; follicular thyroid cancer, which accounts for about 10 to 15 percent of all thyroid cancer cases and generally does not spread beyond the thyroid; medullary cancer, which is an inherited form of thyroid cancer; and anaplastic thyroid cancer, which is the most aggressive form of thyroid cancer and is not usually treatable. Another type of thyroid disease is Graves' disease, or toxic diffuse goiter. This is an autoimmune condition that is known to be the most common cause of hyperthyroidism in the United States and affects about 1 in every 100 people around the world.

The risk of thyroid disease is increased in people who have been exposed to radiation therapies for the head or neck region or those who take certain medications, including lithium, which is commonly used to treat bipolar disorders. A family history of thyroid problems can also factor into the possibility of being affected. If thyroid disease is suspected, a doctor will perform a thyroid-stimulating hormone test, which is a blood test used to evaluate the condition of the thyroid gland. Other laboratory tests may also be recommended to help determine the extent of the abnormality, and a thyroid-imaging scan may also be performed. If a person has a nodule, professionals will most likely take a biopsy to sample the tissue and determine whether or not it is cancerous and, if so, what type of cancer has caused it.

Thyroid disease is often treatable, with treatment protocols varying depending on the type of condition a person has. In some cases, surgery is the recommended course of action, particularly in patients experiencing cancerous growths. In other situations, medication to replace the diminished thyroid hormone or to block the excessive amount of hormone being produced is advised. Radioactive iodine may be given in pill or capsule form to help repair an overactive thyroid in the case of Graves' or to help kill thyroid cancer cells. If a thyroid condition is not addressed, it may lead to serious and life-threatening complications, including seizures, coma, and an irregular heartbeat.

Tamar Burris

See also: Hashimoto's Disease; Hyperthyroidism; Hypothyroidism; Metabolic Disorders; Phenylketonuria

Further Reading

Cleveland Clinic. (2016). Thyroid disease. Retrieved from https://my.clevelandclinic.org /health/diseases_conditions/hic_Hyperthyroidism/hic_ThyrThy_Disease.
Johns Hopkins Medicine. (2016). Thyroid disorders in women. Retrieved from http://www .hopkinsmedicine.org/healthlibrary/conditions/endocrinology/thyroid_disordedi_in _women_85,P00437/.

Khazan, O. (2015, February 9). Sleepy, stressed, or sick? Why thyroid diseases are so common—and still so mysterious. *The Atlantic*. Retrieved from http://www.theatlantic.com/health/archive/2015/02/why-is-one-of-the-most-common-diseases-still-so-mysterious/385256/.

Mayo Clinic. (2015). Hypothyroidism (underactive thyroid). Retrieved from http://www.mayoclinic.org/diseases-conditions/hypothyroidism/symptoms-causes/dxc-20155382.

Miller, J. M., et al. (1983). *Needle Biopsy of the Thyroid: Current Concepts*. Westport, CT: Praeger.

Parangi, S., & Phitayakorn, R. (2010). *Thyroid Disease*. Westport, CT: Greenwood.

U.S. Department of Health and Human Services. Office on Women's Health. (2015). Thyroid disease. Retrieved from http://www.womenshealth.gov/publications/our-publications/fact-sheet/thyroid-disease.html.

TINNITUS

Tinnitus (a Latin term meaning to ring or tinkle) is commonly referred to as a ringing in the ears. It is not a condition but rather a symptom of an underlying problem such as hearing loss or ear injury resulting from a variety of events. Treatment depends on identifying the underlying cause.

Millions of Americans experience tinnitus, characterized by a ringing, buzzing, whistling, hissing, or clicking sound in the ear. Tinnitus can be either subjective or objective. Subjective tinnitus, the most common variety, represents sound that only the person experiencing it can hear. Objective tinnitus, on the other hand, is a less common form that can be perceived by others. For instance, a doctor conducting a physical examination of the ear may observe tinnitus in the nature of sound arising from blood turbulence around the ear or muscle spasms. In any case, tinnitus is actually neurological in origin, an illusion of sound created by neural circuits in the brain and processed by the auditory system. The level of sound varies, and it may affect one or both ears.

Causes of tinnitus include ear problems, chronic health conditions, injuries or conditions that affect the nerves in the ear or the hearing center in the brain, and medications. Tinnitus can be caused by ear problems in the outer, middle, or inner ear. A common cause of the malady is damage to tiny, delicate hairs in the inner ear that move in relation to the pressure of sound waves and send messages to the brain. If the hairs are bent or broken, then they can send incorrect electrical impulses to the brain, causing tinnitus. Earwax blockage in the outer ear is another common cause of tinnitus resulting from irritation of the eardrum. Age-related hearing loss (at around age 60) and exposure to loud noises are likewise common causes. Although less common, head or neck injuries can cause damage to the inner ear, resulting in tinnitus in only one ear. Other less common occurrences of tinnitus result from health conditions such as head and neck tumors, blood vessel diseases, thyroid problems, and hormonal changes. Sometimes, medications used to treat health conditions cause or worsen tinnitus. These medications include high doses of aspirin, certain antibiotics, cancer medications, malaria pills, and some antidepressants.

Depending on the cause, certain treatments may mitigate the effects of tinnitus. For instance, if tinnitus is due to an underlying condition such as earwax, then removing the impacted earwax may reduce its symptoms. Likewise, treatment of underlying heart or vascular conditions or a change in medication may mitigate the effects of tinnitus. Because noise-induced hearing loss is a common cause, it is particularly important to limit exposure to loud noises, such as those from heavy equipment, chainsaws, firearms, and loud music. However, many cases of tinnitus cannot be treated or cured. Therefore, those who suffer chronically may benefit from stress management or counseling.

Linda Tancs

See also: Ear Diseases; Meniere's Disease; Vestibular Diseases

Further Reading

American Speech-Language-Hearing Association. (2016). Tinnitus. Retrieved from http://www.asha.org/public/hearing/Tinnitus/.

American Tinnitus Association. (2016). Understanding the facts. Retrieved from https://www.ata.org/understanding-facts.

Beck, J. (2016, January 21). The sound that comes from nowhere. *The Atlantic*. Retrieved from http://www.theatlantic.com/health/archive/2016/01/the-sound-that-comes-from-nowhere/424932/.

Marder, J. (2013, November 6). Neuroscience may offer hope to millions robbed of silence by tinnitus. *PBS NewsHour*. Retrieved from http://www.pbs.org/newshour/updates/science-july-dec13-tinnitus_11-06/.

Vernon, J. A. (1997). *Tinnitus: Treatment and Relief*. Boston, MA: Allyn & Bacon.

Vestibular Disorders Association. (2015). What is that ringing in my ears? Retrieved from http://vestibular.org/tinnitus.

TOBACCO ADDICTION

Tobacco is a farm-grown plant that can be manufactured into a variety of products, including cigarettes, cigars, and flavored chewing tobaccos. Tobacco is the leading cause of preventable and premature death in the United States. As indicated in a Surgeon General's report, "Cigarettes are responsible for approximately 443,000 deaths—one in every five deaths—each year in the United States" (CDC 2014). Some of the health effects associated with the use or exposure to chemicals released by tobacco products include diseases of the heart, lungs, and eyes; circulation problems; and several forms of cancer. Tobacco, like other drugs, has a tendency to promote addiction due to its properties that change brain chemistry. Despite the many biological sicknesses the product induces, cigarette smokers always find a reason to justify their behavior. A commonly used excuse is that cigarettes release stress. Therefore, working hard to break nicotine dependence remains very difficult.

As noted by the Centers for Disease Control and Prevention (CDC 2016), the total economic cost of smoking in the United States is more than $300 billion a year, and it includes almost $170 billion in direct medical care for adults and more than $156 billion in lost productivity due to premature death and exposure to secondhand smoke. Nearly all tobacco use begins during youth and progresses during young adulthood (CDC 2014). Daily, more than 3,200 children age 18 or younger smoke their first cigarette; nearly 9 out of 10 smokers start before the age of 18 and almost all start by the time they reach 26. If smoking continues at its current rate, 1 out of every 13 of today's children will die prematurely from a smoking-related illness.

Symptoms

Symptoms of tobacco addiction include difficulty breathing, the presence of high blood pressure, tachycardia, persistent coughing, coughing up blood, and having a low exercise tolerance.

Causes

Addiction to cigarettes is the result of a false feeling of relaxation. When nicotine crosses the brain barrier, the pleasurable sensation does not last long. Within a short period of time, smokers want more nicotine. In fact, going without nicotine makes smokers feel tense and stressed out. Another puff of nicotine makes the addicted brain have another pleasure reaction, which is a false feeling of calm.

Addiction to tobacco can cause harmful consequences on individual health, such as heart disease, lung and mouth cancer, tooth decay, bad breath, blood pressure, and stroke.

Tar is the substance responsible for long-standing cigarette addiction.

Carbon monoxide can damage the wall of arteries and encourage fatty buildup. Over time, it can cause hardening of the blood vessels, a condition of oxygen deficiency in lungs and heart, which can easily raise the blood pressure and trigger a heart attack.

The worst common negative effect of cigarettes smoking is lung cancer. Most of the time, the cancer is located in both lungs due to the excessive amount of carbon monoxide that blocks oxygen penetration.

Diagnosis

Tests include a medical history, x-rays, CT scans to localize any tumors or see if any other organs are affected, and other lab tests such as red blood cell count to verify any presence of anemia or other preexisting conditions.

Treatments

Most treatments for tobacco-related illnesses involve surgical removal of the affected organs—for example, the lung. Bypass surgery may be recommended for patients who have experienced a heart attack. Medications such as Zyban (bupropion) and Chantix (varenicline), the nicotine patch, or nicotine gum—which can greatly reduce cravings and double one's chances of success—are often recommended. Other strategies are behavioral modification, avoiding peers who smoke, and support groups.

Some states have laws about tobacco smoking. Current tobacco laws in New York State, for example, prohibit smoking within 15 feet of a building entrance, in or near the entrance of hospitals, in areas of mass public transportation, in places of employment, and in a variety of other locations (New York State Department of Health 2016). Smoking has been prohibited in all public parks, beaches, and pedestrian plazas in New York City. Those found smoking in these areas must pay fines. Stores selling tobacco products are required to have their tobacco sale licenses, as well as "Age of Sale" and "We Card" signs posted on the store wall.

Future

Some future directions in the tobacco movement include getting store owners to remove tobacco ads, relocating tobacco ads so they are not as visible, or most ideally, covering tobacco power walls (a wall usually located at the front of the store containing only tobacco products) with frosted glass doors to reduce the visibility of tobacco products. More immediate goals include providing information about the intent of tobacco companies to get new customers through various ad strategies so that the impact of such ads on youth can be reduced. Smoke-free organizations throughout New York State are working to address issues of outdoor air quality as related to smoking, as well as create smoke-free housing.

Tiffany Crystal Rivera

See also: COPD (Chronic Obstructive Pulmonary Disease); Emphysema; Lung Cancer; Lung Diseases; Oral Cancer; Pneumonia; Pneumothorax; Pollution; Respiratory Diseases; Secondhand Smoke; Substance Abuse

Further Reading

Centers for Disease Control and Prevention (CDC). (2016, February 17). Smoking & tobacco use. Retrieved from http://www.cdc.gov/tobacco/data_statistics/fact_sheets/fast_facts/index.htm#cost.

Centers for Disease Control and Prevention (CDC). (2014). 2014 Surgeon General's report: The health consequences of smoking—50 years of progress. Retrieved from http://www.cdc.gov/tobacco/data_statistics/sgr/50th-anniversary/index.htm.

Centers for Disease Control and Prevention. (2006). Cigarette use among high school students-United States, 1991–2005. *MMWR Morbidity and Mortality Weekly Report*, 55(26), 724–726. Retrieved from http://www.cdc.gov/mmwr/preview/mmwrhtml/mm5526a2.htm.

Ennett, S. T., & Bauman, K. E. (1993). Peer group structure and adolescent cigarette smoking: A social network analysis. *Journal of Health and Social Behavior*, 34(3), 226–236.

National Cancer Institute. (2015). Tobacco. Retrieved from http://www.cancer.gov/about-cancer/causes-prevention/risk/tobacco.

National Institute on Drug Abuse (NIDA). (2012). Tobacco/nicotine. Retrieved from http://www.drugabuse.gov/publications/research-reports/tobacco/nicotine-addictive.

New York State Department of Health. (2016, January). The New York State Tobacco Control Program (TCP). Retrieved from https://www.health.ny.gov/prevention/tobacco _control/program_components.htm.

Perkins K. A., Stitzer, M., & Lerman, C. (2006). Medication screening for smoking cessation: A proposal for new methodologies. *Psychopharmacology*, *184*, 628–636.

TRACHEAL DISORDERS

Often referred to as the windpipe, the trachea is a rigid tube of cartilage rings that provide support and prevent collapse. It starts beneath the larynx, or voice box, and connects to the lungs via the two bronchi (bronchial tubes). With each breath a person takes, it widens and lengthens, providing air flow to and from the lungs. Soft tissue allows the expansion, and a mucous-membrane lining traps microorganisms and other particles.

People of all ages, from infants to older adults, may experience tracheal disorders that severely affect breathing. Inflammation can scar or narrow the trachea, tumors can block it, and injury or birth defects can cause it to become floppy or soft. Common symptoms of tracheal disorders are shortness of breath or difficulty breathing, coughing, hoarseness, wheezing or other abnormal breath sounds, and difficulty swallowing. Depending on the type of disorder, surgery may be required, although stents, chest and breathing exercises, and mild pressure are treatments for a soft or weakened windpipe.

Types of Tracheal Disorders

In general, tracheal disorders fall into two main categories: *stenosis*, or a narrowing, restricts air from reaching the lungs fully and *tracheomalacia*, a structural abnormality in which the trachea's walls become weak or floppy. Rare disorders include tumors that block the airway, occurring mostly in adults, and tracheitis, a serious bacterial infection that primarily affects children.

History

The first references to pediatric tracheomalacia come from the 1930s and 1940s, when clinicians described tracheal obstruction due to congenital abnormalities. The first description of an unusually large adult trachea and bronchi was reported in postmortem findings in 1897, and the first clinical report of an enlarged trachea was in 1932. The use of a bronchoscope, a device that passes through the mouth or nose and through the trachea, was first used to diagnose the condition in 1949, and in the 1950s, case reports began to appear in medical literature.

Symptoms

Regardless of the type, all tracheal disorder symptoms are similar and usually include at least one of the following:

- Wheezing
- Stridor, a high-pitched musical sound that occurs while taking a breath
- Shortness of breath or difficulty breathing
- Coughing, occasionally with blood
- Hoarseness
- Pneumonia or other frequent or recurring upper respiratory infections
- Treatment-resistant asthma
- Bluish skin color or inside mouth or nose, associated with a lack of oxygen
- Difficulty swallowing

Many people are not aware of tracheal stenosis because it can develop over time and be mistaken for other illnesses. Bacterial tracheitis appears as an upper respiratory infection similar to the flu; in addition to those just listed, symptoms of infection and airway obstruction may include a high fever, nasal flaring, and a very deep cough.

Causes and Risk Factors

Tracheal stenosis that is not congenital usually results from scar tissue due to intubation (a breathing tube inserted during a medical procedure) or a tracheostomy (surgical opening in the neck). Other injuries to the throat or tumors pressing on the trachea also cause constriction, as can chronic infections, radiation-therapy side effects, and autoimmune disorders. The causes of tracheomalacia are many and similar, but the most common also include emphysema, gastroesophageal reflux disease (GERD), and inhaling irritants. Tracheomalacia present at birth usually goes away by the time a child reaches two years old, when tracheal cartilage grows and strengthens.

Tumors in the trachea are rare, but most are malignant, and they may develop when cancer spreads from elsewhere in the body. The most common tumor affecting the trachea is a fast-growing squamous cell carcinoma that is more common in men and primarily caused by smoking. Both women and men may develop a slow-growing adenoid cystic carcinoma, usually between the ages of 40 and 60; smoking is not a factor.

Tracheitis, usually affecting only young children, is most commonly caused by a *staphylococcus aureus* bacterial infection, although occasionally also by viruses and allergies.

Diagnosis

Reaching an accurate diagnosis of a tracheal disorder can be difficult because many symptoms occur slowly and are similar to asthma, bronchitis, and other illnesses. After taking a medical history and conducting a physical exam, a doctor may employ one or more tests to diagnose stenosis or tracheomalacia:

- Chest x-rays and PET and CT scans produce images of the airway organs; a dynamic three-dimensional chest CT scan focuses on the suspected stenosis location while a patient inhales and exhales.
- Bronchoscopy and laryngoscopy examine inside the trachea, using tubes often equipped with tiny cameras.

- A biopsy examines a small sample of tracheal tissue under a microscope.
- The pulmonary function test, measuring how much air is inhaled and exhaled, can determine where a blockage might be located.
- The six-minute walk test measures endurance by monitoring a patient's heart rate and oxygen level.

In addition to a tracheal x-ray, bacterial tracheitis diagnostic tools include measuring blood oxygen levels and examining cultures taken from the nose, throat, and trachea in search of bacteria. A doctor also listens to a child's lungs, noting intercostal retractions or muscles between the ribs pulling inward caused by reduced air pressure in the chest—a medical emergency.

Treatments

If an underlying condition causes tracheal stenosis or tracheomalacia, doctors focus on treating the primary cause first. Several surgical options are commonly used for stenosis. One successful treatment is tracheal resection and reconstruction, in which a surgeon removes a constricted section and rejoins the remaining sections. Other options include stent therapy, which is a narrow metal or silicone tube placed in the narrowed trachea to keep it open; tracheal dilation to widen the trachea, with a balloon or surgical instruments, that provides temporary relief and allows surgeons to determine how much of the trachea is affected; and laser surgery, a short-term treatment using a highly focused beam of light that removes scar tissue. If a tumor is the cause, brachytherapy can deliver radiation therapy directly to the tumor cells in the trachea through a bronchoscope.

Tracheomalacia may improve without treatment. But if respiratory infections frequently recur, treatment is indicated. Milder cases are best treated nonsurgically, with continuous positive airway pressure (called CPAP), which applies slight air pressure through a mask during sleep, and chest therapy, which involves deep-breathing exercises and chest-tapping to help break up mucus. More severe tracheomalacia may require the insertion of a stent, which holds open the airway. Surgical interventions are tracheal resection and reconstruction (as discussed earlier), tracheostomy to create an opening in the neck, and tracheoplasty to tighten the loose tissue and prevent collapse of the trachea. In infants and children with severe cases, bronchoscopically performed aortopexy has become a well-established surgical procedure; the aortic arch is fixed to the sternum to help widen the trachea.

Treatment of childhood tracheitis focuses on curing the infection through intravenous antibiotics and keeping the airway open, often with an endotracheal tube connected to a ventilator. The goal is to improve the lung function while fighting the infection.

Prognosis and Outcomes

Successful outcomes rely on accurate diagnoses and appropriate treatment. Currently, when surgery is indicated, tracheal resection and reconstruction is considered the best treatment; it has demonstrated excellent long-term results for adult patients with stenosis, tracheomalacia, and some tumors.

The prognosis for childhood tracheitis depends on the speed treatment was delivered because the condition can be fatal if the trachea becomes completely blocked. Full recovery can be expected with prompt treatment.

Jean Kaplan Teichroew

See also: Asthma; Bronchitis; Swallowing Disorders; Throat Disorders

Further Reading

Brigham and Women's Hospital. (2015, April 4). Tracheal disorders. Retrieved from http://www.brighamandwomens.org/Departments_and_Services/surgery/thoracic-surgery/lung-airway-conditions/tracheal-disorders.aspx?sub=2.

Memorial Sloan Kettering Cancer Center. (2015). About tracheal diseases. Retrieved from https://www.mskcc.org/cancer-care/types/tracheal-diseases/about-tracheal-diseases.

Mount Sinai Hospital. (2015). Tracheal stenosis. Retrieved from http://www.mountsinai.org/patient-care/service-areas/ent/areas-of-care/tracheal-surgery/tracheal-stenosis.

NIH MedlinePlus. (2014, May 14). Tracheal disorders, also called: Windpipe disorders. Retrieved from http://www.nlm.nih.gov/medlineplus/trachealdisorders.html.

UC Neurosensory Disorders Center. (2015). Adult airway disorders. Retrieved from http://ucneurofunctionalcenter.com/types-of-neurosensory-disorders/adult-airway-disorders/.

TUBERCULOSIS

A chronic infectious disease commonly called TB, tuberculosis most often infects the lungs, but it can also involve other organs and parts of the body. The *Mycobacterium tuberculosis* bacteria spreads through the air from people with the active disease. Even when infected, healthy people with good immune systems may not exhibit symptoms, the most common of which are coughing for three weeks or longer, occasionally with blood or sputum; chest pain; weakness; loss of appetite and weight loss; fatigue; fever; and night sweats.

Although individuals of any age, race, and gender can get TB, those with weakened immune systems are at higher risk, as well as residents or travelers in countries with high rates of the disease. Worldwide, TB is a major cause of death and disability. An estimated 8.8 million became infected in 2010 and 1.4 million died, 95 percent of those in developing countries. In the United States in 2010, 11,182 cases were reported, which represents a small decline from the previous year. Both the infection and the disease are treatable and usually curable with antibiotic medications taken for 6 to 12 months.

History

Scientists have discovered evidence of tuberculosis in Egyptian mummies thousands of years old, as well as in ancient Greece and Rome. Identifying the bacteria and developing new drugs have helped control it, but the disease continues to be a lead-ing cause of death around the world.

Symptoms

Individuals with healthy immunity may be unaware of early symptoms, which range from a cough to feeling vaguely ill, appetite and weight loss, and fever and night sweats. When the illness worsens, becoming what's known as active TB, additional symptoms include chest pain, weakness or fatigue, cough lasting at least three weeks, and bloody sputum, which is mucous and saliva.

TB symptoms can affect parts of the body other than the lungs, including lymph node swelling; bone and joint pain; urination pain, blood, or frequency; enlarged mass in both male and female genital organs; rash on the arms or legs; headaches or stiff neck; brain mass; and shortness of breath, dizziness, and prominent neck veins (a symptom affecting the heart).

Causes and Risk Factors

The TB bacteria is spread only from an infected person when it is inhaled into the lungs via airborne droplets, which can take place when someone sneezes, coughs, sings, speaks, or laughs. The infection does not make every individual sick, and some may live with it for many years without illness or spreading it; this is known as latent TB. To develop an active form of the disease, the bacteria must cause an infection after entering a body with an immune system that cannot stop it from growing.

Recently infected individuals face an increased risk of developing TB. Those at risk are often in close contact with immigrants from areas with a high rate of TB; homeless populations; susceptible groups, such as those infected with HIV; and in-jection drug users in hospitals, shelters, and correctional and other facilities.

Those living in poverty and crowded conditions with poor medical care—as well as those with malnutrition; diabetes; HIV/AIDS; end-stage kidney disease; some can-cers and chemotherapy; antirejection drugs for transplanted organs; and medi-cations for psoriasis, rheumatoid arthritis, and Crohn's disease—often have a compromised immune system. The very young and very old do, too, which places them at increased risk.

Diagnosis

A doctor diagnoses TB with a physical examination and a medical history, particu-larly if an individual has been exposed to a population at high risk for infection. The tuberculin skin test is the most common test; a small amount of tuberculin is injected into skin on the forearm. A reaction within 48 to 72 hours usually indi-cates a TB infection. To determine if the infection is active, further tests are called for, including blood tests, chest x-rays, and sputum samples.

Treatments

Although people with latent TB cannot spread the disease, medications are prescribed to prevent the illness from becoming active. Antibiotic medications can cure active TB in most people if the prescribed regimen is carefully followed for at least six months and occasionally up to 12 months. Some TB bacteria are resistant to the standard drugs, making the disease more difficult and expensive to treat. In those cases, a combination of special TB drugs are prescribed. Worldwide, drug-resistant TB is rising, leaving patients with limited and less-effective options for treatment.

Prevention

No single method can prevent the transmission of the TB bacteria. Health officials recommend regular TB skin testing for those who travel to developing countries and work in populations at high risk of infection. A fairly effective vaccine is available for children in areas of the world where the disease is common, but it does not protect adults and it is not recommended for children in the United States.

An individual with active TB can take measures to prevent spreading the disease by staying home, ventilating rooms, covering the mouth, and wearing a mask around other people.

Prognosis and Outcomes

Most people who receive appropriate antibiotic treatment can be cured of tuberculosis, but it usually takes several weeks before a patient is no longer contagious. It is imperative that patients on medication do not stop or modify their treatment, which can allow the bacteria to mutate and become resistant to the standard TB drugs.

David Ajuluchukwu

See also: AIDS (Acquired Immune Deficiency Syndrome); Crohn's Disease; Immune System Disorders; Lung Diseases; Lymphatic Disorders; Pericardial Disorders; Vaccines

Further Reading

Centers for Disease Control and Prevention (CDC). (2015, April 28). Tuberculosis (TB). Retrieved from http://www.cdc.gov/tb.

Foster, D. (2015, October 19). The global toll of drug-resistant tuberculosis. *The Nation, 301*(16), 22–25.

Mayo Clinic. (2014, August 1). Tuberculosis. Retrieved from http://www.mayoclinic.com /health/tuberculosis/DS00372.

National Institute of Allergy and Infectious Diseases. (2015, April 10). Tuberculosis (TB). Retrieved from http://www.niaid.nih.gov/topics/tuberculosis/Pages/Default.aspx.

PDRhealth. (2015). Tuberculosis. Retrieved from http://www.pdrhealth.com/diseases /tuberculosis.

U

ULCERATIVE COLITIS

Ulcerative colitis is a form of inflammatory bowel disease, or IBD, a chronic disease in which the lining of the colon, or large intestine, and rectum become inflamed. It occurs when the immune system mistakes food, bacteria, and intestinal tissue in the colon for foreign substances and attacks them by sending in white blood cells. The result is irritation, swelling, and ulcers, which may be limited to the rectum or affect the entire colon. Symptoms may include intermittent rectal bleeding, cramps, abdominal pain, and diarrhea. The cause is unknown, but research suggests a complex interaction among inherited genes, the immune system, and environmental factors. Found worldwide, the disease may affect as many as 700,000 adults in the United States. It can strike men and women equally at any age, but it is usually diagnosed between the ages of 15 and 30 and in those older than 60, most commonly in people of European origin and particularly those of Ashkenazi Jewish descent. Family history of ulcerative colitis or other immune system disorders are other risk factors. Ulcerative colitis is usually treated with drug therapy or surgery.

Symptoms

Symptoms can develop slowly or attack suddenly, begin as mild and become severe later, or go into remission for months or years. Most people have mild to moderate symptoms, which vary depending on how much of the colon is affected and the severity of inflammation; ulcerative colitis is often classified based on its location.

The most common symptoms include diarrhea with blood or pus; abdominal discomfort or pain; painful or urgent bowel movements; inability to defecate despite urgency; rectal pain; dehydration; nausea or loss of appetite; weight loss; fatigue; fever; anemia, when the body has fewer than normal red blood cells; and failure to grow in children. Other less common symptoms include skin rashes, joint pain, eye irritation, blood clots, and an increased risk for colon cancer.

Causes and Risk Factors

The cause of ulcerative colitis is unknown, but inherited genes, an overactive intestinal immune system, and environmental triggers most likely play a role; infection and diet have not been identified as causes. Substances in the environment may cause the inflammation or stimulate an abnormal immune response. When the body mistakes food, beneficial bacteria, or intestinal tissue as harmful, it releases various chemicals and white blood cells, which cause chronic inflammation in the intestinal lining, damaging it and causing permanent changes over time. In ulcerative colitis, researchers believe, the immune system may not be able return to a normal response. As many as 20 percent of people with ulcerative colitis have a close relative with the disease. Other risk factors include people ages 15 to 35 and over 60 and Caucasians, especially Ashkenazi Jews, who face a greater risk.

Diagnosis

Diagnostic procedures for ulcerative colitis include a physical examination of symptoms such as abdominal pain, swelling, or tenderness; rectal bleeding; and diarrhea—as well as personal and family medical histories.

Endoscopies of the large intestine are most accurate for diagnosing ulcerative colitis and ruling out other illnesses or conditions: A colonoscopy examines the entire colon, while a flexible sigmoidoscopy examines its lower third; both can show irritated and swollen tissue, ulcers, and abnormal growths. In addition, a biopsy examines samples of rectal or intestinal tissues with a microscope. Other lab tests include blood tests for anemia; inflammation or infection somewhere in the body; indications of ongoing inflammation; indication of low albumin, a protein common with severe ulcerative colitis; and stool tests to detect white blood cells and rule out other diseases, parasites, or infection. Emerging diagnostic techniques include video capsule endoscopy, a swallowed capsule containing a camera that takes pictures and sends them to a recorder while traveling through the intestines, and CT and MRI enterography, noninvasive imaging tests that are considered more sensitive for detecting inflammation.

Treatments

The extent and severity of ulcerative colitis are factors in the treatment options. Aside from surgically removing the colon for severe forms of the disease, no cure exists. The goals of treatment are to better regulate the immune system, control and prevent attacks, and help the colon heal. Medications include anti-inflammatory drugs and immunosuppressants, which suppress the immune system response that triggers inflammation. Other medications may include antibiotics to prevent or control infection, antidiarrheal medications, pain relievers, and iron supplements.

No diet has been found to slow, treat, or cure ulcerative colitis, although some foods can aggravate active symptoms. But good nutrition and a balanced diet rich in fruits, vegetables, grains, lean meats, beans, fish, eggs, and nuts and low in saturated fats and high cholesterol can help reduce symptoms, replace lost nutrients, and promote healing.

Prevention

There is no known way to prevent ulcerative colitis.

Prognosis and Outcomes

The course of ulcerative colitis is unpredictable: About 50 percent of people have mild symptoms, some have long remission periods after a single attack, and others develop a chronic debilitating or life-threatening complications. Those with more severe forms of the disease do not respond as well to medications; surgical removal of the entire colon is the only known cure. The risk of colon cancer increases each decade after the disease is diagnosed. Most people experience remission with medication treatment, which about 80 percent are able to maintain.

Future

Active research in ulcerative colitis is examining causes and mechanisms of inflammation. Scientists have also discovered genetic differences that may identify certain people who may respond differently to medications. Improvements in surgical procedures to make them safer and more effective are being developed, as are medications with fewer side effects.

Ray Marks

See also: Crohn's Disease; Immune System Disorders; Inflammatory Bowel Disease

Further Reading

Crohn's & Colitis Foundation of America. (2015). What is ulcerative colitis? Retrieved from http://www.ccfa.org/what-are-crohns-and-colitis/what-is-ulcerative-colitis/.

Mayo Clinic. (2014, September 9). Ulcerative colitis. Retrieved from http://www.mayoclinic.org/diseases-conditions/ulcerative-colitis/basics/definition/CON-20043763.

National Institute of Diabetes and Digestive and Kidney Diseases. (2014, September 3). Ulcerative colitis. Retrieved from http://www.niddk.nih.gov/health-information/health-topics/digestive-diseases/ulcerative-colitis/Pages/facts.aspx.

Saibil, F. (2011). *Crohn's Disease and Ulcerative Colitis: Everything You Need to Know: The Complete Practical Guide.* Ontario, Canada: Firefly Books.

URETHRAL CANCER

Urethral cancer, when present as a primary disease, is a relatively rare health condition in which the cells lining the urethra—a structure that transports urine to the bladder—become malignant or cancerous.

African Americans suffer from urethral cancer at higher rates than whites. It is three times more common in males than females. It occurs at any age but most commonly after age 70.

Types

The different types of urethral cancer that can occur are squamous cell carcinoma, adenocarcinoma, and transitional cell carcinoma. Squamous cell carcinoma is the most common type.

Five stages are used to describe urethral cancer:

Stage 0 or carcinoma in situ refers to the presence of abnormal cells in the lining of the urethra.

Stage A is where the cancer has developed and spread beneath the lining of the urethra.

Stage B is where the cancer is found in the muscle around the urethra.

Stage C is where the cancer has spread beyond the urethra

In stage D, the cancer may have spread to nearby lymph nodes in the pelvis and groin, which is stage D1; and in stage D2, it spreads to distant lymph nodes in other body parts such as the liver or lungs.

Symptoms and Signs

The presence of blood in the urine may be due to urethral cancer, as may trouble with urination. Other problems may include the presence of urethral discharge and having a lump in the area of the perineum, penis, or groin. Swelling in the groin, incontinence, or frequent night urination may also indicate the presence of a urethral cancer problem.

Key Causes and Risk Factors

The presence of bladder cancer can increase the risk for urethral cancer, as can the presence of an infectious disease, such as human papillomavirus (HPV). Other problems such as frequent urinary tract infections may predispose a person to urethral cancer. Very rarely, arsenic ingestion has been cited as increasing the risk for primary urethral cancer (Guidos, Mydlo, Donohoe, & Powell 2015).

Diagnosis

A person's medical history, physical examination of the pelvis and rectum, and special tests to examine the urethra and bladder cells for abnormality in the lab, as well as urine cytology tests and content tests, may be used to help diagnose urethral cancer. Blood tests plus CT scans, cystoscopy, or a procedure known as ureteroscopy—which involves the use of a thin tube with a light at the end as well as a lens for viewing the structures and taking tissue samples or biopsies that can be viewed under a microscope—may be used.

Treatment

Treatment will depend on the type of cancer, the extent of the cancer, the health status of the individual, and the individual's age, among other factors. Treatment may involve various forms of surgery, radiation, and chemotherapy, plus drug therapy.

Prognosis

The outcome of treatment will depend on the site of the cancer, how far the cancer has spread, whether the patient is male or female, the patient's general health, and what is reasonable with surgery or radiation treatment. If not diagnosed early, this form of cancer can spread quite quickly to surrounding lymph node tissues. The cancer can also reoccur after treatment.

Ray Marks

See also: HPV (Human Papillomavirus); Squamous Cell Carcinoma; Urethral Disorders

Further Reading

Guidos, J., Myldo, J. H., Donohoe, J. M., & Powell, C. (2015). Urethral cancer treatment & management. Retrieved from http://emedicine.medscape.com/article/451496-treatment.

Lynch Jr., D. F. (2003). Carcinoma of the urethra. In *Holland-Frei Cancer Medicine I. Holland-Frei Cancer Medicine I.* Edited by D. W. Kufe, R. E. Pollock, and R. R. Weichselbaum, et al. Hamilton, Ontario: BC Decker.

Mydlo, J. (2010). *Penile and Urethral Cancer: An Issue of Urologic Clinics.* Philadelphia, PA: Saunders-Elsevier.

National Cancer Institute. (2014). Urethral cancer treatment. Retrieved from http://www.cancer.gov/types/urethral/patient/urethral-treatment-pdq.

Urethral Cancer. (2011). Urethral cancer—Causes, symptoms, and treatment. Retrieved from http://urethralcancer.net.

Varricchio, C. G. (2004). *A Cancer Source Book for Nurses.* Burlington, MA: Jones & Bartlett Learning.

URETHRAL DISORDERS

The urethra delivers urine from the bladder to the outside of the body. In women, it sits above the vagina and measures about 1.5 to 2 inches, ending at the vulva, or external genital organs. In men, the urethra measures about eight inches and ends at the tip of the penis.

Commonly diagnosed urethral disorders include urethral stricture, scarring that narrows the urethra, found mostly in men; urethral syndrome, inflammation or irritation more common in women; urethritis, inflammation of the urethra in both sexes; and diverticulum, a condition of small, bulging pouches forming next to the urethra, also more common in women. Other disorders include lesions, which are polyps, cysts, warts, masses, and other noncancerous irregular growths, and urethral cancer, or malignant cells in the urethral tissues.

Symptoms of most urethral disorders are similar: difficulty or pain while passing urine, blood in the urine, increased urgency to urinate, and discharge. Illness, injury, or aging are common causes of these disorders. Depending on the type, doctors treat urethral disorders with medications, including antibiotics, and surgery, if needed. Most people who receive treatment have significant improvement.

Symptoms

Women and men experience similar symptoms of urethral disorders, including painful urination or difficulty passing urine, pain or discomfort during sex, blood in the urine (as well as semen in men), discharge, pain or pressure low in the abdomen, more frequent urination, or feeling increased urgency.

In addition, symptoms more specific to scarring from urethral stricture are reduced urine output; a spraying, slow, or blocked urine stream; incomplete bladder emptying; and inability to void. Urinary tract infections are also common.

With urethral syndrome, additional specific symptoms may include a burning sensation during urination, difficulty urinating after intercourse, and swelling or tenderness in the groin. In men, symptoms may cause swollen testicles, ejaculation pain, blood in the semen, and discharge from the penis. A painful episode involves voluntary tightening of the pelvic muscles and involuntary spasms.

Urethritis can also cause itching, pain, or discomfort even while not urinating. Some people with diverticulum experience recurrent cystitis or urinary tract infections, as well as vaginal discharge, urinary retention, and incontinence. Symptoms of diverticulum may be intermittent or even disappear temporarily. Lesions can cause the same symptoms as other urethral disorders, primarily pain or a burning sensation during urination.

Causes

Although occasionally doctors cannot find a cause, a urethral stricture is usually the result of an accident or injury such as a broken pelvis, and some men are born with a urethra that does not develop correctly. Other causes include the placement of a urethral catheter, endoscope, or other foreign body as well as difficulty following prostate surgery or kidney stone removal. Sexually transmitted diseases and untreated urinary tract infections are infrequent causes. Men who have had urethritis or an enlarged prostrate have an increased risk of developing a stricture.

By definition, urethral syndrome presents no evident cause. So the many possibilities that cause or increase the risk of development include undetected infections of the bladder or kidneys (bacterial or viral); caffeinated foods and drinks; radiation and chemotherapy; irritation—particularly in women—from sensitivity to douches or feminine hygiene sprays, bubble baths, perfumes, soaps, contraceptive gels, condoms, sanitary napkins, tampons, and diaphragms; unprotected sexual activity; sexually transmitted infections; medications that limit the ability to fight infection; and a narrow urethra.

Urethritis is most often caused by bacteria, viruses, or fungi present on the skin that enter the urethral opening, including bacteria that cause gonorrhea, chlamydia, and other sexually transmitted diseases and *E. coli* from stool. Urethral diverticulum is due to repeat infections, although childbirth and congenital conditions may play a role. This disorder is most common in women between the ages of 40 and 70. Noncancerous lesions in the urethra can affect anyone. They are caused by infections, viruses, abscesses, accidents, and injuries (including from medical tools), and rarely, they appear as health issues at birth.

Diagnosis

To diagnose a urethral stricture, a doctor first feels the urethra for lumps. A cystoscope, or flexible viewing tube, inserted into the penis gives a closer look, and an x-ray using contrast (radiopaque) dye, called a retrograde urethrogram, may be required to further define the location and size of the stricture.

A doctor may prescribe further tests as well: measuring the rate of flow, urinalysis to determine if bacteria are present, measuring the size of the urethral opening, and testing for gonorrhea and chlamydia.

A diagnosis of urethral syndrome results after ruling out viral and bacterial infections and other disorders or illnesses. Further diagnostic tools include a medical history, a physical exam, a urine sample, and possibly a blood sample or pelvic ultrasound and, if necessary, viewing the urethra with a cystoscope.

Similarly, urethral diverticulum diagnosis requires many of the same tests, minus the blood sample and pelvic ultrasound. Instead, a variety of radiologic imaging may be applied, as well as endoscopic examination of the urethra, including the voiding cystourethrogram (VCUG), and tests to study incontinence.

Diagnosing urethritis requires a physical exam, including of the genital organs, abdomen, and rectum; urine tests for sexually transmitted and other bacteria; and a lab analysis of any discharge to identify the infecting agent. A cystoscope is used also to diagnose noncancerous urethral lesions, as is a VCUG, which is an x-ray study of the bladder and urethra performed while the bladder is emptying.

Treatments

The first-line treatment of a urethral stricture is dilation, or gradually stretching and widening the urethra. A urethrotomy, or cutting open the stricture, may be indicated to provide relief. Depending on its severity, surgical procedures can remove the stricture and rebuild the urethra.

Medications used to treat urethral syndrome include antibiotics if undetected infections are suspected, anesthetics, antispasmodics to reduce bladder spasms, antidepressants, muscle relaxants, and alpha blockers, which also relax muscles. Dilating or surgically widening the urethra is indicated if constriction from an injury, inflammation, or scar tissue is the cause. For those whose symptoms are from failure to relax pelvic muscles during urination, biofeedback has shown some promise.

Urethritis can be treated and cured with antibiotics or antiviral mediations. Identifying the bacteria or virus that causes urethritis can take several days, so doctors usually begin treatment with antibiotics, which is the most common treatment.

Surgery is the preferred treatment for urethral diverticulum, but not all urethral diverticula require it, especially without noticeable symptoms. Several surgical options can remove or close the pockets if necessary. Lesions in the urethra without symptoms may not need treatment. But if they cause blockage, pain, or infection, treatment includes removal via cystourethroscopy, a minimally invasive technique or by cauterization. Sexually transmitted lesions can be controlled with antibiotics, but they often return and require further treatment.

Prevention

Urethral stricture is not completely preventable, except when sexually transmitted infections are the cause. The consistent use of protection during sexual contact is the best preventive measure. Practicing safe sex is also recommended as a method to prevent urethral syndrome, urethritis, and noncancerous lesions.

Care can be taken to avoid any products, including acidic foods, or behavior that irritate the urethra and cause urethral syndrome and urethritis. In addition, getting tested and treated for sexually transmitted infections, urinating immediately after intercourse, and consuming plenty of fluids can reduce the risk factors.

Prognosis and Outcome

Treatment of urethral stricture is usually successful. Left untreated, however, the risk increases of developing urinary infections and the inability to urinate due to urethral blockage. But even after surgery, urethral strictures may return, making repeated surgery necessary. Urethritis can be treated quickly with medication. The effects of untreated urethritis include infection spreading elsewhere in the urinary tract and eventually damaging reproductive organs. The symptoms of urethral syndrome often improve with medical treatment as women age, but they remain a lifelong disorder that may require additional treatment. Because comparatively little is known about untreated urethral diverticulum, doctors recommend continual monitoring, particularly for those who have not had surgery. Even following surgery, the disorder may recur or new pockets appear, which may require further treatment.

Jean Kaplan Teichroew

See also: Diverticular Disease; Urethral Cancer; Urinary Tract Infections

Further Reading

MedlinePlus. (2015, May 12). Urethral disorders. Retrieved from http://www.nlm.nih.gov/medlineplus/urethraldisorders.html.

Merck Manual. (2015). Urethritis. Retrieved from https://www.merckmanuals.com/home/kidney-and-urinary-tract-disorders/urinary-tract-infections-uti/urethritis.

Urology Care Foundation. (2015, May 4). Benign urethral lesions in adults. Retrieved from http://www.urologyhealth.org/urologic-conditions/benign-%28not-cancerous%29-uretheral-lesions.

Urology Care Foundation. (2015). Urethral diverticulum. Retrieved from http://www.urologyhealth.org/urologic-conditions/uretheral-diverticulum.

Urology Care Foundation. (2015, June 4). Urethral stricture disease. Retrieved from http://www.urologyhealth.org/urologic-conditions/urethral-stricture-disease.

URINARY INCONTINENCE

Urinary incontinence, or the involuntary loss of bladder control, is a common hygienic or social problem. It can range from mild—the occasional accidental leakage of urine while running or sneezing—to a sudden urge to urinate without enough time to reach a toilet. Doctors recognize different types of incontinence, and the causes vary widely, sometimes making diagnosis difficult. Correctly identifying the cause, as well as the type and severity of the incontinence, determines the treatment that will be most effective. Treatments range from behavioral changes to medication to intervention or surgery.

Incontinence can happen to anyone, but it is more common in adults older than 50. It is estimated that up to 13 million people in the United States are affected. It is usually not a serious health problem, but if untreated, it can lead to skin rashes, sores, and infections and urinary tract infections. Some types are more common in women and others in men. Although it is more common among older women, it is not a normal process of aging.

Symptoms

Difficulty controlling urination is the main symptom of urinary incontinence. But symptoms vary based on the type. *Stress incontinence* is leaking a small or moderate amount of urine during exercise, lifting, sneezing, or other physical activity or sudden pressure and, occasionally, during no movement at all. *Urge incontinence*, also called overactive bladder, is the frequent and sudden uncontrollable need to urinate, even while asleep. *Mixed incontinence* involves experiencing the symptoms of both stress and urge incontinence. *Overflow incontinence*, an overfilled bladder causing uncontrollable leakage, is characterized by feeling unable to completely empty the bladder. *Functional incontinence* is normal urine control, but the inability to get to a toilet in time, usually due to a physical condition or disease that limits mobility.

Causes and Risk Factors

The muscles in the bladder, which stores urine, tighten to move urine into the urethra, which relaxes its sphincter muscles to allow urine to leave the body. When the bladder muscles are weak or overactive or the sphincter muscles weaken and relax without warning, incontinence occurs.

Urinary incontinence is a symptom of an underlying condition, rather than a disease itself. Many factors can stimulate the bladder and increase the volume of urine, including spicy, sweet, or acidic foods such as citrus fruits; constipation; smoking; alcoholic and carbonated beverages, as well as coffee and tea with and without caffeine; plus some cardiac, blood pressure, and muscle relaxant medications; artificial sweeteners; and very large doses of vitamins B and C.

Medical causes include urinary tract infections, tumors, and stones; diabetes; and Alzheimer's disease. Nerve damage resulting from Parkinson's disease, multiple sclerosis, spinal cord injury, or a stroke can affect bladder control, as can arthritis and other illnesses that limit mobility.

Women have incontinence twice as often as men, due in part to the anatomy of their urinary tract and from vaginal infections or irritations, as well as the physical changes accompanying pregnancy, childbirth, hysterectomy, menopause, and aging bladder muscles. Men are at risk when they have an enlarged prostate gland blocking the urethra and other prostate problems.

It is not an inevitable risk factor, but aging causes general weakening of bladder and urethra muscles, as well as the amount of urine a bladder can hold. Excess weight and obesity increase pressure on these muscles, which often causes weakening. Individuals with neurological diseases and disorders also face an increased risk of incontinence.

Diagnosis

To diagnose the correct type of urinary incontinence, a doctor takes a medical history, asks about symptoms, and conducts a physical exam. This may include a cough stress test that observes the urethra and the loss of urine and the identification of medical or physical underlying conditions.

Patients may keep a bladder diary for up to a week, recording fluid intake, as well as times and amounts of urination and episodes of incontinence. Further diagnostic tests include a urine sample, examined for bacteria or blood, and a measurement of how completely the bladder can empty.

Among more specialized tests are ultrasound or x-ray images of the bladder, kidneys, and pelvic organs; urodynamic tests measuring pressure in the bladder and the flow of urine; cystogram, a dye that helps identify abnormalities in the urinary tract; and cystoscopy, a tiny camera inserted on a tube that examines inside the urethra and bladder.

Treatment

The type of urinary incontinence, its severity, and underlying cause determine the most effective treatment strategy. Treating the underlying medical cause also treats the incontinence. Behavioral changes are usually recommended, such as bladder training, carefully managing consumption of liquids and acidic foods, quitting smoking, losing weight or adding physical activity, and practicing Kegel exercises that strengthen the pelvic floor muscles. Biofeedback or electrical stimulation may aid in learning how to regain control of these muscles.

A variety of medications are commonly prescribed to treat incontinence and can calm an overactive bladder, increase the amount of urine the bladder can hold, help it empty more easily and completely, and lessen leakage. Women may be prescribed topical estrogen, and men may take medication to shrink an enlarged prostate.

Medical and interventional devices are designed for men or women, based on the type and cause of incontinence. Surgery may be performed if other treatments have failed or when symptoms are severe. In general, these techniques help keep the urethra closed or provide support to the urethra and bladder.

Prevention

While it's not always preventable, it is possible to decrease risk factors not associated with neurological or other medical causes: practicing Kegel exercises, maintaining a healthy body weight, avoiding food and drink irritants, and avoiding tobacco.

Prognosis and Outcomes

Urinary incontinence is under diagnosed and underreported, but most types are treatable. High cure rates of medical and surgical treatment options also provide an excellent prognosis. Depending on the underlying cause, the outcome can rest on the compliance of a patient to make behavioral changes. Symptoms do not generally disappear without some intervention, but effective treatments are available.

Future

The National Institute of Diabetes and Digestive and Kidney Diseases (NIDDK) is sponsoring a consortium of urologists and urogynecologists who evaluate treatment methods for stress and mixed incontinence in women to determine which have the best short- and long-term outcomes. Ongoing studies focus on treatments for urge incontinence and minimally invasive treatments for stress incontinence in women (NIDDK 2013a). The NIDDK has also formed a consortium to conduct clinical trials looking at surgical and drug therapies.

Jean Kaplan Teichroew

See also: Bladder Diseases; Kidney Diseases; Urinary Tract Disorders

Further Reading

Mayo Clinic. (2014, August 7). Urinary incontinence. Retrieved from http://www.mayoclinic.org/diseases-conditions/urinary-incontinence/basics/definition/con-20037883.

Newman, D., & Wein, A. (2008). *Managing & Treating Urinary Incontinence,* 2nd ed. Baltimore, MD: Health Professions Press.

National Institute of Diabetes and Digestive and Kidney Diseases (NIDDK). (2013, April 12). Urinary incontinence in men. Retrieved from http://www.niddk.nih.gov/health-information/health-topics/urologic-disease/urinary-incontinence-in-men/Pages/facts.aspx#cause.

National Institute of Diabetes and Digestive and Kidney Diseases (NIDDK). (2013a, September 18). Urinary incontinence in women. Retrieved from http://www.niddk.nih.gov/health-information/health-topics/urologic-disease/urinary-incontinence-women/Pages/facts.aspx.

National Institute on Aging. (2015, January 22). Urinary incontinence. Retrieved from https://www.nia.nih.gov/health/publication/urinary-incontinence.

URINARY TRACT INFECTIONS

Overview

A urinary tract infection refers to an infection of the tract or tube that carries wastes and water, including the kidneys and their ureters, the bladder, and urethra.

These infections are very common, especially among women, although everyone is at risk, including those with spinal cord injuries, people with HIV or taking immunosuppressant system medications, and pregnant women. Other people who tend to get them are those who have catheters. They can affect people of all ages, including children.

Symptoms, Key Causes, and Risk Factors

A common symptom is frequent urination, having cloudy or bloody urine, and pain on urination. Other symptoms include pain in the back; having a mild fever; lethargy; or chills, nausea, or vomiting. The infection is caused by viruses, fungi, or bacteria in the region of the urinary tract.

Diagnosis

Various forms of scanning, special x-rays called an intravenous pyelogram, and urine tests may help to diagnose the problem. Blood tests, a physical exam (including a pelvic exam), and a medical history may all be helpful.

A cystoscopy involving the use of a thin, flexible tube with a tiny camera on its end that is passed through the urethra into the bladder can detect problems in the bladder that might be causing the infection.

Treatment

The most common form of treatment is medication, especially antibiotics. Sometimes, a person with this condition has to be hospitalized.

Prognosis

Most urinary tract infections are not serious, but on occasion, they can cause prolonged kidney infections that can be life-threatening. They can reoccur even if treated successfully.

Ray Marks

See also: Kidney Diseases; Urethral Cancer; Urethral Disorders; Urinary Incontinence

Further Reading

Mayo Clinic. (2015). Urinary tract infections. Retrieved from http://www.mayoclinic.org /diseases-conditions/urinary-tract-infection/basics/definition/con-20037892.

MedlinePlus (2015). Urinary tract infections: Adults. Retrieved from http://www.nlm.nih .gov/medlineplus/ency/article/000521.htm.

National Institute of Diabetes and Digestive and Kidney Diseases (NIDDK). (2015). Urinary tract infections in adults. Retrieved from http://kidney.niddk.nih.gov/Kudiseases /pubs/utiadult/.

UTERINE CANCER

Like other organs in the body, the uterus—a female, pear-shaped organ located in the lower pelvic region and lined by a tissue called the endometrium and associated with fertility, carrying the fetus, and giving birth—can become cancerous. Some of these cancerous tumors may not be dangerous and are nonmalignant, while others can be life-threatening and can spread to other organs or tissues. It is also termed *endometrial cancer*.

Types of Uterine or Endometrial Cancer

Nearly all endometrial cancers are endometrial adenocarcinomas, meaning they arise from glandular uterine tissue (Emedicinehealth 2015). Those that originate in muscle or connective tissue are called uterine sarcomas. A subtype of endometrial adenocarcinomas known as adenosquamous carcinoma is derived from cells that are located on the surface of the cervix—the bottom part of the uterus—or the skin. Other subtypes include papillary serous adenocarcinomas and clear cell carcinomas. Most common are endometrial adenocarcinomas.

Symptoms

Common symptoms of uterine cancer include the presence of pain during sexual intercourse or urination or both, bleeding, and/or the presence of uterine discharge.

Key Causes and Risk Factors

Risk factors include endometrial overgrowth, obesity, pelvic radiation, a family history, not having given birth, menopause after age 55 years of age, estrogen therapy, and having a history of Lynch syndrome—a form of inherited colorectal cancer.

Diagnosis

Pelvic examinations, a medical history, x-rays, tissue biopsies, and ultrasound or magnetic resonance image scanning may be helpful.

Treatment

Common treatment approaches include surgery, hormone therapy, chemotherapy, and radiation therapy, depending on the severity of the cancer or the stage of the cancer and the extent to which it has spread.

Prognosis

The prognosis or outcome of uterine cancer generally depends on the stage of the cancer and timely intervention as this form of cancer is highly curable.

Prevention

No specific form of prevention is documented, but keeping a healthy weight, being physically active, and taking birth control pills might be helpful.

Ray Marks

See also: Bleeding Disorders; Reproductive Disorders; Sexually Transmitted Diseases; Uterine Diseases; Women's Health

Further Reading

Centers for Disease Control and Prevention. (2015). Uterine cancer. Retrieved from http://www.cdc.gov/cancer/uterine/index.htm.

Emedicinehealth. (2015). Endometrial cancer. Retrieved from http://www.emedicinehealth.com/endometrial_cancer/article_em.htm.

MedicineNet.com. (2016). Cancer of the uterus (uterine cancer or endometrial cancer). Retrieved from http://www.medicinenet.com/uterine_cancer/article.htm.

Diaz-Montes, T. P. (2009). *Johns Hopkins Patients' Guide to Uterine Cancer.* Burlington, MA: Jones & Bartlett Learning.

Dizon, D. S. (2010). *100 Questions & Answers about Uterine Cancer.* Burlington, MA: Jones & Bartlett Learning.

Mayo Clinic. (2015). Endometrial cancer. Retrieved from http://www.mayoclinic.org/diseases-conditions/endometrial-cancer/basics/definition/CON-20033696.

National Cancer Institute. (2015). Endometrial cancer treatment. Retrieved from http://www.cancer.gov/cancertopics/pdq/treatment/endometrial/Patient/page1.

UTERINE DISEASES

The term *uterine diseases* refers to any disease affecting the uterus or womb—the structure where a baby develops. Examples of uterine diseases are uterine cancer; uterine fibroids; endometriosis, where uterine tissue spreads from inside the uterus to outside; and uterine prolapse. The most serious condition is uterine cancer.

Symptoms

Common symptoms of the presence of a uterine problem are bleeding and pain. Others are weight loss, fever, and cramps. A woman with one of these conditions may experience irregular menstrual cycles.

Key Causes and Risk Factors

The causes are not always clear. Factors such as overweight, smoking history, and older age may play a role, as may use of birth control pills, genetics, and hormone imbalances.

Diagnosis and Treatment

A medical history; a physical examination, including a pelvic exam; x-rays; and scanning tests such as ultrasound may be used to diagnose a uterine problem. Treatment will vary depending on the problem and characteristics of the patient. This can include surgery, nonsurgical interventions, pain medication, hormone therapy, and radiation therapy.

Prognosis and Prevention

The outcome will depend on the nature of the condition and its severity. In some cases, the affected individual may become infertile or experience a miscarriage. It does not seem that uterine conditions are readily preventable, but early diagnosis and treatment is recommended.

Ray Marks

See also: Bleeding Disorders; Reproductive Disorders; Sexually Transmitted Diseases; Uterine Cancer; Women's Health

Further Reading

Agency for Healthcare Research and Quality (AHRQ). (2015). Common uterine conditions. Retrieved from http://archive.ahrq.gov/consumer/uterine1.htm.

Diaz-Montes, T. P. (2009). *Johns Hopkins Patients' Guide to Uterine Cancer*. Burlington, MA: Jones & Bartlett Learning.

Dizon, D. S. (2010). *100 Questions & Answers about Uterine Cancer*. Burlington, MA: Jones & Bartlett Learning.

Mayo Clinic. (2015). Andenomyosis. Retrieved from http://www.mayoclinic.org/diseases -conditions/adenomyosis/basics/definition/con-20024740.

Mayo Clinic. (2015). Endometrial cancer. Retrieved from http://www.mayoclinic.org/diseases -conditions/endometrial-cancer/basics/definition/con-20033696.

Mayo Clinic. (2015). Uterine prolapse. Retrieved from http://www.mayoclinic.org/diseases -conditions/uterine-prolapse/basics/definition/con-20027708.

V

VACCINES

Vaccines help people safely reduce the risk of infection that causes disease. They work with the body's immune system, or natural defenses, to help it develop immunity to illness and disease. Most vaccines are given orally, or they are injected into under the skin or into a muscle. Vaccines do not cause illnesses, but a vaccine may cause fever or aching at the site of the injection, a normal side effect as the body builds immunity; rarely are the side effects severe. They also prevent outbreaks of disease and save lives, including the lives of those who can't receive vaccinations.

How Vaccines Work

The body's immune system naturally fights infection—or the invading and multiplying bacteria or viruses that cause illnesses—and other harmful or foreign substances called pathogens. Once the body successfully fights a pathogen, creating immunity, its cells can recognize a disease and fight it again if necessary. The pathogens that cause infection and illness are those not recognized naturally by the body, so vaccines "teach the immune system" how to recognize and eliminate them.

Vaccines create immunity by imitating an infection, creating a safe version of the infection that causes the same response to destroy pathogens. Triggering the immune response, a vaccine equips the body to fight off actual infection and allows it to react the same way to future exposures of pathogens. Most vaccines given in childhood produce immunity from about 90 to 100 percent of the time.

Over time, vaccines have continued to help prevent many dangerous and deadly diseases, including chickenpox, diphtheria, hepatitis A and B, influenza (flu), human papillomavirus (HPV), Japanese encephalitis, measles, meningococcal diseases (meningitis), mumps, pertussis (whooping cough), pneumococcal diseases (including pneumonia), polio, rabies, rotavirus (childhood diarrhea), rubella (German measles), shingles, tetanus, tuberculosis (TB), typhoid fever, and yellow fever.

Vaccines protect large populations by way of herd immunity. After a large enough group of individuals is immunized, a disease has little or no opportunity to affect even those who are not immunized. The bacteria or viruses die out eventually because they will not have enough hosts to infect. This works to protect infants; older adults; those with certain allergies, compromised immune systems, and underlying illnesses; and others who cannot be vaccinated.

Types of Vaccines

A vaccine is a small dose of an antigen, or a molecule that triggers the immune response. Usually injected, most vaccines have two parts: The antigen is the disease the body learns to recognize, and the adjuvant responds to the antigen as an infection, which helps create immunity.

Live attenuated, or weakened, vaccines effectively fight viruses such as measles, mumps, and chickenpox. Containing a version of the live virus, this type of vaccine is weakened so that it can't cause a disease. As the closest things to a natural infection, these are considered good triggers of the immune system. Inactivated vaccines, such as those for polio, hepatitis A, and rabies, are produced with inactive or dead viruses. They trigger a weaker response in the immune system so several additional doses, or booster shots, are necessary to maintain immunity.

Toxoid vaccines fight bacteria that secrete toxins, or harmful chemicals. The toxins are weakened to avoid illness, and they are used when a bacterial toxin such as diphtheria or tetanus is the cause of illness.

Subunit vaccines include only the antigens that best stimulate the immune system, rather than the entire microbe. Conjugate vaccines fight the bacteria that have antigens with an outer coating of polysaccharides, or sugar-like substances. This coating disguises the antigen, which makes it difficult for an immature immune system to recognize, so these vaccines link the polysaccharides to antigens that the immune system responds to well. These two types work against hepatitis B, influenza, *Haemophilus influenzae* Type B (Hib), pertussis, pneumococcal, HPV, and meningococcal.

Still in the experimental phase is the DNA vaccine. Once a microbe's genes are analyzed, scientists may attempt to create a vaccine against it. Ultimately, the body's cells make the vaccine by creating the antigens needed to stimulate the immune system. Another experimental vaccine is the recombinant vector vaccine, which uses a weakened virus or bacterium to introduce microbial DNA to cells of the body. The goal is to cause a harmless bacterium to imitate a harmful microbe and provoke an immune response. Researchers are working on developing such vaccines for HIV, rabies, and measles.

Prevention Successes

Before a vaccine was developed for polio, the disease paralyzed up to 20,000 people in the United States every year. The vaccine, introduced in 1955, helped eliminate the disease from the Western hemisphere. Widespread use of the measles vaccine, first tested in 1958, has reduced the infection nearly 100 percent in the United States. Common in other countries, the highly contagious measles virus can spread rapidly where people are not vaccinated. In other parts of the world, vaccines are not always available widely, and many deaths occur from vaccine-preventable diseases. When these diseases enter the United States, they put anyone who is not vaccinated at high risk.

There has recently been controversy about parents who choose not to vaccinate their children due to fears of side effects. Nearly all pediatricians and other physicians state that the risk of children contracting serious diseases, with lasting effects, far outstrips the very small risks of experiencing side effects.

Future

Research continues to develop vaccines for dangerous diseases, HIV, malaria, and tuberculosis for adults. Scientists are also working to design vaccines for cancer, which they hope will reduce the growing rates of a common cause of death. Currently, the vaccine against HPV, the human papillomavirus, is, in fact, a vaccine that can prevent cervical cancer as well as oral cancers and other types of cancers.

Ray Marks

See also: Autism; Hepatitis; HPV (Human Papillomavirus); Meningitis; Polio and Post-Polio Syndrome; Rheumatic Fever; Sexually Transmitted Diseases; Shingles; Tuberculosis; Whooping Cough

Further Reading

Centers for Disease Control and Prevention (2012, March 8). How vaccines prevent diseases. Retrieved from http://www.cdc.gov/vaccines/parents/vaccine-decision/prevent -diseases.html.
National Institute of Allergy and Infectious Diseases. (2015, July 30). Vaccines. Retrieved from http://www.niaid.nih.gov/topics/vaccines/Pages/Default.aspx.
Vaccines.gov. (2015). Basics. Retrieved from http://www.vaccines.gov/.

VAGINAL DISEASES

Most women are found to experience vaginal problems at some point. The most common problem—vaginal infection, or vaginitis—is an inflammation of the vagina. Among these very common vaginal conditions are vaginal yeast infections, trichomoniasis, and bacterial vaginosis. Vaginal disorders can also include cancer of the vaginal area or vulvar cancer.

Symptoms

The symptoms of most vaginal infections include vaginal itching; the presence of a thick, white vaginal discharge; pain and redness; burning; soreness; swelling; and general irritation of the vaginal area.

Key Causes and Risk Factors

Some women are at higher risk of developing vaginal diseases; among these are women who are sexually active with multiple partners as well as women with weakened immune systems. Other provoking factors may be sensitivity to vaginal sprays, douches, spermicides, soaps, detergents, and fabric softeners that cause burning, itching, and discharge, even if no infection is present. Some women experience vaginal irritation as a result of low estrogen levels during breast-feeding and/or after menopause. Other risk factors are regular douching or using water or a medicated solution to cleanse the vagina and cervix. Health problems linked to douching include bacterial vaginosis, pelvic inflammatory disease, sexually transmitted infections, and vaginal irritations.

Diagnosis

Vaginal problems may be detected during a regular pelvic exam. A sample of vaginal fluid may be taken for laboratory examination to detect different infections. Blood and urine tests may also be conducted. A Pap test, or a collection of a sample of cells from the cervix, is used to test for any abnormalities or early cell changes that may become cancerous. Vulvar cancer may be diagnosed through a biopsy, where cells or tissues are removed and viewed under a microscope.

Treatment

Treatments for vaginal diseases depend on the cause. They may include antibiotics or other medicines. If cancer is the cause, they also may include surgery, radiation therapy, chemotherapy, or laser therapy.

Prognosis

The prognosis depends on the cause and reduction of risk factors, if possible. Without treatment, symptoms of vaginitis can worsen.

Prevention

Women who often get yeast infections may want to avoid clothing that increases their irritation. They should avoid chemicals that are irritating, practice safe sex, and avoid douching.

Ray Marks

See also: Abdominal Diseases; Ovarian Cancer; Pelvic Inflammatory Disease; Reproductive Disorders; Sexually Transmitted Diseases; Urinary Tract Infections; Women's Health

Further Reading

Centers for Disease Control and Prevention. (2010). Diseases characterized by vaginal discharge. Retrieved from http://www.cdc.gov/std/treatment/2010/vaginal-discharge.htm.

Eunice Kennedy Shriver National Institute of Child Health and Development. (2014). How is vaginitis treated? Retrieved from http://www.nichd.nih.gov/health/topics/vaginitis/conditioninfo/Pages/treatments.aspx.

Eunice Kennedy Shriver National Institute of Child Health and Development. (2014). What causes vaginitis? Retrieved from http://www.nichd.nih.gov/health/topics/vaginitis/conditioninfo/Pages/causes.aspx.

Mayo Clinic. (2015). Vagina: What's normal, what's not. http://www.mayoclinic.org/healthy
-lifestyle/womens-health/in-depth/vagina/art-20046562.

Rankin, L. (2010). *What's Up Down There? Questions You'd Only Ask Your Gynecologist if She Was Your Best Friend.* London: St. Martin's Griffin.

Stewart, E. G. (2002). *The V Book: A Doctor's Guide to Complete Vulvovaginal Health.* New York: Bantam.

VASCULAR DISORDERS

The term *vascular disease* refers to any condition that abnormally affects the circulatory system. The heart and the blood that flows through a system of blood vessels is called the circulatory system. The main types of blood vessels are arteries that carry blood away from the heart, while veins return blood to the heart.

Vascular disease includes diseases of the arteries, veins, and lymph vessels, plus blood disorders that affect circulation. The following are some examples of these conditions: aneurysms, arterial blockages, disease of the carotid artery of the heart, and peripheral vascular diseases.

Any of these problems can cause severe disability and death and can strike anyone, at any age, often without warning. Vascular disease can affect many different parts of the body—including the heart, brain, and legs—and is extremely serious. The condition may lead to a stroke, a heart attack, or blood clots.

Symptoms

Symptoms of leg artery disease include leg numbness or weakness, coldness in the lower leg or foot, cramping pains in the leg muscles on exertion, and sores on the feet or lower legs that do not heal. Other signs may include changes in the color of the leg, decreased or absent pulses, large protruding veins, hair loss on the legs, and changes in the color or thickness of the toenails. Signs and symptoms of stroke are vision loss, speech loss, weakness, numbness, and paralysis.

Key Causes and Risk Factors

Vascular disease is mainly caused by hardening of the arteries. Risk factors include smoking, an unhealthy diet, lack of exercise, diabetes, high blood pressure, high cholesterol, and stress.

Diagnosis

Diagnosis is based on a medical history, dye injection into the arteries that are then x-rayed, ultrasound imaging tests, brain scans, and blood tests.

Treatment

Treatments may range from recommending changes in the diet and increasing or beginning exercise to moderately invasive treatments such as placing a vascular stent to open a blocked artery or vein. In severe cases, a surgical bypass may be necessary to address blocked arteries, particularly in the heart. Medication may also be prescribed to help blood flow more easily and to reduce the buildup of plaque on artery and vein walls.

Prognosis

The prognosis depends on the cause of the problem, its severity, and location, as well as duration. Minimizing the risk factors will be especially helpful at all stages.

Prevention

Avoid smoking or tobacco usage, adopt healthy eating habits, exercise regularly, and reduce high blood pressure and cholesterol levels. Also keeping diabetes under control and reducing stress will help.

Ray Marks

See also: Angina; Arrhythmias/Dysrhythmias; Atherosclerosis; Cardiomyopathy; Circulation Disorders; Coronary Artery Disease; Heart Diseases; Hypertension; Peripheral Arterial Disorders; Venous Disorders

Further Reading

Cleveland Clinic. (2015). Vascular disease overview. Retrieved from https://my.clevelandclinic.org/services/heart/disorders/vascular-disease.

Dean, S., & Satiani, B. (2013). *Color Atlas and Synopsis of Vascular Disease.* Columbus, OH: McGraw-Hill Education.

Jaff, M. R., & White, C. J. (2011). *Vascular Disease: Diagnostic and Therapeutic Approaches.* Minneapolis, MN: CardioText Publishing.

Stanford Health Care. (2015). Types of peripheral vascular disease. Retrieved from https://stanfordhealthcare.org/medical-conditions/blood-heart-circulation/peripheral-vascular-disease/types.html.

Vascular Cures. (2014). What is vascular disease? Retrieved from http://vasculardisease.org/about-vascular-disease.

VENOUS DISORDERS

Chronic venous disorders, or venous insufficiency, refers to the blockage in the circulation of the veins due to trauma, inflammation, or valve problems or blood clots that block blood flow, mainly from the legs to the heart. It leads to pain, most commonly of the lower legs, plus swelling of the legs.

Symptoms

There may be no symptoms, but especially if symptoms are present in the legs, these may include fatigue, throbbing, ankle or leg swelling, and itching; later on, the development of varicose veins, muscle cramps, and possibly blood clots or a breakdown of the skin due to bleeding from the varicose veins may occur.

Key Causes and Risk Factors

Family history, increasing age, being female, and being involved in prolonged standing or sitting may be risk factors. Having a history of deep vein thrombosis or high blood pressure, as well as smoking and a sedentary lifestyle, are risk factors.

Diagnosis

Physical examination, as well as the use of duplex ultrasound scanning to examine vein blood flow, venograms or vein x-rays, or MRI or CT scans may be helpful.

Treatment

Treatments aim at reducing the symptoms and include exercise, elevating the legs, compression bandaging, paying attention to diet and lifestyle, and selected medications.

Other treatments are sclerotherapy, or having a chemical injected into the affected varicose veins so blocked veins are scarred and no longer used. Ablation is a similar procedure that uses a catheter to destroy the varicose veins. Others are vein stripping to remove individual veins through surgery. Bypass surgery to reroute blood flow and valve repair or angioplasty and stenting may be used to minimize vein blockages.

Prognosis and Prevention

In severe cases, ulcers can form on the bottom of the legs and can cause considerable disability. Prevention or lessening venous disorders includes not smoking, exercising regularly, and not sitting or standing for long periods of time.

Ray Marks

See also: Deep Vein Thrombosis; Physical Activity; Thrombophlebitis

Further Reading

Bergan, J. J., & Bunke-Paquette, N., eds. (2014). *The Vein Book*. New York: Oxford University Press.

Cleveland Clinic. (2015). Chronic vein insufficiency. Retrieved from https://my.clevelandclinic.org/services/heart/disorders/arterial-and-vascular-disease/chronic-venous-insufficiency.

England, T., & Nasim, A., eds. (2014). *ABC of Arterial and Venous Disease*. London: Blackwell.

Gloviczki, P., et al. (2009). *Handbook of Venous Disorders*. London: Hodder Arnold Publishers.

Vascular Disease Foundation. (2014). What is chronic vein insufficiency? Retrieved from http://vasculardisease.org/flyers/chronic-venous-insufficiency-flyer.pdf.

Vascular Web. (2014). Chronic vein insufficiency. Retrieved from http://www.vascularweb
.org/vascularhealth/pages/chronic-venous-insufficiency.aspx.

VESTIBULAR DISEASES

Vestibular disorders, also termed vestibular balance disorders, are disorders of both
the brain and inner ear or vestibule that cause balance or unsteadiness problems
that can lead to falls and walking problems.

Symptoms and Causes

Symptoms include dizziness, nausea, hearing loss, a spinning or floating sensation,
confusion, and visual problems, as well as anxiety and fatigue. A variety of problems or infections as well as injuries to the ear, the central nervous system, the eye,
or the proprioceptive systems can produce vestibular symptoms.

Diagnosis and Treatments

Diagnosis may include a medical examination, as well as CT scans, ultrasound tests, or
MRI scans and hearing and blood tests. An eye exam and postural exam may be conducted as well. Treatments depend on the cause and could involve physical therapy to
assist with improving walking ability and other functions of daily living. Medical
and dietary changes may be recommended. Occasionally, surgery of the ear may
be required.

Scientists supported by the National Institute on Deafness and other Communication Disorders are testing vestibular prostheses, or miniature devices designed to
regulate functioning of balance organs in the inner ear in order to reduce dizziness.
They are also studying the effectiveness of different types of exercises and other approaches to treat balance disorders.

Ray Marks

See also: Ear Diseases; Meniere's Disease; Tinnitus

Further Reading

Blakely, B., & Siegel, M.. (1997). *Feeling Dizzy Understanding and Treating Dizziness, Vertigo,
and Other Balance Disorders*. Hoboken, NJ: John Wiley & Sons.
Cleveland Clinic. (2014). Vestibular and balance disorders. Retrieved from http://my
.clevelandclinic.org/services/head-neck/departments-centers/vestibular-balance
-disorders.
Hickey, S. (2011). *Finding Balance: Healing from a Decade of Vestibular Disorders*. New York:
Demos Health.
Vestibular Disorders Association. (2015). About vestibular disorders. Retrieved from http://
vestibular.org/understanding-vestibular-disorder.
Wazen, J., & Mitchell, D. (2004). *Dizzy: What You Need to Know about Managing and Treat-
ing Balance Disorders*. New York: Touchstone Books.
Wright, W. (2014). *Dizziness and Vertigo: A Simple Guide to Figuring It Out*. Switzerland: Wise
Media Group.

W

WATERBORNE DISEASES

Overview

Waterborne or related diseases are those that arise from ingesting water that is contaminated in some way or coming into contact with contaminated water. Examples of waterborne diseases include typhoid fever, cholera, malaria, guinea worm disease, and shigellosis—all diseases that mostly harm the digestive system.

Chemicals in the water such as arsenic can cause painful skin lesions that can lead to skin, lung, bladder, and kidney cancer.

Signs, Symptoms, Causes, and Risk Factors

Common symptoms are diarrhea. Microorganisms and chemicals in water people drink may contribute to one or more waterborne diseases. People with compromised immune systems such as those with HIV/AIDS may be at higher risk for one or more waterborne infections.

Diagnosis and Treatment

A personal history and a physical exam and laboratory tests may help to formulate a diagnosis. A person who is infected as a result of a waterborne illness may have to be hospitalized. Antibiotics may be prescribed as indicated. Many deaths in developing countries occur as a result of unsafe drinking water; thus, prevention is strongly indicated.

Prognosis or Outcome

It is possible to recover from one of more of these waterborne infections, but these can still reduce quality of life.

Prevention

Sanitation, proper personal hygiene, and a safe drinking water supply can prevent most waterborne infections. Supplying people with clean drinkable water and improving sanitation will help reduce this problem.

Ray Marks

See also: Malaria; Parasitic Diseases; Public Health

Further Reading

Centers for Disease Control and Prevention. (2015). Water-related diseases and contaminants in public water systems. Retrieved from http://www.cdc.gov/healthywater/drinking /public/water_diseases.html.

Hunter, P. (1997). *Waterborne Disease: Epidemiology and Ecology*. Hoboken, NJ: John Wiley & Sons.

Lenntech, at the Technical University of Delft, the Netherlands. (2015). Waterborne diseases: General information. Retrieved from http://www.lenntech.com/library/diseases /diseases/waterborne-diseases.htm.

UNICEF. (2014). Common water and sanitation-related diseases. Retrieved from http://www .unicef.org/wash/index_wes_related.html.

World Health Organization. (2015). Water-related diseases. Water sanitation health. Retrieved from http://www.who.int/water_sanitation_health/diseases/en/.

WHOOPING COUGH

Whooping cough, also called pertussis, arises due to an infection within the respiratory system that results in severe intermittent coughing lasting one to three weeks, but it can last 6 to 10 weeks in severe cases. Children younger than six months and children 11 to 18 years of age may be vulnerable. A vaccine is available to prevent this condition. Adults may have whooping cough in a milder form. Some children need to be hospitalized because they are susceptible to pneumonia. The problem usually starts in a milder form and progresses to become more severe. The condition has been rare in the United States, but it is now increasing in frequency due to some children not receiving vaccines.

Signs and Symptoms

The child may have a runny nose, red watery eyes, severe intermittent dry cough attacks, violent and rapid coughing, choking spells, nasal congestion, and sneezing and coughing spells, as well as vomiting and a blue or red face. When the child tries to take a breath, a "whooping" noise is heard, leading to the name.

Causes and Risk Factors

Whooping cough is caused the bacterium *Bordetella pertussis* (or *B. pertussis*) that infects the top of the throat. Whooping cough bacteria can be transmitted by others through tiny droplets being passed in the air as they laugh, cough, or sneeze. Risk factors are low immunity and the fact that the vaccine wears off after childhood. Many babies diagnosed with whooping cough were infected by parents, older siblings, or other caregivers who might not even know they have the disease (Centers for Disease Control and Prevention 2014). Symptoms may depend on whether the vaccine has been given or not and how active it is. Generally, the cough worsens over time, even though the cold symptoms may lessen.

Diagnostic Procedures

Blood tests, a physical exam, a nose or throat culture, and chest x-rays can confirm the diagnosis.

Treatment

Antibiotics can help to treat the condition, which is highly contagious. Cough medicines may be of little help.

Prognosis or Outcome

Data show about 75 percent of children younger than six months of age may need to be hospitalized if they have whooping cough because the condition can be life-threatening. With good care, most affected individuals will recover, but this could be dependent on the vaccine and how effective it is. It is important to be vaccinated because other possible complications include breathing difficulties, periods of apnea or breathlessness, and needing to use oxygen during a coughing spell, along with dehydration.

Prevention

The condition can be prevented by the use of DTaP immunization given before a child's sixth birthday and getting all the required shots. Children ages 11 to 18 can now receive a booster shot called Tdap, ideally at 11 or 12 years of age. Pregnant women should get vaccinated in their third trimester. Everyone around a baby should have had an up-to-date whooping cough vaccination.

Ray Marks

See also: Pneumonia; Respiratory Diseases; Vaccines

Further Reading

Centers for Disease Control and Prevention. (2014). Help protect babies from whooping cough. Mayo Clinic. Retrieved from http://www.mayoclinic.org/diseases-conditions /whooping-cough/basics/definition/con-20023295.

Centers for Disease Control and Prevention. (2015). About pertussis. Retrieved from http:// www.cdc.gov/pertussis/about/.

Cleveland Clinic. (2015). Whooping cough: Pertussis. http://my.clevelandclinic.org/health /diseases_conditions/hic-whooping-cough-pertussis.

Johns Hopkins Medicine Health Library. (2015). Whooping cough. Retrieved from http:// www.hopkinsmedicine.org/healthlibrary/conditions/adult/infectious_diseases /whooping_cough_pertussis_in_adults_85,P00622/.

WILSON'S DISEASE

Wilson's disease is a rare inherited disorder involving the accumulation of high copper levels in the liver and other organs and body systems, including the nervous system, kidneys, and eyes. It can cause serious harm because it is poisonous, but if detected and treated early on, people diagnosed as having Wilson's disease can expect to live normal, healthy lives.

Although copper is a vital mineral to the body when present in small amounts and is found in most foods, in Wilson's disease, the liver fails to release or excrete excessive copper from the body. This causes a buildup of excessive amounts of copper in the liver, plus liver damage and liver scar tissue, as well as liver failure. Once excessive copper enters the bloodstream, which transports copper to other areas of the body, the affected person can experience severe damage, scarring, and dysfunction of other vital organs, such as the brain, eyes, and kidneys, and maybe premature death.

Wilson's disease is a genetic disorder caused by a recessive, defective gene from both parents. That is, it only occurs among those with a biological mother and father who both carry the defective gene for the disorder. It is most common in people of Eastern European and Southern Italian descent and affects about 1 in 30,000 individuals of any race or ethnicity.

Signs and Symptoms

Wilson's disease is present at birth, but the symptoms usually occur later on between the ages of 6 and 20 years and can begin as late as age 40. The most characteristic sign is a rusty brown ring around the cornea of the eye called the Kayser-Fleischer ring. This can be seen only through an eye exam. Symptoms include abdominal pain, abdominal swelling, and jaundice, and the disease first attacks the liver, the central nervous system, or both. Over time, signs similar to those of chronic liver disease occur, including swelling of the liver or spleen, fluid buildup in the legs, a tendency to bruise easily, and fatigue.

Neurological problems that can arise include muscle stiffness or rigidity; behavioral problems; tremors or uncontrolled movements; speech, swallowing, or physical coordination; and clumsiness problems. Other problems may include premature arthritis or osteoporosis, anemia, depression, nausea, slower blood clotting, joint pain, high protein, carbohydrate and uric acid levels in the urine, and a low white cell or platelet count.

Causes and Risk Factors

The disease is an inherited one, so having parents who carry the gene puts a person at risk, and this can cause excess release of copper into the bloodstream and possible neurological symptoms if people with this disease cannot release copper from the liver at a normal rate.

Diagnosis

Wilson's disease is diagnosed through a physical examination and laboratory tests, including blood tests to examine copper levels, 24-hour urine tests, liver biopsy tests, brain scans, and a test to see if the individual carries the defective gene. A special eye test using a slit lamp can help to detect the presence of Kayser-Fleischer rings in the eyes.

Treatment

Wilson's disease requires lifelong treatment to reduce and control the amount of copper in the body. The initial treatment involves removing excess copper and reducing copper intake, as well as applying treatments for any liver- or central nervous system–related problems.

Maintenance therapy then begins when symptoms improve and tests show copper levels are safe. This typically involves taking zinc and low doses of either d-penicillamine or trientine hydrochloride to help remove copper from the tissues. Blood and urine should be monitored periodically to ensure copper is maintained at a safe level.

People with Wilson's disease should reduce their dietary copper intake—including not eating shellfish or liver, mushrooms, nuts, dried fruit, and chocolate—and should have their drinking water checked for copper content; they should not take multivitamins containing copper.

Patients may be helped by taking vitamin B6, and those presenting with acute liver failure due to Wilson's disease might be considered for liver transplantation, which effectively cures this disease and has a long-term survival rate of about 80 percent.

Prognosis or Outcome

If the disease is diagnosed early on, and treated, the prognosis is positive.

Prevention

There are no prevention approaches at present, but genetic testing and early diagnosis may help.

Future

The National Institute of Diabetes and Digestive and Kidney Diseases conducts research in this area and is examining the effect of a new anti-copper drug called tetrathiomolybdate. A trial has shown this to be effective in removing copper with less risk of neurological problems than trientine hydrochloride.

Ray Marks

See also: Genetics and Genomics; Liver Diseases

Further Reading

American Liver Foundation. (2013). Wilson disease. Retrieved from http://www.liverfoun dation.org/abouttheliver/info/wilson/.

Mayo Clinic. (2011). Wilson's disease. Retrieved from http://www.mayoclinic.org/diseases -conditions/wilsons-disease/basics/definition/con-20043499.

National Institute of Diabetes and Digestive and Kidney Diseases. (2015). What is Wilson's disease? Retrieved from http://digestive.niddk.nih.gov/ddiseases/pubs/wilson.

Rosenblum, L. (2013). Wilson's disease. Retrieved from http://www.lifescript.com/health /a-z/conditions_a-z/conditions/w/wilsons_disease.aspx?gclid=CNeCxv6OzLsCFbB9O godVmkAsg&trans=1&du=1&ef_id=UcyOMQAAAACU6Qfa:20131225193334:s.

Wilson Disease Association. (2013). About Wilson disease. Retrieved from http://www .wilsonsdisease.org/about-wilsondisease.php.

WOMEN'S HEALTH

Some health issues affect women differently than men. Women may require necessary care that is different from men, even though the symptoms may be similar between women and men. It is important to note that some of the conditions may also affect women more severely than men. According to the Eunice Kennedy Shriver National Institute of Child Health and Human Development (2012b), several leading health issues or conditions affect women differently than men: (1) alcohol abuse, (2) heart disease, (3) mental health, (4) osteoarthritis, (5) sexually transmitted diseases/sexually transmitted infections (STDs/STIs), and (6) stress.

Alcohol Abuse

Men are more likely to become dependent on alcohol; however, women's dependency on alcohol increases their risk for injuries, violence, breast cancer, heart disease, liver diseases, and fetal alcohol syndrome, where an infant born to a mother who is actively drinking during pregnancy will suffer brain damage and have difficulties learning (NIH 2012). Excessive alcohol use for women is defined as four or more drinks on an occasion or more than seven drinks a week (Centers for Disease Control and Prevention [CDC] 2015b).

Heart Disease

Although coronary heart disease is a leading cause of death for both women and men, it is the leading cause of death for women (American Heart Association 2016). Women are more likely to die following a heart attack than men. Even with an increase in public awareness, treatment to control heart attacks for women lacks behind men when it comes to both at the primary care and emergency care levels. It is reported that one in every four deaths for women is due to heart disease (CDC, 2015a). It has also been reported that more research needs to be done on women and heart disease because recommendations and treatment can be much improved, instead of basing it on research done primarily on men, as has been done in the past.

Mental Health

The most common mental health problem for women is depression, where women show more signs and are diagnosed at a higher rate than men (NIH 2012).

As reported by the CDC (2010), the majority of adults with, or without, mental health symptoms believe that living normal lives is possible with the help of treatment.

Osteoarthritis

Osteoarthritis is a type of arthritis in which one experiences joint pain, stiffness, and swelling, mostly affecting knees, hips, hands, and spine, which in turn may lead to physical disability (NIH 2012). More women are affected by this condition than men. Currently, there is no cure for osteoarthritis, and the specific causes are not known (CDC 2011b).

Sexually Transmitted Diseases/Sexually Transmitted Infections (STDs/STIs)

Some STDs/STIs symptoms are not treated in women because it is confused with less serious conditions (NIH 2012). In the United States, each year at least 24,000 women experience infertility due to cases of untreated STDs/STIs. Infertility can be prevented if treatment is sought early for STDs/STIs (CDC 2011a).

Stress

More women are reporting that they are feeling stressed (NIH 2012). Symptoms of stress may include loss of appetite, loss of interest in normal activities, anger, feeling powerless, and having trouble concentrating (CDC 2012).

It is important for women to take care of themselves by eating healthily, exercising, and getting sufficient sleep. Spending time with family and friends is a great way to connect with others. Understanding how some of the health issues affect women differently from men is a significant way to live a healthy life. Health practitioners should be consulted for how to achieve a healthy lifestyle. It is also important for women, and indeed all people, to take an active role in their own health care by asking questions and educating themselves on issues affecting them.

Susana Leong

See also: Alcoholism; Breast Cancer; Cardiovascular Disease; Cervical Cancer; Eating Disorders; HPV (Human Papillomavirus); Irritable Bowel Syndrome; Men's Health; Mental Disorders; Osteoarthritis; Osteoporosis; Ovarian Cancer; Reproductive Disorders; Sexually Transmitted Diseases; Stress

Further Reading

American Heart Association. (2014). Gender-specific research improves accuracy of heart disease diagnosis in women. American Heart Association Scientific Statement. Retrieved from http://newsroom.heart.org/news/gender-specific-research-improves-accuracy-of -heart-disease-diagnosis-in-women.

American Heart Association. (2016). About heart disease in women. Retrieved from https:// www.goredforwomen.org/home/about-heart-disease-in-women.

Centers for Disease Control and Prevention. (2010). Attitudes toward mental illness: 35 states, District of Columbia, and Puerto Rico, 2007. Retrieved from http://www.cdc.gov /mmwr/preview/mmwrhtml/mm5920a3.htm.

Centers for Disease Control and Prevention. (2011a). 10 ways STDs impact women differently from men. Retrieved from http://www.cdc.gov/std/health-disparities/stds-women -042011.pdf.

Centers for Disease Control and Prevention. (2011b). Osteoarthritis. Retrieved from http:// www.cdc.gov/arthritis/basics/osteoarthritis.htm.

Centers for Disease Control and Prevention. (2015a). Women and heart disease fact sheet. Retrieved from http://www.cdc.gov/dhdsp/data_statistics/fact_sheets/fs_women_heart .htm.

Centers for Disease Control and Prevention. (2015b, November 16). Alcohol and public health: Frequently asked questions. Retrieved from http://www.cdc.gov/alcohol/faqs .htm.

Centers for Disease Control and Prevention (CDC). (2012, December 19). Managing stress. Retrieved from http://www.cdc.gov/features/handlingstress.

Eunice Kennedy Shriver National Institute of Child Health and Human Development. (2012a). What health issues or conditions are specific to women only? Retrieved from https://www.nichd.nih.gov/health/topics/womenshealth/conditioninfo/pages /whatconditions.aspx.

Eunice Kennedy Shriver National Institute of Child Health and Human Development. (2012b). What health issues or conditions affect women differently than men? Retrieved from https://www.nichd.nih.gov/health/topics/womenshealth/conditioninfo /pages/howconditions.aspx.

Kolander, C., Ballard, D., & Chandler, C. (2013). *Contemporary Women's Health: Issues for Today and the Future*. Columbus, OH: McGraw-Hill Education.

Womenshealth.gov. (2015). Healthy aging. Retrieved from http://www.womenshealth.gov /aging/diseases-conditions/.

WORLD HEALTH ORGANIZATION

The World Health Organization (WHO) is a branch of the United Nations that oversees the health conditions of the world. It provides public health leadership and oversight to numerous communities across the globe.

Located in Geneva, Switzerland, WHO provides resources and know-how to all countries that belong to the United Nations and focuses on serious health issues that can be prevented or reduced in severity.

Data from the World Health Organization show that chronic disease is the major cause of premature death around the world, even in countries with a high rate of infectious diseases.

This organization works to reduce the problems associated with chronic diseases and to foster long, healthy lives for citizens in all countries because many chronic conditions are largely preventable, such as tobacco use, HIV/AIDS, and maternal ill health. Obesity, infectious diseases, heart disease, and diabetes are among the many topics of interest to WHO.

The WHO website provides the following information about its activities.

1. It promotes healthy living, such as improving diet, increasing physical activity, and refraining from smoking. It works to promote healthy societies, especially for poor and disadvantaged populations.
2. It works to prevent premature deaths and excess disability due to chronic diseases.
3. It uses the latest available knowledge to treat chronic diseases effectively and make treatments available to all, especially those in the poorest settings.
4. It provides appropriate care by facilitating resource development and disseminating educational information.

Ray Marks

See also: Access to Health Services; Centers for Disease Control and Prevention (CDC); Food Guides from the USDA; Health; National Institute of Health (NIH); Poverty; Public Health

Further Reading

Council on Foreign Relations. (2014). Global Governance Monitor: Public health. Retrieved from   http://www.cfr.org/global-governance/global-governance-monitor/p18985#! /public-health.

Lee, K., & Fang, J (2012). *Historical Dictionary of the World Health Organization.* Lanham, MD: Scarecrow Press.

Renwick, D., & Johnson, T. (2014). The World Health Organization. Council on Foreign Relations. Retrieved from http://www.cfr.org/public-health-threats-and-pandemics /world-health-organization-/p20003.

Roemer, M. I. (1993). *National Health Systems of the World: The Issues.* New York: Oxford University Press.

World Health Organization. (2015). The role of WHO in public health. Retrieved from http://www.who.int/about/role/en/.

Recommended Resources

BOOKS

General Health and Chronic Disease

Lieberman, D. (2014). *The Story of the Human Body: Evolution, Health, and Disease*. New York: Vintage.

Lorig, K., et al. (2012). *Living a Healthy Life with Chronic Conditions: Self-Management of Heart Disease, Arthritis, Diabetes, Depression, Asthma, Bronchitis, Emphysema and Other Physical and Mental Health Conditions*, 4th ed. Boulder, CO: Bull Publishing Co.

Schulz, A. J., & Mullings, L. (2006). *Gender, Race, Class, and Health*. Hoboken, NJ: John Wiley and Sons, Inc.

The Toolkit for Active Living with Chronic Conditions. (2015). Boulder, CO: Bull Publishing Co.

Chronic Diseases and Disorders

Alcoholism and Addiction

Kuhar, M. (2011). *The Addicted Brain*. Upper Saddle River, NJ: Pearson Education.

Leukefeld, C., Gullotta, T. P., Ramos, J., & Staton-Tindall, M. (Eds.). (2009). *Issues in Children's and Families' Lives: Adolescent Substance Abuse: Evidence-Based Approaches to Prevention and Treatment*. New York: Springer-Verlag.

Ludwig, A. M. (1989). *Understanding the Alcoholic's Mind: The Nature of Craving and How to Control It*. New York: Oxford University Press.

Alzheimer's Disease

Petersen, R. (Ed.). (2002). *Mayo Clinic on Alzheimer's Disease*. (2002). Rochester, MN: Mayo Clinic, 2002.

Poirier, J., & Gauthier, S. (2014). *Alzheimer's Disease: The Complete Introduction (Your Health)*. Toronto: Dundurn.

Arthritis

Lorig, K., & Fries, J. F. (2006). *The Arthritis Helpbook: A Tested Self-Management Program for Coping with Arthritis and Fibromyalgia*, 6th ed. New York: Da Capo Press.

Shlotzhauer, T. L. (2014). *Living with Rheumatoid Arthritis*, 3rd ed. Baltimore, MD: Johns Hopkins University Press.

Asthma and Allergies

Adams, F. (2006). *The Asthma Sourcebook*, 3rd ed. New York: McGraw-Hill.
Fanta, C. H., Cristiano, L. M., & Haver, K. E., with N. Waring. (2003). *The Harvard Medical School Guide to Taking Control of Asthma: A Comprehensive Prevention and Treatment Plan for You and Your Family.* New York: Free Press.

Back Pain

Moore, J., Lorig, K., Von Korff, M., González, V., & Laurent, D. (1999). *The Back Pain Helpbook.* New York: Perseus Books.

Bipolar Disorder

Braun, S. R. (2007). *A Guide to Bipolar Disorder.* American College of Physicians. Potomac, MD: Conrad and Associates.
Jamison, K. R. (2009). *An Unquiet Mind.* New York: Vintage Books.
Miklowitz, D. J. (2011). *The Bipolar Disorder Survival Guide: What You and Your Family Need to Know*, 2nd ed. New York: Guilford Press.
Mondimore, F. M. (2006). *Bipolar Disorder: A Guide for Patients and Families*, 2nd ed. Baltimore, MD: Johns Hopkins University Press.

Cancer

DeVita, V. T., Jr., with DeVita-Raeburn, E. (2015). *The Death of Cancer: After 50 Years on the Front Lines of Medicine, a Pioneering Oncologist Reveals Why the War on Cancer Is Winnable & How We Can Get There.* New York: Sarah Crichton Books/Farrar Straus and Giroux.
Feuerstein, M., & Findley, P. (2006). *The Cancer Survivor's Guide: The Essential Handbook to Life after Cancer.* New York: Marlowe & Co.
Mukherjee, S. (2010). *The Emperor of All Maladies: A Biography of Cancer.* New York: Scribner.

Crohn's Disease and Ulcerative Colitis

Sklar, J., & Sklar, M. (2007). *The First Year: Crohn's Disease and Ulcerative Colitis: An Essential Guide for the Newly Diagnosed.* Boston: Da Capo Press.

Cystic Fibrosis

Orenstein, D. M., & Spahr, J. E. (2012). *Cystic Fibrosis: A Guide for Patient and Family.* Philadelphia: Lippincott/Williams & Wilkins.

Depression and Anxiety

Burns, D. D. (2008). *Feeling Good: The New Mood Therapy.* New York: Harper.
Solomon, A. (2001). *The Noonday Demon: An Atlas of Depression.* New York: Scribner.
Wilson, R. (2009). *Don't Panic: Taking Control of Anxiety Attacks*, 3rd ed. New York: Harper Perennial.

Diabetes

American Diabetes Association Complete Guide to Diabetes: The Ultimate Home Reference from the Diabetes Experts. (2011). Alexandria, VA: American Diabetes Association.
Mayo Clinic. (2014). The Essential Diabetes Book. New York: Time Home Entertainment

Eating Disorders

Costin, C. (2012). Eight Keys to Recovery from an Eating Disorder: Effective Strategies from Therapeutic Practice and Personal Experience. New York: W. W. Norton & Co.

Epilepsy

Wyllie, E. (2008). Epilepsy: Information for You and Those Who Care about You. Cleveland, OH: Cleveland Clinic Press.

Gastrointestinal Disorders

Sonnenburg, E. (2015). The Good Gut. New York: Penguin Publishing Group.

Health Disparities for Racial and Ethnic Groups

Byrd, W. M., & Clayton, L. A. (2000). An American Health Dilemma: A Medical History of African Americans and the Problem of Race: Beginnings to 1900 (Vol. 1). New York: Routledge.
LaVeist, T. A., & Isaac, L. A. (Eds.). (2013). Race, Ethnicity, and Health: A Public Health Reader. Hoboken, NJ: John Wiley and Sons, Inc.
Smedley, B. D., Stith, A., & Nelson, A. R., with Committee on Understanding and Eliminating Racial and Ethnic Disparities in Health Care. (Eds.). (2003). Unequal Treatment: Confronting Racial and Ethnic Disparities in Health Care. Washington, DC: The National Academies Press.

Heart Disease

Cohen, B. M. (2008). Coronary Heart Disease: A Guide to Diagnosis and Treatment. Omaha, NE: Addicus Books.
Cohen, T. J. (2010). A Patient's Guide to Heart Rhythm Problems. Baltimore, MD: Johns Hopkins University Press.
Esselstyn, C. B., Jr. (2008). Prevent and Reverse Heart Disease: The Revolutionary, Scientifically Proven, Nutrition-Based Cure. New York: Avery.
Granato, J. E. (2008). Living with Coronary Heart Disease: A Guide for Patients and Families (A Johns Hopkins Press Health Book). Baltimore, MD: Johns Hopkins University Press.
Kasper, E. K., & Knudson, M. (2010). Living Well with Heart Failure, the Misnamed, Misunderstood Condition. Baltimore, MD: Johns Hopkins University Press.

HIV

Webel, A. R., et al. (2016). Living a Healthy Life with HIV, 4th ed. Boulder, CO: Bull Publishing Co.

Kidney Disease

Hunt, W. A. (2011). *Kidney Disease: A Guide for Living.* Baltimore, MD: The Johns Hopkins University Press.

Lupus

Thomas, D. E., Jr. (2014). *The Lupus Encyclopedia: A Comprehensive Guide for Patients and Families.* Baltimore, MD: Johns Hopkins University Press.

Lymphoma

Adler, E. M. (2015). *Living with Lymphoma: A Patient's Guide,* 2nd ed. Baltimore, MD: Johns Hopkins, UP 2015.

Multiple Sclerosis

Furney, K. O. F. (2009). *When the Diagnosis Is Multiple Sclerosis: Help, Hope, and Insights from an Affected Physician.* Baltimore, MD: Johns Hopkins University Press.

Osteoporosis

Hodgson, S. (2003). *Mayo Clinic on Osteoporosis: Keeping Bones Healthy and Strong and Reducing the Risk of Fracture.* Rochester, MN: Mayo Clinic.

Overweight and Obesity

Lustig, R. H. (2013). *Fat Chance: Beating the Odds against Sugar, Processed Food, Obesity, and Disease.* New York: Hudson Street Press.

Power, M. L., & Schulkin, J. (2009). *The Evolution of Obesity.* Baltimore, MD: Johns Hopkins University Press.

Taubes, G. (2011). *Why We Get Fat and What to Do about It.* New York: Alfred A. Knopf.

Parkinson's Disease

Weiner, W. J., Shulman, L. M., & Lang, A. E. (2013). *Parkinson's Disease: A Complete Guide for Patients and Families,* 3rd ed. Baltimore, MD: Johns Hopkins University Press.

Post-Polio Syndrome

Halstead, L. S. (2015). *Managing Post-Polio: A Guide to Living and Aging Well with Post-Polio Syndrome.* Washington, DC: MedStar NRH Press.

SELECTED AUTHORITATIVE HEALTH WEBSITES

The following websites are excellent resources for up-to-date information on diseases, disorders, treatment, research, statistics, and other helpful knowledge. These sites are created and maintained by a number of entities, including:

- The U.S. government
- Organizations of physicians and health specialists
- Medical schools or major hospitals and other health care facilities
- Organizations and foundations that support the study of and treatment for particular diseases, such as cancer.

This is by no means an exhaustive list, and it includes only those websites that provide information on a number of diseases, conditions, or disorders. It does not include organizations that focus on one or a few related diseases, which also can be extremely helpful.

GENERAL (THE SITE COVERS A WIDE RANGE OF DISEASES AND CONDITIONS)

The Centers for Disease Control and Prevention (CDC).
(Diseases and Conditions, Prevention of Illness, Publications.)
http://www.cdc.gov/

Center for Managing Chronic Disease.
University of Michigan School of Public Health.
http://cmcd.sph.umich.edu/

Cleveland Clinic.
Publications and information for patients.
http://my.clevelandclinic.org/health

Familydoctor.org
A publication of the American Academy of Family Physicians.
http://familydoctor.org/familydoctor/en.html

Healthfinder.gov.
Provides health information from various government sites.
http://healthfinder.gov/

Johns Hopkins University Medicine.
Health Library for patients.
http://www.hopkinsmedicine.org/healthlibrary/atoz/s/

Kids' Health.
Children's health and illnesses.
http://kidshealth.org/

Mayo Clinic.
Information on a wide variety of illnesses and conditions.
http://www.mayoclinic.org/patient-care-and-health-information.

MedlinePlus. U.S. National Library of Medicine.
Health Information from a number of sources, both government and other organizations.
https://www.nlm.nih.gov/medlineplus/
https://www.nlm.nih.gov/medlineplus/spanish/

NIH Senior Health.
Information from the government's National Institute on Aging (NIA) and the National Library of Medicine (NLM).
http://nihseniorhealth.gov/

Patient Education Center.
Content developed exclusively by Harvard Health Publications, the media and publishing division of the Harvard Medical School of Harvard University.
http://www.patienteducationcenter.org

Stanford Medicine Patient Education.
Stanford University.
http://patienteducation.stanford.edu/materials

University of California at San Francisco.
A-Z listing of conditions.
https://www.ucsfhealth.org/conditions/all.html

World Health Organization.
http://www.who.int/en.

Types of Diseases

The diseases listed have been chosen for the informational content on their websites, where a number of diseases, disorders, and treatments are explained. (There are other excellent associations and organizations that offer support and information about diseases or disorders but may not have as many types of information sources.)

Alcoholism and Addiction

Alcoholics Anonymous
http://www.aa.org/

National Institute on Alcohol Abuse and Alcoholism (NIAAA)
http://www.niaaa.nih.gov/

Alzheimer's Disease

Alzheimer's Association
Alzheimer's Association National Office

Arthritis

Arthritis Foundation
http://www.arthritis.org/

Asthma and Allergies

Asthma and Allergy Foundation of America
http://www.aafa.org/page/welcome.aspx

American Academy of Allergy, Asthma, and Immunology
http://www.aaaai.org/conditions-and-treatments/asthma

Bleeding Disorders

National Hemophilia Foundation
(includes other bleeding disorders)
https://www.hemophilia.org/Bleeding-Disorders/Types-of-Bleeding-Disorders

American Society of Hematology
Blood Disorders
http://www.hematology.org/Patients/Blood-Disorders.aspx

Cancer

American Cancer Society
All types of cancer; Spanish and Asian language versions available
http://www.cancer.org/index

The National Cancer Institute
http://www.cancer.gov

Diabetes

American Diabetes Association
http://www.diabetes.org/

Heart and Cardiovascular Diseases

American Heart Association
http://www.heart.org/HEARTORG/

Kidney Diseases

National Kidney Foundation
https://www.kidney.org/kidneydisease

Liver Diseases

American Liver Foundation
http://www.liverfoundation.org/

Lung and Respiratory Diseases

American Lung Association
http://www.lung.org/

Hearing Disorders

American Hearing Research Foundation
http://american-hearing.org/disorders/

Genetic Diseases

Genetic Disease Foundation
http://www.geneticdiseasefoundation.org/genetic-diseases/

Genetics Home Reference
https://ghr.nlm.nih.gov/

HIV

HIV In Site
University of California at San Francisco (comprehensive information on HIV and AIDS)
http://hivinsite.ucsf.edu/

Leukemia and Lymphoma

Leukemia & Lymphoma Society (LLS)
Information on blood cancers
http://www.lls.org/disease-information

Mental Health Disorders

American Academy of Child and Adolescent Psychiatry (AACAP)
http://www.aacap.org

National Alliance on Mental Illness (NAMI)
https://www.nami.org/Learn-More/Mental-Health-Conditions

The National Institute of Mental Health (NIMH)
Disorders and Conditions Health Topics
http://www.nimh.nih.gov/health/index.shtml

Multiple Sclerosis

National Multiple Sclerosis Society
http://www.nationalmssociety.org/What-is-MS

Neurological Disorders

National Institute of Neurological Disorders and Stroke (NINDS)
Disorders A-Z
http://www.ninds.nih.gov/disorders/disorder_index.htm

Seeing Disorders

Bright Focus Foundation
Alzheimer's disease, macular degeneration, and glaucoma
http://www.brightfocus.org/about

American Federation for the Blind
http://www.afb.org/info/living-with-vision-loss/eye-conditions/12

Skin Diseases

American Academy of Dermatology
https://www.aad.org/public/diseases

Stroke

American Stroke Association
http://www.strokeassociation.org/STROKEORG/

Index

Entries in **bold** denote main entries in the Encyclopedia

About the Editor and Contributors

EDITOR

Jean Kaplan Teichroew, MA, is an editor and writer as well as vice president of communications at the Anxiety and Depression Association of America (ADAA). Prior to working at ADAA, she was the editorial director of the Discovery Education division at Discovery Communications Inc. and a senior features editor of *WORLD* magazine at the National Geographic Society. She holds a master's degree in folklore from Indiana University, Bloomington, and a bachelor's degree in anthropology from the University of California, Berkeley.

ABOUT THE CONTRIBUTORS

David Ajuluchukwu is department chair and associate professor and chair of health and physical education and gerontological studies at York College, City University of New York, Jamaica, New York.

Megan Aronson, MA, CHES, CHWC, is a health promotion coordinator for federal occupational health. She helps with health promotion outreach, health education workshops, health fairs, and health coaching for federal employees. She is a Certified Health Education Specialist and Certified Health and Wellness Coach with a master's in health education from Teachers College at Columbia University. She has also worked at Baruch College, New York-Presbyterian Hospital, and the French Ministry of Education.

Linda R. Barley is a professor of health promotion and gerontology at York College, The City University of New York. She has published extensively on health promotion for older adults and program planning and program assessment.

Roy Benaroch, MD, is clinical assistant professor of pediatrics at Emory University and a pediatrician with a private practice in Roswell, Georgia. He completed an undergraduate degree in biomedical engineering at Tulane University and medical school and his residency at Emory University.

Barbara A. Brehm, EdD, is a professor in the department of exercise and sport studies at Smith College in Northampton, Massachusetts, where she teaches nutrition and health and sports nutrition, as well as seminars in nutrition literacy and women's health. She received her undergraduate degree from Duke University, graduating Phi Beta Kappa, summa cum laude. Her doctoral degree is from the program in applied physiology, Teacher's College, Columbia University. She also studied science writing at the Columbia University School of Journalism.

Tamar Burris is founder and president of Tab Writers, Inc., a curriculum and educational writing company based in northern California, and a former writer/editor with ABC-CLIO. She is also a featured blogger for *Prevent,* an online program designed to help individuals with prediabetes make healthier lifestyle choices, as well as a contributing writer to a local parenting magazine in Humboldt County, California. Burris holds a master's in education from the University of California, Santa Barbara.

Karen Jeanne Coleman, EdD, CHES (community health education specialist), is a former adjunct assistant professor at Teachers College, Columbia University, New York, and Northern Michigan University, Marquette, Michigan. She holds a doctorate from Columbia University, Teachers College, New York. Her research interests, in which she has also published, include bereavement, children's coping with loss and change, and life review for hospice patients.

Andrea D'Souza, BSW, BA, is a social worker in the community engagement and mental health field in Toronto, Canada. She has a passion for applying mindfulness-based interventions, expressive arts, narrative ideas, and body-based approaches in her work with women and youth who have experienced trauma and mental health and addictions issues. She also works with newcomer populations and leads a mindful yoga group for individuals living with schizophrenia.

Renee Dubie is a freelance writer who has written about a diverse array of subjects, including health. She earned a BA in philosophy from the University of California, Santa Barbara, and an MA in political science from San Diego State University.

Kim Masters-Evans is a freelance writer specializing in scientific topics. She has authored dozens of reference books, textbook lessons, and encyclopedia articles for students at the high school and undergraduate levels. Her published works include *Energy: Supplies, Sustainability, and Costs*; *The Environment: A Revolution in Attitudes*; and *Space Exploration: Triumphs and Tragedies*. She is also a licensed professional engineer with two decades of experience in the field of environmental engineering. Evans holds a BS in chemical engineering from Tennessee Technological University.

Christina M. Girod is a freelance writer and editor in educational multimedia. She formerly worked in elementary education and speech pathology in public schools. Her published works include writing and editing extensive articles for ABC-CLIO and the Gale Group. Girod graduated with a BA in speech and hearing sciences from the University of California, Santa Barbara, and has earned teaching credentials through Chapman University.

Cathy Hogstrom Stiller has a master's degree in health education and has worked for the American Cancer Society as a community mission manager in Queens, New York.

Sukhminder Kaur is currently a doctoral candidate in the health education program at Teachers College, Columbia University.

William D. Kernan, EdD, MPA, MCHES, is associate professor and chair of public health at William Paterson University in Wayne, New Jersey. His published research studies include "Searching for and Making Meaning after Breast Cancer: Prevalence, Patterns, and Negative Affect" (2009); "Health-Related Barriers to Learning among Graduate Students"

(2011); and "Linking Learning and Health: A Pilot Study of Medical Student's Perceptions of the Academic Impact of Various Health Issues" (2008). He has also worked on health-related projects internationally for the United Nations' World Food Program and in the U.S. Peace Corps. He holds a doctorate in health education from Columbia University. His research interests include social epidemiology, food systems/food insecurity, and substance-abuse prevention.

Brad Lang writes about and researches public health issues.

Susana Leong earned her doctorate and master's degrees in health and behavior studies from Columbia University, and her bachelor's degree from the University of California, Berkeley. Dr. Leong is an adjunct assistant professor in the department of physiological nursing at the University of California, San Francisco. Her research interests include eating disorders, nutrition, Type 2 diabetes, and college health services.

Evelyn B. Kelly, PhD, is a medical writer and professor of education at Saint Leo University Ocala Education Center in Ocala, Florida.

Angela Libal is a science writer. She has published more than 400 articles dealing with animal husbandry, biology, and environmental science on various educational websites, as well as several books, including Ferguson's *Field Guides to Finding a New Career: Science*. Her areas of interest include the intersection of the natural sciences, religious and ethnological history, and folklore. She holds a BA from Sarah Lawrence College.

Howard MacLennan, DO, Captain, serves in the U.S. Army as a family medicine physician. He graduated with a bachelor's of science degree in genetics and molecular biology from Iowa State University and received his DO degree from the University of New England College of Osteopathic Medicine. (Any views expressed by Howard MacLennan in this work are those of the author and do not reflect the official policy or position of the Department of the Army, Department of Defense, or the U.S. government.)

Ray Marks, EdD, is a clinical professor of health promotion at the City University of New York, York College, and an adjunct professor of health education at Columbia University, Teachers College, New York. His published works include *Health Literacy and School-Based Education* (2012) and "Childhood, Adolescent and Adult Obesity: An Analysis of Related Health Outcomes and Their Prevention" in *Frontiers in Clinical Medicine* (2015). Marks holds a doctorate in health education from Columbia University, Teachers College, and an MS in physical therapy from the University of Alberta.

James A. Martinez, EdD, MPH, is an assistant clinical professor with the School of Public Health at Loma Linda University in Loma Linda, California. He teaches GIS for Public Health Practice and the integrated public health core coursework. He is also a population health project manager with the Wholeness Institute at Loma Linda University Health. Prior to this, he served as an epidemiologist at the Los Angeles County, Department of Public Health. James holds a master's degree in epidemiology and a doctorate in health education from Columbia University, New York. His research interests include patient-physician communications, health-disparities reduction, chronic diseases prevention, and integrating technology and mobile solutions for improving patient outcomes.

Gloria Shine McNamara, PhD, is an assistant professor of nutrition and health sciences at the City University of New York–Borough of Manhattan Community College. Her published works include, among others, "Impact of Socio-Environmental Factors on College Students' Vending Food and Beverage Purchasing Behaviors" (*Food Studies*, 2014) and "College Students' Self-Regulation of Motoric Flexibility: The Effects of Modeling and Self-Evaluation" In *The International Journal of Sport and Society*. McNamara is a registered dietitian and NYS-certified nutritionist. She has also served as the director of NYC Department of Health's Project LEAN and Maimonides Medical Center's WIC Program. McNamara holds a doctorate in health education and behaviors from the Graduate Center of the City University of New York. Her research interests include self-regulation of and environmental supports for health behaviors pertaining to diet and exercise.

David E. Newton, EdD, has been a freelance writer of nonfiction books and ancillary materials for nearly 55 years. He has published more than 400 textbooks, research manuals, trade books, encyclopedias, and encyclopedia articles as well as lab manuals, problems books, and other publications. He has also been an updating and consulting editor on a number of books and reference works. Newton was formerly a teacher of high school science and mathematics in Grand Rapids, Michigan; professor of chemistry and physics at Salem State College; and adjunct professor at the University of San Francisco. His interest is in the social, political, economic, and other aspects of science and technology. He holds a doctorate in science education from Harvard University and a master's degree in education from the University of Michigan.

Betty Perez-Rivera, MS, EdD, MCHES, is the director of health literacy/patient and family education at NYU Langone Medical Center, working to transform, centralize, and standardize patient and family education practices throughout the enterprise. Dr. Perez-Rivera has more than 20 years of experience in health management and health education, providing services to individuals and families from diverse ethnic and socioeconomic backgrounds. Dr. Perez-Rivera was previously the director of the East Harlem Asthma Center of Excellence, a Mayor Bloomberg and Manhattan Borough President Scott Stringer initiative to reduce health disparities for children with asthma and their families. She earned a master's degree and a doctoral degree in health and behavior studies from Teachers College, Columbia University, and was selected as the first postdoctoral Fellow in Health Disparities at Teachers College, Columbia University.

Tiffany Crystal Rivera, MA, is vice president of health education and recruitment at the Institute of Education for the Care of Chronic Diseases, providing educational resources and sustainable skills to diverse populations. She was the Manhattan Borough Coordinator for the NYC Coalition for a Smoke-Free City, working with elected officials to pass anti-tobacco legislation. She has presented at several national conferences and conducted professional and community workshops and trainings to promote multidisciplinary approaches to care throughout New York City.

Christine L. B. Selby, PhD, is an associate professor of psychology at Husson University in Bangor, Maine, and she maintains a part-time private practice as a licensed psychologist, where she specializes in eating disorders and sport psychology. She is the author of *Chilling Out: The Psychology of Relaxation*, which is part of ABC-CLIO's Psychology in Everyday Life series. Dr. Selby is past-president of the Division of Exercise and Sport Psychology of the

American Psychological Association and is the co-founder and co-chair of the Eating Disorder Special Interest Group of the Association of Applied Sport Psychology. Selby holds a master's in athletic counseling from Springfield College and a doctorate in counseling psychology from the University of North Texas.

Dena Simmons is a doctoral candidate at Teachers College, Columbia University.

Patricia A. McGarry-Strizak, RN, MPH, is the health and safety trainer at the Massachusetts Coalition for Occupational Safety and Health and the organization's lead trainer with The New England Consortium in Lowell, Massachusetts. She received her BSN from Dominican College, Orangeburg, New York, and an MPH with a concentration in health care policy and administration from Brooklyn College, Brooklyn, New York. An emergency responder, she has studied and responded to Super Storm Sandy and the World Trade Center attack on September 11, 2001, both in New York City, as well as a number of other natural and human-made emergency incidents.

A. J. Smuskiewicz is a freelance writer and editor with more than 20 years of experience specializing in science and medicine. Before becoming a writer, he worked as a laboratory and field biologist. He has written numerous educational articles and books for adults and children.

Nelda Street is an editorial professional specializing in complementary and alternative medicine, personal growth, and evidence-based self-help psychology subject matters, including dialectical behavior therapy, acceptance and commitment therapy, mindfulness-based stress reduction, and compassion-focused therapy. Throughout the years, she has edited scores of books for many publishers.

Leah Sultan-Khan, EdD, is the patient and family education coordinator at Toronto General Hospital in Ontario, Canada. She is a Certified Health Education Specialist with 15 years combined health promotion experience working within the community, hospital, and government sectors. She holds a doctorate in health education from Columbia University and a master's in comparative, international, and development education from the University of Toronto. Her passion is to promote the health and well-being for all people by empowering them with knowledge and skills to achieve their best level of wellness.

Linda Tancs is lawyer-turned-content developer, editor, and communications consultant. Tancs holds a master of laws degree from Columbia University School of Law, a doctorate in law from Seton Hall University School of Law, and a bachelor of arts degree in communication from Rutgers University in New Brunswick.

Rachel Torres, EdD, is an assistant professor for the department of health education at the Borough of Manhattan Community College. Dr. Torres received her MPH in an interdisciplinary program with a focus on sociomedical sciences from Columbia University Mailman School of Public Health. Her EdD in health education with an emphasis on health promotion and disease prevention is from Teachers College, Columbia University. Her overall research goal is to reduce health disparities and improve outcomes across diverse populations through a dual focus on the health care system and patients.

Tim J. Watts is a content development librarian at Kansas State University, where he is responsible for reference and content development.

Micaela A. Young graduated from Smith College, where she studied biology and exercise science.